Recent Advances in Antibody Therapeutics

Recent Advances in Antibody Therapeutics

Editor

Yong-Seok Heo

MDPI • Basel • Beijing • Wuhan • Barcelona • Belgrade • Manchester • Tokyo • Cluj • Tianjin

Editor
Yong-Seok Heo
Konkuk University
Korea

Editorial Office
MDPI
St. Alban-Anlage 66
4052 Basel, Switzerland

This is a reprint of articles from the Special Issue published online in the open access journal *International Journal of Molecular Sciences* (ISSN 1422-0067) (available at: https://www.mdpi.com/journal/ijms/special_issues/Antibody_Therapeutics).

For citation purposes, cite each article independently as indicated on the article page online and as indicated below:

LastName, A.A.; LastName, B.B.; LastName, C.C. Article Title. *Journal Name* **Year**, *Volume Number*, Page Range.

ISBN 978-3-0365-4353-6 (Hbk)
ISBN 978-3-0365-4354-3 (PDF)

Contents

About the Editor vii

Yong-Seok Heo
Recent Advances in Antibody Therapeutics
Reprinted from: *Int. J. Mol. Sci.* **2022**, *23*, 3690, doi:10.3390/ijms23073690 1

Heesu Chae, Seulki Cho, Munsik Jeong, Kiyoung Kwon, Dongwook Choi, Jaeyoung Lee, Woosuk Nam, Jisu Hong, Jiwoo Lee, Seonjoo Yoon and Hyojeong Hong
Improvement of Biophysical Properties and Affinity of a Human Anti-L1CAM Therapeutic Antibody through Antibody Engineering Based on Computational Methods
Reprinted from: *Int. J. Mol. Sci.* **2021**, *22*, 6696, doi:10.3390/ijms22136696 5

Se-Young Lee, Deok-Han Ko, Min-Jeong Son, Jeong-Ah Kim, Keunok Jung and Yong-Sung Kim
Affinity M aturation o f a T -Cell R eceptor-Like A ntibody S pecific fo r a Cytomegalovirus pp65-Derived Peptide Presented by HLA-A*02:01
Reprinted from: *Int. J. Mol. Sci.* **2021**, *22*, 2349, doi:10.3390/ijms22052349 21

Yu Jung Kim, Min Ho Lee, Se-Ra Lee, Hyo-Young Chung, Kwangmin Kim, Tae Gyu Lee and Dae Young Kim
Neutralizing Human Antibodies against Severe Acute Respiratory Syndrome Coronavirus 2 Isolated from a Human Synthetic Fab Phage Display Library
Reprinted from: *Int. J. Mol. Sci.* **2021**, *22*, 1913, doi:10.3390/ijms22041913 33

Dong-Hoon Yeom, Yo-Seob Lee, Ilhwan Ryu, Sunju Lee, Byungje Sung, Han-Byul Lee, Dongin Kim, Jin-Hyung Ahn, Eunsin Ha, Yong-Soo Choi, Sang Hoon Lee and Weon-Kyoo You
ABL001, a Bispecific Antibody Targeting VEGF and DLL4, with Chemotherapy, Synergistically Inhibits Tumor Progression in Xenograft Models
Reprinted from: *Int. J. Mol. Sci.* **2020**, *22*, 241, doi:10.3390/ijms22010241 51

Soo Bin Park, Sun-Jick Kim, Sang Woo Cho, Cheol Yong Choi and Sangho Lee
Blocking of the IL-33/ST2 Signaling Axis by a Single-Chain Antibody Variable Fragment (scFv) Specific to IL-33 with a Defined Epitope
Reprinted from: *Int. J. Mol. Sci.* **2020**, *21*, 6953, doi:10.3390/ijms21186953 65

Yuko Abe, Yasuhiko Suga, Kiyoharu Fukushima, Hayase Ohata, Takayuki Niitsu, Hiroshi Nabeshima, Yasuharu Nagahama, Hiroshi Kida and Atsushi Kumanogoh
Advances and Challenges of Antibody Therapeutics for Severe Bronchial Asthma
Reprinted from: *Int. J. Mol. Sci.* **2021**, *23*, 83, doi:10.3390/ijms23010083 79

Maria Gabriella Donà, Paola Di Bonito, Maria Vincenza Chiantore, Carla Amici and Luisa Accardi
Targeting Human Papillomavirus-Associated Cancer by Oncoprotein-Specific Recombinant Antibodies
Reprinted from: *Int. J. Mol. Sci.* **2021**, *22*, 9143, doi:10.3390/ijms22179143 95

Aida Kouhi, Vyshnavi Pachipulusu, Talya Kapenstein, Peisheng Hu, Alan L. Epstein and Leslie A. Khawli
Brain Disposition of Antibody-Based Therapeutics: Dogma, Approaches and Perspectives
Reprinted from: *Int. J. Mol. Sci.* **2021**, *22*, 6442, doi:10.3390/ijms22126442 117

Eunhye Ji and Sahmin Lee
Antibody-Based Therapeutics for Atherosclerosis and Cardiovascular Diseases
Reprinted from: *Int. J. Mol. Sci.* **2021**, *22*, 5770, doi:10.3390/ijms22115770 . . . . **141**

Ames C. Register, Somayeh S. Tarighat and Ho Young Lee
Bioassay Development for Bispecific Antibodies—Challenges and Opportunities
Reprinted from: *Int. J. Mol. Sci.* **2021**, *22*, 5350, doi:10.3390/ijms22105350 . . . . **157**

Chih-Wei Lin and Richard A. Lerner
Antibody Libraries as Tools to Discover Functional Antibodies and Receptor Pleiotropism
Reprinted from: *Int. J. Mol. Sci.* **2021**, *22*, 4123, doi:10.3390/ijms22084123 . . . . **177**

Man-Seok Ju and Sang Taek Jung
Antigen Design for Successful Isolation of Highly Challenging Therapeutic Anti-GPCR Antibodies
Reprinted from: *Int. J. Mol. Sci.* **2020**, *21*, 8240, doi:10.3390/ijms21218240 . . . . **189**

Olga Bednova and Jeffrey V. Leyton
Targeted Molecular Therapeutics for Bladder Cancer—A New Option beyond the Mixed Fortunes of Immune Checkpoint Inhibitors?
Reprinted from: *Int. J. Mol. Sci.* **2020**, *21*, 7268, doi:10.3390/ijms21197268 . . . . **203**

About the Editor

Yong-Seok Heo

Yong-Seok Heo is currently a professor of chemistry, Konkuk University, Korea. He received his Bachelor's degree in 1996, Master's degree in 1999, and Ph.D. in 2005 at Seoul National University in chemistry, studying the structural biology of MAPK signaling. He joined LG chem. In 1999 and CrystalGenomics in 2000 as a research scientist for structure-based drug discovery. He joined Konkuk university in 2006 as a professor in the department of chemistry. His research focuses on the mechanism of action of biologics, including therapeutic antibodies. He has unveiled the molecular mechanisms underlying the therapeutic efficacies of antibody drugs used in cancer immunotherapy and to treat inflammatory autoimmune diseases. He is a member of the board of director of Korean Society for Structural Biology and editorial board of BioDesign.

International Journal of *Molecular Sciences*

MDPI

Editorial

Recent Advances in Antibody Therapeutics

Yong-Seok Heo

Department of Chemistry, Konkuk University, 120 Neungdong-ro, Gwangjin-gu, Seoul 05029, Korea; ysheo@konkuk.ac.kr; Tel.: +82-2-450-3408; Fax: +82-2-3436-5382

Antibody-based therapeutics have achieved unprecedented success in treating various diseases, including cancers, immune disorders, and infectious diseases. Since the approval of OKT3 in 1986, more than 100 antibody-based drugs have been approved by the FDA. In this Special Issue, "Recent Advances in Antibody Therapeutics", promising discoveries and developments of this most prevalent biologics are presented. In addition, the review articles covering the clinical and technical advances for antibody usage and discovery could provide valuable insight into applications by clinicians and scientists in this field.

As an antibody discovery is advanced to preclinical development, it is essential to consider its biophysical properties to determine whether it can be successfully developed into an efficacious drug. Chae et al. reported the successful result for improving biophysical properties of an antibody against the L1 cell adhesion molecule for cancer therapy [1]. In this study, one of the variants derived by a computer-aided method demonstrated reduced aggregation propensity, increased stability, higher purification yield, lower pI, higher affinity, and greater in vivo anti-tumor efficacy, leading to a promising candidate antibody for preclinical development.

T-cell immune responses are initiated by the interaction between the T-cell receptor (TCR) and peptide-HLA complex. In January 2022, the U.S. Food and Drug Administration (FDA) approved KIMMTRAK (tebentafusp-tebn), which is the first T-cell receptor (TCR) therapeutics fused with an anti-CD3 T-cell engaging scFv. The approval of this biologic verified TCR-based protein engineering as a valuable therapeutic modality. Lee et al. reported a TCR-like antibody specific for HLA-A*02:01 in complex with a peptide derived from human cytomegalovirus (CMV) pp65 protein [2]. The binding affinity was matured by sequential mutagenesis of complementarity-determining regions using yeast surface display technology for its application to the diagnostics and therapeutics of CMV infection.

The FDA has approved several monoclonal antibodies neutralizing the SARS-CoV-2 virus for treating COVID-19. Kim et al. discovered human monoclonal antibodies that neutralize SARS-CoV-2 through the phage display method against the receptor-binding domain (RBD) of the SARS-CoV-2 spike protein [3]. Some of them elicit cross-reactivity with the SARS-CoV spike protein and neutralize activities on pseudo-typed and authentic SARS-CoV-2 viruses, anticipating their therapeutic and diagnostic application against SARS-CoV-2.

Bispecific antibodies against two distinct antigens have been extensively explored for therapeutic purposes. Due to a biophysical bridge between two targets by simultaneous binding, bispecific antibodies can achieve specific therapeutic efficacy with multiple MoA. Yeom et al. reported a bispecific antibody targeting VEGF and DLL4, eliciting more potent anti-angiogenic activity than investigational antibodies targeting VEGF or DLL4 alone [4]. In addition, the combination of this bispecific antibody with paclitaxel or irinotecan synergistically inhibited tumor progression in xenograft models.

A significant number of the antibodies in clinical use target interleukins (ILs) or their receptors for treating chronic inflammatory diseases, including psoriasis, rheumatoid arthritis, Castleman disease, atopic dermatitis, and asthma. Park et al. discovered a single-chain antibody variable fragment (scFv) against interleukin 33 (IL-33) to block its binding to the suppressor of tumorigenicity 2 (ST2) receptor using the phage display library [5].

Citation: Heo, Y.-S. Recent Advances in Antibody Therapeutics. *Int. J. Mol. Sci.* **2022**, *23*, 3690. https://doi.org/10.3390/ijms23073690

Received: 2 March 2022
Accepted: 25 March 2022
Published: 28 March 2022

Downregulation of IL-33-mediated signaling has been recognized as a therapeutic strategy to prevent allergic inflammation and chronic diseases such as asthma, atopic dermatitis, and allergic rhinitis asthma. The antibody fragment in this study can be further engineered and improved for therapeutic application.

Abe et al. recently reviewed the therapeutic antibodies in clinical use for treating severe asthma, including omalizumab, mepolizumab, reslizumab, benralizumab, and dupilumab, describing their distinct mechanisms of action, achievements, and limitations [6]. They also emphasized the importance of biomarkers for the clinical prediction of good responders to each antibody therapy. They summarized new potential targets for asthma treatment, including thymic stromal lymphopoietin (TSLP), IL-25, IL-33, IL-13, and chemokines, with investigational antibodies against them. Further studies to fully understand the pathogenesis and clarify the effects of each antibody type in asthma endotypes will guide decision-making regarding appropriate antibody therapeutics with improved efficacy.

Donà et al. reviewed the state of the art of the therapeutic antibodies targeting human papillomavirus (HPV) oncoproteins developed so far in different formats and outlined their mechanisms of action [7]. Cervical cancer is by far the most common HPV-related disease. To date, as there is no treatment for HPV itself, an infection could cause abnormal cell changes that might lead to cancer. Given that the global burden of HPV-associated cancers is unacceptably high, antibody-based therapies can be a promising strategy for fighting HPV-associated cancers in parallel with vaccination.

Kouhi et al. reviewed the various methods currently used for antibody delivery to the central nervous system (CNS) at the preclinical stage and the underlying mechanisms of blood–brain barrier (BBB) penetration, with the description of the recent efforts to improve or modulate antibody distribution and disposition into the brain [8]. Very recently, the FDA approved the first BBB-penetrating antibody, aducanumab, for Alzheimer's disease treatment. Further development in this field can revolutionize the treatment of diseases of the CNS.

Ji et al. reviewed the recent findings on the preclinical and clinical studies of therapeutic antibodies in atherosclerosis and their underlying mechanism of action targeting LDL and cytokines [9]. In clinical trials, many antibodies targeting PCSK9, TNFα, IL-1β, IL-6, IL-17, and IL-12/23 have shown ambivalent results, with some cases showing significant alleviation of symptoms and others experiencing adverse events such as the aggravation of cardiovascular diseases. Further studies to fully understand the exact mechanism of action of the target molecules would be very helpful in overcoming the side effects or applying the appropriate treatment.

Register et al. reviewed recent advances and case studies of bioassay development for different types of bispecific antibodies [10]. As bispecific antibodies have complicated mechanisms of action, diverse structural variations, and dual-target binding, developing a bioassay method is challenging. The detailed description of the diverse bioassay technologies and case studies in this review article can provide insight into designing strategies for developing and characterizing bispecific antibodies.

Lin et al. reviewed current findings and applications to identify functional antibodies, especially agonist antibodies capable of activating cell-signaling cascades, selected from combinatorial antibody libraries [11]. This review suggests that the use of phenotypic screening with combinatorial antibody libraries shows great promise in allowing the identification of receptor pleiotropism and the selection of antibodies capable of modulating the differentiation, growth, and function of cells.

Despite the high value of G-protein-coupled receptors (GPCRs) as a therapeutic target, only two antibodies targeting GPCR, erenumab and mogamulizumab, have been approved by the FDA. One of the main reasons for the slow development of therapeutic antibodies against this attractive drug target is the difficulty in preparing functional GPCR antigens. Ju et al. reviewed various successful technologies to prepare active GPCR antigens that enable the isolation of therapeutic antibodies to proceed toward clinical validation [12].

The treatment of bladder cancer has advanced rapidly since the approval of immune-checkpoint inhibitors. Bednova et al. reviewed recent clinical trials of targeted therapeutics, including the antibody-drug conjugates (ADCs) enfortumab vedotin and sacituzumab govitecan, for patients with metastatic bladder cancer [13]. In addition, they described the cost-effectiveness of these targeted molecular therapeutics relative to the antibody drugs blocking immune checkpoints PD-1 and PD-L1.

The five research articles and eight reviews published within this Special Issue, "Recent Advances in Antibody Therapeutics", are excellent studies of the advances made in the field of therapeutic antibodies for treating various diseases. I want to thank all the authors and reviewers for their contributions and the editor, Sydney Tang, for outstanding dedication and professionalism throughout this Special Issue.

Funding: Konkuk University, 2021.

Acknowledgments: This paper was supported by Konkuk University in 2021.

Conflicts of Interest: The author declares no conflict of interest.

References

1. Chae, H.; Cho, S.; Jeong, M.; Kwon, K.; Choi, D.; Lee, J.; Nam, W.; Hong, J.; Lee, J.; Yoon, S.; et al. Improvement of Biophysical Properties and Affinity of a Human Anti-L1CAM Therapeutic Antibody through Antibody Engineering Based on Computational Methods. *Int. J. Mol. Sci.* **2021**, *22*, 6696. [CrossRef] [PubMed]
2. Lee, S.Y.; Ko, D.H.; Son, M.J.; Kim, J.A.; Jung, K.; Kim, Y.S. Affinity Maturation of a T-Cell Receptor-Like Antibody Specific for a Cytomegalovirus pp65-Derived Peptide Presented by HLA-A*02:01. *Int. J. Mol. Sci.* **2021**, *22*, 2349. [CrossRef] [PubMed]
3. Kim, Y.J.; Lee, M.H.; Lee, S.R.; Chung, H.Y.; Kim, K.; Lee, T.G.; Kim, D.Y. Neutralizing Human Antibodies against Severe Acute Respiratory Syndrome Coronavirus 2 Isolated from a Human Synthetic Fab Phage Display Library. *Int. J. Mol. Sci.* **2021**, *22*, 1913. [CrossRef] [PubMed]
4. Yeom, D.H.; Lee, Y.S.; Ryu, I.; Lee, S.; Sung, B.; Lee, H.B.; Kim, D.; Ahn, J.H.; Ha, E.; Cho, Y.S.; et al. ABL001, a Bispecific Antibody Targeting VEGF and DLL4, with Chemotherapy, Synergistically Inhibits Tumor Progression in Xenograft Models. *Int. J. Mol. Sci.* **2021**, *22*, 241. [CrossRef] [PubMed]
5. Park, S.B.; Kim, S.J.; Cho, S.W.; Choi, C.Y.; Lee, S. Blocking of the IL-33/ST2 Signaling Axis by a Single-Chain Antibody Variable Fragment (scFv) Specific to IL-33 with a Defined Epitope. *Int. J. Mol. Sci.* **2021**, *21*, 6953. [CrossRef] [PubMed]
6. Abe, Y.; Suga, Y.; Fukushima, K.; Ohata, H.; Niitsu, T.; Nabeshima, H.; Nagahama, Y.; Kida, H.; Kumanogoh, A. Advances and Challenges of Antibody Therapeutics for Severe Bronchial Asthma. *Int. J. Mol. Sci.* **2021**, *23*, 83. [CrossRef] [PubMed]
7. Donà, M.G.; Di Bonito, P.; Chiantore, M.V.; Amici, C.; Accardi, L. Targeting Human Papillomavirus-Associated Cancer by Oncoprotein-Specific Recombinant Antibodies. *Int. J. Mol. Sci.* **2021**, *22*, 9143. [CrossRef] [PubMed]
8. Kouhi, A.; Pachipulusu, V.; Kapenstein, T.; Hu, P.; Epstein, A.L.; Khawli, L.A. Brain Disposition of Antibody-Based Therapeutics: Dogma, Approaches and Perspectives. *Int. J. Mol. Sci.* **2021**, *22*, 6442. [CrossRef] [PubMed]
9. Ji, E.; Lee, S. Antibody-Based Therapeutics for Atherosclerosis and Cardiovascular Diseases. *Int. J. Mol. Sci.* **2021**, *22*, 5770. [CrossRef] [PubMed]
10. Register, A.C.; Tarighat, S.S.; Lee, H.Y. Bioassay Development for Bispecific Antibodies-Challenges and Opportunities. *Int. J. Mol. Sci.* **2021**, *22*, 5350. [CrossRef] [PubMed]
11. Lin, C.W.; Lerner, R.A. Antibody Libraries as Tools to Discover Functional Antibodies and Receptor Pleiotropism. *Int. J. Mol. Sci.* **2021**, *22*, 4123. [CrossRef] [PubMed]
12. Ju, M.S.; Jung, S.T. Antigen Design for Successful Isolation of Highly Challenging Therapeutic Anti-GPCR Antibodies. *Int. J. Mol. Sci.* **2021**, *21*, 8240. [CrossRef] [PubMed]
13. Bednova, O.; Leyton, J.V. Targeted Molecular Therapeutics for Bladder Cancer-A New Option beyond the Mixed Fortunes of Immune Checkpoint Inhibitors? *Int. J. Mol. Sci.* **2021**, *21*, 7268. [CrossRef] [PubMed]

International Journal of
Molecular Sciences

Article

Improvement of Biophysical Properties and Affinity of a Human Anti-L1CAM Therapeutic Antibody through Antibody Engineering Based on Computational Methods

Heesu Chae [1,2], Seulki Cho [3], Munsik Jeong [1], Kiyoung Kwon [1], Dongwook Choi [4], Jaeyoung Lee [2], Woosuk Nam [2], Jisu Hong [1], Jiwoo Lee [1], Seonjoo Yoon [2,*] and Hyojeong Hong [1,3,*]

1 Department of Systems Immunology, Kangwon National University, Chuncheon 24341, Korea; chs@apitbio.com (H.C.); anstlrj@kangwon.ac.kr (M.J.); gykwon@kangwon.ac.kr (K.K.); ghdwltn55@kangwon.ac.kr (J.H.); snm04062@kangwon.ac.kr (J.L.)
2 APIT BIO Inc., B910, Munjeongdong Tera Tower, 167 Songpa-daero, Songpa-gu, Seoul 05855, Korea; liy5999@apitbio.com (J.L.); wsnam@apitbio.com (W.N.)
3 Institute of Bioscience and Biotechnology, Kangwon National University, Chuncheon 24341, Korea; seul8502@naver.com
4 Division of Drug Process Development, New Drug Development Center, Osong Medical Innovation Foundation, Chungcheongbuk-do, Cheongju-si 28160, Korea; dwchoi@kbiohealth.kr
* Correspondence: yoonsj@apitbio.com (S.Y.); hjhong@kangwon.ac.kr (H.H.); Tel.: +82-10-2305-9704 (S.Y.); +82-10-5430-0480 (H.H.)

Abstract: The biophysical properties of therapeutic antibodies influence their manufacturability, efficacy, and safety. To develop an anti-cancer antibody, we previously generated a human monoclonal antibody (Ab417) that specifically binds to L1 cell adhesion molecule with a high affinity, and we validated its anti-tumor activity and mechanism of action in human cholangiocarcinoma xenograft models. In the present study, we aimed to improve the biophysical properties of Ab417. We designed 20 variants of Ab417 with reduced aggregation propensity, less potential post-translational modification (PTM) motifs, and the lowest predicted immunogenicity using computational methods. Next, we constructed these variants to analyze their expression levels and antigen-binding activities. One variant (Ab612)—which contains six substitutions for reduced surface hydrophobicity, removal of PTM, and change to the germline residue—exhibited an increased expression level and antigen-binding activity compared to Ab417. In further studies, compared to Ab417, Ab612 showed improved biophysical properties, including reduced aggregation propensity, increased stability, higher purification yield, lower pI, higher affinity, and greater in vivo anti-tumor efficacy. Additionally, we generated a highly productive and stable research cell bank (RCB) and scaled up the production process to 50 L, yielding 6.6 g/L of Ab612. The RCB will be used for preclinical development of Ab612.

Keywords: therapeutic antibody; anti-cancer antibody; antibody engineering; biophysical properties; computational methods; research cell bank

Citation: Chae, H.; Cho, S.; Jeong, M.; Kwon, K.; Choi, D.; Lee, J.; Nam, W.; Hong, J.; Lee, J.; Yoon, S.; et al. Improvement of Biophysical Properties and Affinity of a Human Anti-L1CAM Therapeutic Antibody through Antibody Engineering Based on Computational Methods. *Int. J. Mol. Sci.* **2021**, *22*, 6696. https://doi.org/10.3390/ijms22136696

Academic Editor: Yong-Seok Heo

Received: 31 May 2021
Accepted: 19 June 2021
Published: 22 June 2021

1. Introduction

Therapeutic monoclonal antibodies (mAb) are the leading class of drugs on the biopharmaceutical market, largely due to their high specificity, affinity, potency, and their long in vivo half-life. Since approval of the first mAb (OKT3) in 1983, 79 therapeutic antibodies have been approved by FDA and are currently on the market, including 30 mAbs for cancer treatment [1]. Innovations in antibody engineering technologies—such as humanization of murine mAbs, phage display and transgenic mice for generating fully human mAbs, Fc engineering, antibody-drug conjugates, and bispecific antibodies—have contributed to the development of these important drugs [2–9]. Therapeutic antibody discovery and development starts with early candidates (hits), followed by selection of advanced candidates (leads). A critical element of antibody development is termed chemistry, manufacturing, and controls (CMC), which includes construction of an antibody-producing cell line, development of a manufacturing process, and development of suitable analytical methods to validate the antibody's safety and efficacy [10–12].

During the manufacturing process, including cell culture and downstream processing, therapeutic antibodies are at risk of physical and chemical degradation through multiple pathways [13]. Degradation may affect antigen binding, decrease antibody efficacy, or even lead to immunogenic products [14–16]. Protein aggregation is the most common and substantial type of physical degradation associated with therapeutic antibodies [13,17,18]. High concentrations are associated with increased protein–protein interaction frequency, which proportionally increases the opportunity for aggregation formation. Changes in extrinsic conditions—including pH, salt, temperature, shaking, and viscosity—can also promote protein–protein associations that can lead to aggregation events [13,19–22].

Post-translational modifications (PTMs) may also cause problems during therapeutic antibody development. For example, asparagine (Asn) deamidation, the most common pathway for the chemical degradation of therapeutic antibodies, results from hydrolysis of the amide side-chain of Asn, which cumulatively produces a heterogeneous mixture of aspartate (Asp) and isoAsp at the affected position [23,24]. Asn residues are more prone to deamidation when they are in a solvent-accessible region or are followed by a small or flexible residue, such as serine (Ser) or glycine (Gly). Asn deamidation can affect function if it occurs at a binding interface, such as the complementarity determining regions (CDRs) of an antibody molecule [19,23,25]. Another PTM, Asp isomerization, involves the non-enzymatic interconversion of Asp and isoAsp residues [19]. Asp isomerization may occur more commonly when Asp is followed by Ser, Gly, or Asp; it can affect protein function when it occurs in CDRs; and it can potentially result in fragmentation [26,27].

Each mAb has unique biophysical properties, mainly due to differences in the CDR residues and framework scaffolds. Thus, the identification of degradation-prone or unstable regions early in antibody development could allow for re-engineering of leads. This approach is aided by computational modeling tools that predict regions susceptible to physical and chemical degradation [28–30]. To develop a therapeutic antibody with anti-tumor activity, we previously isolated a human mAb (Ab4) that specifically binds to human and rodent L1 cell adhesion molecule (L1CAM) from a human naïve Fab library using phage display [31]. We next generated an affinity-matured version (Ab417) of this hit through site-directed mutagenesis of CDR residues, and we validated its anti-tumor efficacy and mechanism of action in rodent models [31,32].

In the present study, we aimed to improve the biophysical properties of the lead antibody (Ab417). We analyzed the heavy (VH) and light (VL) chain sequences and the three-dimensional (3D) model of Ab417, using computational methods to identify potential PTMs and to calculate aggregation propensities. Next, we designed 20 variants of Ab417 with reduced aggregation propensity, fewer potential PTM motifs, and the lowest predicted immunogenicity. We constructed these Ab417 variants and analyzed their expression levels and antigen-binding activities. One variant (Ab612), which was generated by substituting the four VH residues and two VL residues of Ab417, exhibited a higher expression level and higher antigen-binding activity compared to Ab417. Further studies demonstrated that compared to Ab417, Ab612 also showed higher productivity, improved biophysical properties, and a higher affinity and in vivo anti-tumor efficacy. For the preclinical development of Ab612, we generated a highly productive and stable research cell bank (RCB), and scaled up the production process to 50 L, which yielded 6.6 g/L of the antibody. Ab612 is now considered a candidate antibody to progress to preclinical development.

2. Results

2.1. Design and Selection of an Ab417 Variant with Improved Biophysical Properties

To design Ab417 variants with reduced aggregation propensity and increased stability, we first aligned the VH and VK sequences of Ab417 with a set of human germline genes and screened for potential PTMs, while constructing a structural model of the Fv of Ab417. Secondly, we calculated the sequence- and structure-based aggregation propensities to identify aggregation hotspots and made substitutions with the aim of reducing the aggregation propensity and improving the stability, using Lonza's AggreSolve^{TM} in silico tools. We evaluated the aggregation propensity by analyzing regions outside the CDRs with high aggregation propensity, screening for positions with potentially problematic PTMs, identifying positions that were out of line with a conserved consensus in the human germline genes, and screening for solvent-exposed aliphatic or hydrophobic residues. Thirdly, we screened the engineered sequences of Ab417 for Th epitopes using Epibase^{TM} in silico tools to ensure that aggregation-reducing substitutions would not increase the immunogenic potential. Finally, we designed 19 Ab417 variants with engineered VH and VK (Figure S1).

To select the Ab417 variants with improved biophysical properties, the genes coding for the VH and VK of the variants were synthesized and individually subcloned into the heavy and light chain expression plasmids, respectively. Then, the variant combinations were introduced into HEK293F cells for transient expression. After six days of cell cultivation, the culture supernatants were analyzed by quantitative ELISA and indirect ELISA. The results revealed that the variant H3L7 exhibited a higher expression level and retained the same antigen binding activity compared to Ab417. In contrast, the other variants with higher expression levels exhibited lower antigen-binding activities compared to Ab417 (data not shown).

The sequence differences between Ab417 and H3L7 include two substitutions in the VL of H3L7 (I31S and V96S) and four in the VH (R16G, D54E, K76A, and P88A), as shown in Figure 1. The substitutions I31S and V96S in the VL were designed to reduce the surface hydrophobicity in the light chain CDR1 (LCDR1) and LCDR3, respectively. The substitutions in the VH—R16G in the FR1 and K76A in the FR3—were designed to reduce the number of positive charges. Compared to other therapeutic antibodies on the market, Ab417 has a high isoelectric point (pI, 9.6), and large numbers of positive charges may cause the antibody to readily interact with any negatively charged molecules. The D54E substitution was designed to remove two potential PTMs (deamidation and isomerization) in the heavy chain CDR2 (HCDR2) without affecting the binding affinity. The P88A substitution was included because all of the most similar germline genes contain an alanine instead of proline at position 88 of the VH.

A

VL residue substitution	
I31S	Reduced surface hydrophobicity
V96P(V96S/S96P)	Reduced surface hydrophobicity/ Substitution to germline residue
VH residue substitution	
R16G	Reduced positive charge
D54E	PTM removal
K76A	Reduced positive charge
P88A	Substitution to germline residue

B

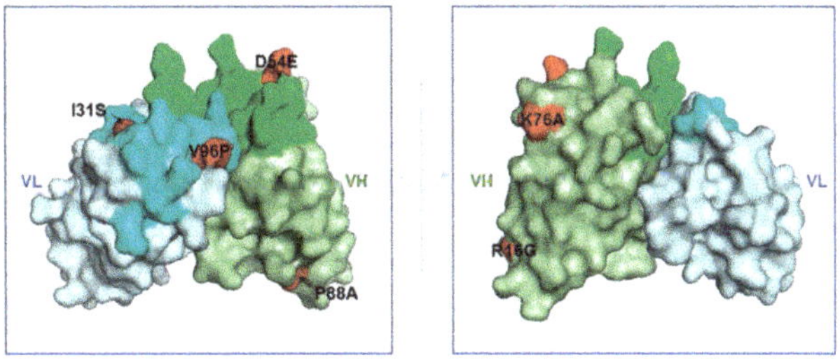

Figure 1. Schematic representation of the substitutions of Ab417 for improved biophysical properties. (**A**) Design of the VL and VH residue substitutions. (**B**) The 3D model of Ab417. The I31S and V96P in the VL and the R16G, D54E, K76A, and P88A in the VH are shown in red. Gray, VL; Green, VH; Lime, LCDR; Light green, HCDR.

To further improve the variant H3L7, we substituted Pro96 for Ser96 in the LCDR3 to reduce the flexibility of the LCDR3 loop. The LCDR3 of Ab417 has a length of 10 residues rather than 9, with no conserved proline residue at position at 95a, and also has two flexible glycine residues. The resulting H3L7 variant (Ab612), as well as Ab417, were transiently expressed in HEK293F cells. Analysis of the culture supernatants by ELISA revealed that the expression levels and antigen-binding activities of Ab612 were higher than those of Ab417 (data not shown). Therefore, Ab612 was selected for further studies.

2.2. Expression Analysis and Optimization of Purification Process of Ab417 and Ab612

To precisely compare the expression levels between Ab417 and Ab612, each antibody was expressed using the ExpiCHO-S transient expression system, and the culture supernatant was subjected to quantitative ELISA. The results indicated that the expression level of Ab612 was 2.6-fold higher than that of Ab417 (Figure 2A).

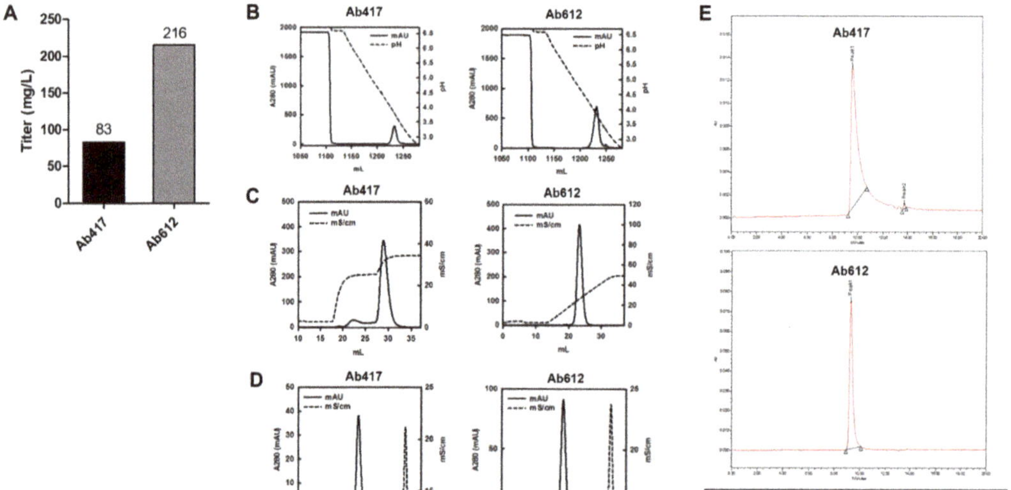

	RT	Height	Area	% Area
Ab417	9.59	12482	409313	98.72
Ab612	9.3	75454	1350835	100

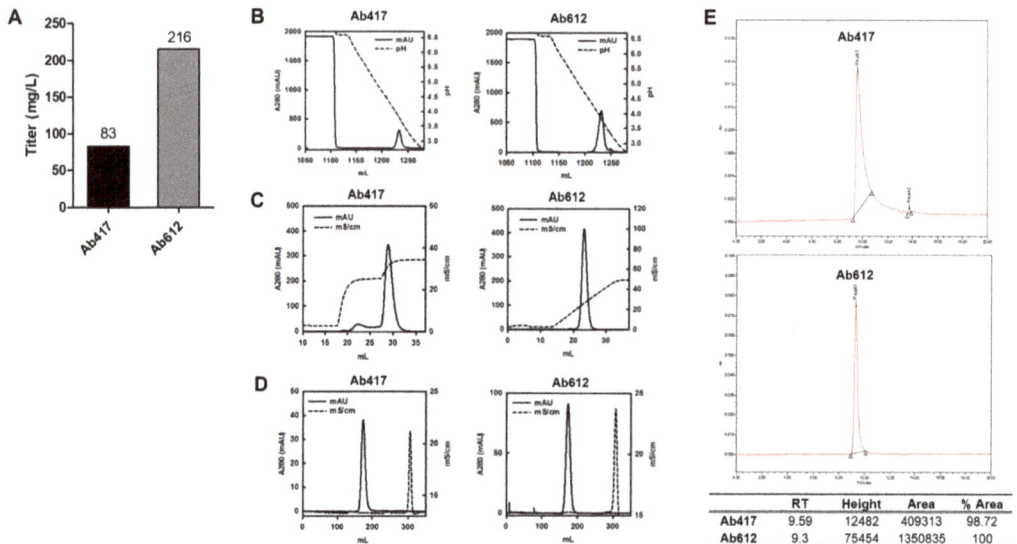

Figure 2. (**A**) Expression levels of antibodies using the ExpiCHO transient expression system. (**B**,**C**) Ab417 and Ab612 were purified by protein A affinity chromatography (**B**) and CIEX by stepwise gradient elution and linear gradient elution, respectively (**C**). (**D**) Final polishing was conducted using SEC. (**E**) SEC-HPLC of each antibody was performed to determine the purity and homogeneity following purification.

To compare the quality of the produced antibodies, Ab417 and Ab612 were purified from the culture supernatants via three purification steps using Protein A affinity chromatography, cation-exchange chromatography (CIEX), and size exclusion chromatography (SEC) (Figure 2B–D). In the case of Ab417, high-molecular-weight aggregates could be separated from the IgG monomer by stepwise gradient elution in CIEX because they were not separated by linear gradient elution. On the other hand, Ab612 was eluted as a single peak by linear gradient elution (Figure 2C). After SEC, the purification yields of Ab417 and Ab612 were 43% and 61%, respectively, indicating that the purification yield of Ab612 was 40% higher compared to that of Ab417. SEC-HPLC was conducted to validate the purity and homogeneity of the purified antibody. A fraction of fragmented Ab417 was detected, whereas fragmented Ab612 was not detected (Figure 2E).

2.3. Thermal Stability of Ab417 and Ab612

To assess the thermal stability of Ab417 and Ab612, the purified antibodies were evaluated by dynamic light scattering (DLS) while increasing the temperature from 30 °C to 80 °C. The aggregation starting point was 74 °C for Ab417 and 77 °C for Ab612 (Figure 3), indicating that Ab612 exhibited increased thermal stability compared to Ab417. Taken together with the analyses of expression and purification processing, these results demonstrate that compared to Ab417, Ab612 showed improved biophysical properties, including increased productivity, reduced aggregation propensity and fragmentation, and increased thermal stability.

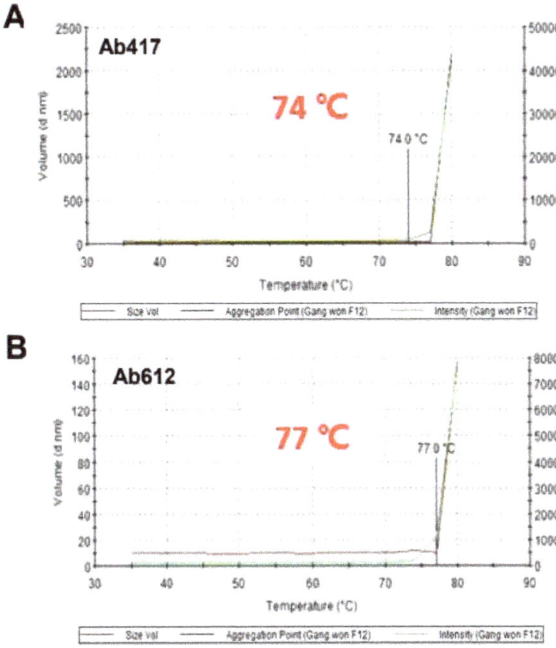

Antibody	Aggregation point (°C)
Ab417	74
Ab612	77

Figure 3. Assessment of thermal stability of Ab417 (**A**) and Ab612 (**B**) by DLS. The blue line indicates the starting point of protein aggregation.

2.4. Affinity and pI Values of Ab417 and Ab612

To compare the antigen-binding affinities of Ab417 and Ab612, we determined the affinities of the purified antibodies using both competitive ELISA and bio-layer interferometry (BLI) with Octet Red384. We measured the affinities for both human and mouse L1CAM because Ab417 is cross-reactive with rodent L1CAM [31]. In a competitive ELISA, the affinities (KD) of Ab417 and Ab612 for human L1CAM were 0.50 nM and 0.26 nM, respectively (Figure 4A), while both antibodies showed the same affinity for mouse L1CAM (KD, 0.12 nM) (Figure 4B). As determined by BLI, the affinities of Ab417 and Ab612 for human L1CAM were 0.26 nM and 0.11 nM, respectively, while the antibodies showed identical affinities for mouse L1CAM (KD, 0.10 nM) (Figure 4C). These results indicated that Ab612 exhibited a 2-fold higher affinity for human L1CAM compared to Ab417, but not an increased affinity for mouse L1CAM. This demonstrated that the increased affinity of Ab612 was due to an increased intrinsic affinity, but not to its improved biophysical properties.

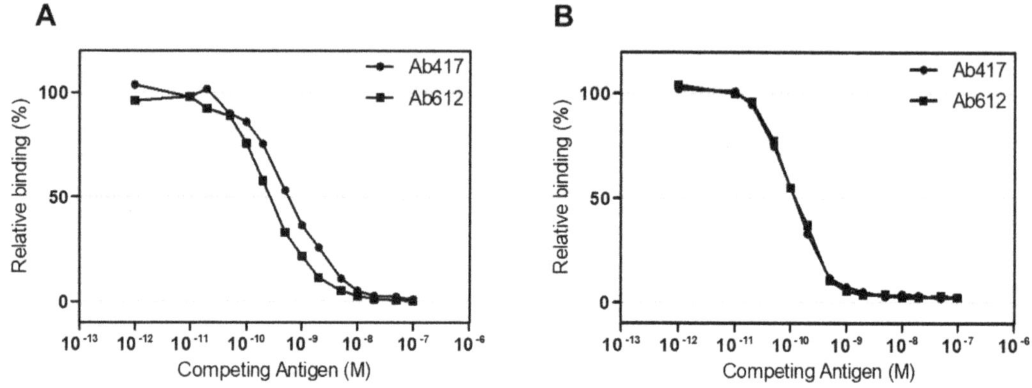

C

Antigen	Antibody	KD (M)	kon(1/Ms)	kdis(1/s)	Full R^2
Human L1CAM	Ab417	2.63E-10	3.59E+05	9.45E-05	0.99
	Ab612	1.05E-10	3.13E+05	3.28E-05	0.99
Mouse L1CAM	Ab417	1.08E-10	2.44E+05	2.64E-05	0.99
	Ab612	9.6E-11	2.42E+05	1.30E-05	0.99

Figure 4. Determination of the affinities of Ab417 and Ab612 for hL1-s1 (**A**) and mL1-s1 (**B**) by competitive ELISA and the Octet system (**C**). Kon, rate of association; Kdis, rate of dissociation; Full R^2, estimate of the goodness of the curve fit.

In the VH of Ab417, two positively charged amino acid residues (Arg16 and Lys76) were substituted with Gly16 and Ala76 to construct Ab612. Thus, we measured the pI of the purified antibodies by capillary isoelectric focusing (cIEF). As expected, the pI of Ab612 (9.25) was lower than that of Ab417 (9.62) (Figure S2).

2.5. In Vivo Anti-Tumor Activities of Ab417 and Ab612

Since we confirmed that Ab612 showed improved biophysical properties and affinity compared to Ab417, we next investigated its in vivo anti-tumor efficacy in a cholangiocarcinoma xenograft nude mouse model where Ab417 inhibited tumor cell proliferation.Balb/c nude mice (n = 8) bearing Choi-Ck xenografts were i.v. injected with Ab417 or Ab612 (10 mg/kg) or vehicle three times per week for three weeks, and the tumor volume and body weights were measured. At 22 days after the first injection, tumor tissues were removed and weighed. Compared to the control, Ab417 and Ab612 resulted in tumor growth inhibition of 55.5% and 78.2%, respectively, based on mean tumor weight, while not affecting body weight (Figure 5A–D). These results indicated that Ab612 exhibited enhanced anti-tumor efficacy compared to Ab417 in the cholangiocarcinoma model.

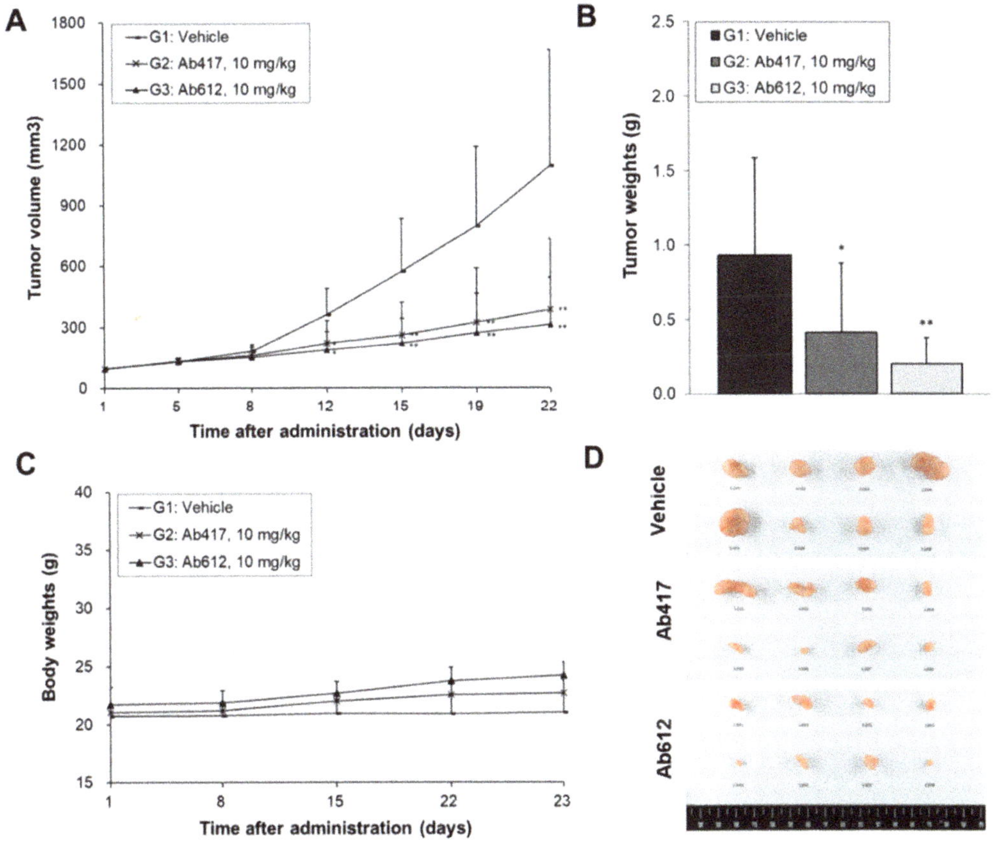

Figure 5. Anti-tumor efficacy of Ab612 compared with Ab417 in a Choi-Ck cholangiocarcinoma xenograft nude mouse model ($n = 8$). When the tumor volume reached an average of 100 mm^3, dosing (10 mpk) was initiated 3 times weekly for 22 days. Mean tumor volume (**A**), tumor weight (**B**), and body weight (**C**) are shown. (**D**) Photographs of the resected tumors at the end of the experiment. Each point represents the mean ± SD. * $p < 0.05$, ** $p < 0.01$, significant difference from the isotype control group by Dunnett's t-test.

2.6. Generation of an RCB for Preclinical Development of Ab612

To initiate the preclinical development of Ab612, stable and high-producing Chinese hamster ovary (CHO) cell clones were generated according to the regulatory guidelines. Figure 6A presents the overall scheme for RCB development. Briefly, the heavy and light chain genes were codon-optimized and cloned into the manufacturer's expression vector, followed by transfection into CHO-K1 host cells. The transfected cells were seeded in 96-well plates (96 WPs) to prepare mini pools. These mini pools were gradually screened from 96 WPs to 24 WPs, cell culture plates (TPPs), and 125 mL shake flasks, based on the titer. Finally, the top 8 mini pools were selected. Next, 117 monoclones were isolated from the 8 mini pools by limiting dilution and were gradually screened from 96 WPs to 24 WPs, TPPs, and shake flasks, according to the titer. After the top 10 clones were amplified for RCB building, the top 8 RCBs were selected based on a fed-batch assay, including antibody purification using Protein A, and quality analysis by UPLC-MS, SEC, and CIEF (data not shown). Finally, the top RCB (006-M71-14), which showed the highest cell line stability, was incubated for 11 days, and then passaged every 3 days until passage 23 (p23). Over this time, the titer and cell-specific productivity (Qp) were measured by PA-HPLC. As shown in Figure 6B, the titers of RCB 006-M71-14 were 3120 (p3), 2577 (p11), 2891 (p18), and

2798 mg/mL (p23), and the Qps were 30.98 (p3), 32.38 (p11), 30.65 (p18), and 29.15 (p23) pg/cell/day. These results indicated that the RCB stably maintained its high productivity during the 80 days of culture.

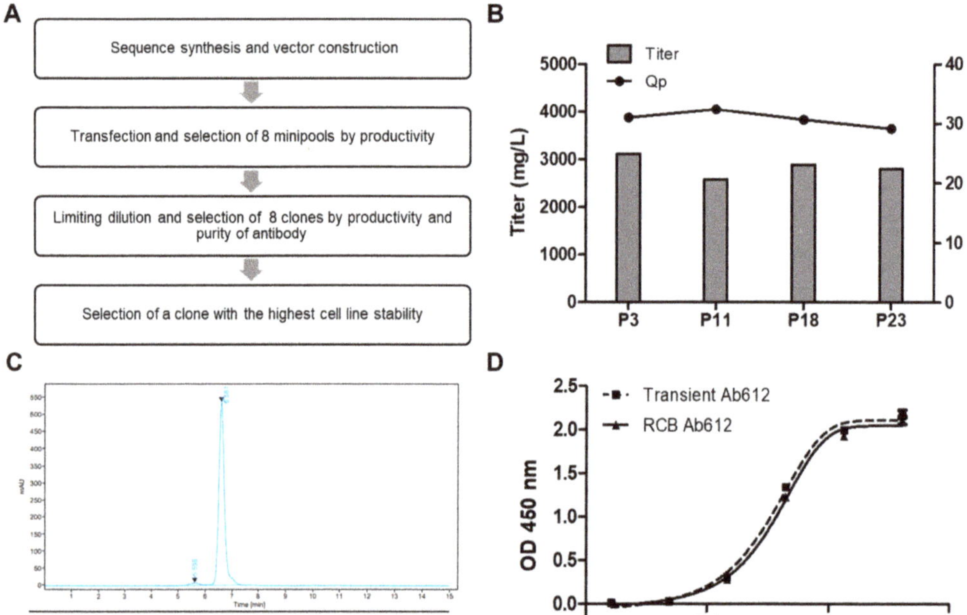

	Retention time (min)	Area %
peak1 (Polymer)	5.59	2.47
peak2 (Monomer)	6.58	97.53

Figure 6. (**A**) Schematic diagram showing the generation of a research cell bank (RCB). (**B**) Ab612 titer was measured to assess the expression level, and Qp was calculated as PCD = (pg/cell/day) using PA-HPLC. (**C**) The purity of Ab612 produced from the RCB was analyzed by SEC-HPLC after purification. (**D**) Ag binding activity was determined by sandwich ELISA.

To assess the quality of the product from RCB 006-M71-14, Ab612 was purified from the culture supernatants by Protein A affinity chromatography and analyzed by SEC-HPLC. The percentages of IgG monomer and high-molecular-weight aggregates of Ab612 were 97.53% and 2.47%, respectively, with no fragmented antibody detected (Figure 6C). Additionally, the purified Ab612 exhibited the same antigen-binding activity as that from transient expression in ExpiCHO-S cells in a sandwich ELISA (Figure 6D). Finally, to test scalability, the fed-batch of the RCB was separately scaled up to 3.7 L and 50 L. After 14 days of cultivation, the titers of 3.7 L and 50 L cultures were determined to be 6.3 and 6.6 g/L, respectively. This demonstrated that the RCB was highly productive and stable, and thus it will be suitable to produce material for preclinical toxicology studies and clinical studies.

3. Discussion

The early phase of drug discovery is focused on antibody selection based on specificity, affinity, and functional properties. However, as an antibody is advanced into preclinical development, it is important to consider its biophysical properties to determine whether it can be successfully developed into an efficacious drug. The biophysical properties of a therapeutic antibody can critically influence its late-stage developability, which requires high-level expression, high solubility, conformational and colloidal stability, low polyspecificity, and low immunogenicity [33].

In our previous attempt to develop a therapeutic antibody with anti-tumor activity, we isolated a human mAb that cross-reacts with rodent L1CAM from a human naïve antibody library, and we then generated an affinity-matured version (Ab417) of this hit and validated its anti-tumor efficacy and mechanism of action in rodent models [31,32]. In the present study, we attempted to optimize Ab417 by improving its biophysical properties.

We designed 19 variants with reduced aggregation propensity, fewer potential PTM motifs, and lower predicted immunogenicity using computational methods. Subsequently, we constructed these variants to analyze their expression levels and antigen-binding activities. The Ab417 variant H3L7 exhibited a higher expression level compared to Ab417.

Therefore, we further changed a residue in the LCDR3 of H3V7 to generate an even more improved variant (Ab612) with higher productivity and antigen-binding affinity. The Ab612 showed 2.6-fold higher productivity and improved biophysical properties, such as 1.4-fold increased purification yield, greater stability, lower aggregation propensity, 2-fold higher affinity for human L1CAM, and enhanced in vivo anti-tumor efficacy. Moreover, for the preclinical development of Ab612, we successfully generated a highly productive and stable research cell bank (RCB) and confirmed the scalability of the production process to a pilot scale.

Overall, the present results demonstrate that we successfully improved the biophysical properties and affinity of Ab417, generating an optimized antibody (Ab612). Ab612 is considered a promising candidate antibody for preclinical development.

4. Materials and Methods

4.1. Design of Ab417 Variants with Improved Biophysical Properties

4.1.1. Sequence Analysis for Potential PTMs

Multiple alignments of Ab4 and Ab417 sequences to human germline sequences were generated using MAFFT [34], and entries in each alignment were ordered according to the sequence identity to the parental sequence. The antibody sequences were analyzed for potential PTMs such as Asn deamidation, Asp isomerization, N- and O-glycosylation, and oxidation.

4.1.2. Construction and Comparison of 3D Models of Ab417 and Its Variants

Structural models of the Fv-region for Ab417, and variants thereof, were generated using Lonza Biologics' modeling platform. Candidate structural template fragments for the FR and CDRs, as well as the full Fv, were scored, ranked, and selected from the antibody database based on their sequence identity to the target, as well as qualitative crystallographic measures (Å) of the template structure. In order to structurally align the CDRs to the FR templates, five residues on either side of the CDR were included in the CDR template. An alignment of the fragments was generated based on overlapping segments and a structural sequence alignment using MODELLER. An ensemble of structures that satisfy the conformational restraints derived from the set of aligned structural templates was created by simulated annealing and conjugation gradient optimization procedures. One or more model structures were selected from this ensemble based on an energy score derived from the quality of the protein structure and satisfaction of the conformational restraints. The models were inspected, and the side chains of the positions which differ between the target and template were optimized using a side chain optimization algorithm and energy minimized. A suite of visualization and computational tools were used to assess the conformational variability of the CDRs, as well as the core and local packing of the domains and regions and surface analysis to select one or more preferred models.

To assess the impact of different substitutions on affinity and stability, a number of structural criteria, including the solvent accessibility, local atomic packing, and location of the substitution relative to the predicted antigen-binding interface or the Fv dimer interface, electrostatic effects, and hydrogen bonding patterns, were used.

4.1.3. Calculation of Aggregation Propensity and Assessment of Potential Substitutions

Aggregation hotspots were identified based on the sequence and structure of antibodies using Lonza's AggreSolve™ in silico tools. The intrinsic aggregation propensity score, A_{res}, was calculated for overlapping 7-mer peptides, and the score was calculated over an entire amino acid sequence to generate A_{tot}. In addition, S_{res}, which reflects the aggregation propensity of a 7-mer peptide from its folded state, was calculated by applying the conformational correction to the intrinsic aggregation propensity profile [35]. A summary score, S_{tot}, was calculated based on the position-specific S_{res}. In addition, given that non-specific protein-protein interactions can be caused by aggregation-prone hotspots on the protein's surface, the surface aggregation propensity per position, Tres, was calculated. A summary score, T_{tot}, was calculated based on the position-specific Tres descriptors.

All positions outside the CDRs that were part of the hot spots were assessed based on their potential impact on binding affinity and stability. Each position was classified as either Neutral, Critical, or Contributing. A neutral position means that substituting another amino acid at this position should not affect binding affinity or stability negatively. A contributing position means that a substitution can be made, but the position may contribute to binding affinity or stability. A critical position means that the position risks a decreased binding affinity or stability, and therefore parental amino acid must be retained.

4.1.4. Analysis of Th Epitopes

The epitopes or clusters of adjoining epitopes of Ab417 and engineered variants were analyzed using Epibase™ for substitutions that would remove or reduce binding to HLA allotypes to the greatest extent possible, with a focus on the HLA-DR allotypes, because these are known to express at a higher level than the other allotypes DQ and DP [36]. Human germline sequences were not considered to be immunogenic as they are found in the pool of circulating antibodies. The substitutions in the engineered antibodies were analyzed for all chosen HLA allotypes (DRB1, DR3/4/5, DQ, and DP).

4.2. Construction of Expression Plasmids and Transient Expression of Antibodies

The genes coding for the VH or VL of the variants were synthesized and subcloned into the EcoRI-ApaI or HindIII-BsiWI sites of the expression plasmid (pCMV-dhfrC) containing the human Cγ1 or Cκ gene to construct heavy or light chain expression plasmid, respectively, as described previously [31].

For transient expression of antibodies, HEK293F cells (Gibco, Thermo Fisher Scientific, Waltham, MA, USA) or ExpiCHO™ cells (Thermo Fisher Scientific, Waltham, MA, USA) were grown in FreeStyle 293 Expression medium (Gibco, Thermo Fisher Scientific, Waltham, MA, USA) at 8% CO_2, 37 °C, 125 rpm or in ExpiCHO Expression medium (Thermo Fisher Scientific, Waltham, MA, USA) at 5% CO_2, 37 °C, 110 rpm on a shaker. For transfection, the heavy and light chain expression plasmids (two vector system) or expression plasmid containing heavy and light chain (one vector system) were introduced into HEK293F using polyethyleneimine (Polysciences) or ExpiCHO™ cells (Thermo Fisher Scientific, Waltham, MA, USA) using the ExpiCHO Expression System. On day 6 post-transfection, the cell culture supernatant was centrifuged, filtered using a bottle top filter (0.22 µm PES, Sartorius, Germany), and subjected to quantitative ELISA and indirect ELISA to analyze the expression level and antigen binding activity.

4.3. ELISAs

A quantitative ELISA was performed to determine the concentration of antibodies. Anti-human IgG kappa antibody (Invitrogen, Waltham, MA, USA) was coated on the 96-well immunoplate (Thermo Fisher Scientific, Waltham, MA, USA) at 4 °C overnight. After blocking with 2% skim milk in 0.05% PBST (PBS with 0.05% tween 20), a standard IgG sample (400 ng/mL) or cell culture supernatant serially diluted in 0.1% PBA was added to each well and incubated at 37 °C for 1 h. The bound antibody was detected using anti-human IgG Fc-HRP (1:10,000 (*v*/*v*); Invitrogen, Waltham, MA), as described previously [31].

An indirect ELISA was performed to determine the antigen binding activity of the antibody. Purified human recombinant L1CAM (hL1-s1) and mouse recombinant L1CAM (mL1-s1) were prepared as described previously [31]. hL1-s1 or mL1-s1 (100 ng/well) was coated on each well at 4 °C overnight. Serially diluted cell culture supernatant or antibody was incubated with the hL1-s1 or mL1-S1 at 37 °C for 1 h. The bound antibody was detected using anti-human IgG(Fc-specific)-HRP (1:10,000, Invitrogen, Waltham, MA, USA).

A competitive ELISA was performed to determine the antigen-binding affinity of the antibody. hL1-s1 or mL1-s1 (100 ng/well) were coated on each well at 4 °C for 12 h. Ab417 or Ab612 antibody (10 ng/mL) in 0.1% PBA solution was pre-incubated with various concentrations (10^{-12}~10^{-7} M) of hL1-s1 or mL1-s1 as a competing antigen at 37 °C for 3 h. The reaction mixture was added to each well coated with the hL1-s1 or mL1-s1, and indirect ELISA was carried out. Affinity (KD) was defined as the antigen concentration required to inhibit 50% of the antigen-binding activity.

A sandwich ELISA was performed to compare the antigen-binding activities of the Ab612 antibody samples produced from the transient expression and the RCB culture. Anti-human Fc antibody (Invitrogen, Waltham, MA, USA, 100 ng/well) was coated on each well at 4 °C overnight. Ab417 or Ab612 (50 ng/mL) was added to each well, incubated at 37 °C for 1 h, and further incubated with hL1-s1 serially diluted from 4 μg/mL at 37 °C for 1 h. The hL1-s1 captured by Ab417 or Ab612 was incubated with mouse anti-s1 antibody KR127 [37] at 37 °C for 1 h. The bound KR127 antibody was detected using anti-mouse IgG(Fc-specific)-HRP (1:10,000, Invitrogen, Waltham, MA, USA).

4.4. Purification of Antibodies

Ab417 and Ab612 were purified using a Protein A affinity column. Harvested Cell Culture Fluid (HCCF) containing a monoclonal antibody was loaded on to pre-packed protein A column (HiTrap MabSelect™ Sure, Cytiva, Marlborough, MA, USA) equilibrated with binding buffer (20 mM sodium citrate, pH 6.0). The column was then re-equilibrated with binding buffer followed by a wash step at pH 6.0 and finally elution with sodium citrate buffer at pH 6.0 and 2.5 (gradient elution). The gradient elution experiments were carried out using a 30 column volume (CV) linear gradient from 0% to 100% buffer B (20 mM sodium citrate, pH 6.0). For virus inactivation, the elution fraction was incubated at 4 °C for 1 h and then neutralized with 1 M Tris-HCl (pH 9.0) to minimize the effect on the structure of the antibody under low pH conditions. The column was then regenerated and sanitized using 0.5 N NaOH.

Desalting chromatography (HiPrep™ 26/10 Desalting, Cytiva, Marlborough, MA, USA) was performed to replace the buffer in the primary purified product (affinity eluate) suitable for the loading condition (50 mM Na-Acetate, pH 5.0). Further purification of Ab417 and Ab612 was performed using cation-exchange chromatography. The sample was applied to a HiTrap Capto SP column (Cytiva, Marlborough, MA, USA) and eluted with a linear gradient of 0 to 500 mM NaCl, 30 CV.

Pooled fractions were further concentrated using Amicon Ultra-4 Centrifugal Filter Unit with Ultracel-10 membrane (Merck Millipore, Burlington, MA, USA). A concentrated protein sample was loaded onto the HiLoad Superdex 200 pg column (Cytiva, Marlborough, MA, USA) equilibrated with Phosphate-buffered saline (PBS) buffer at the rate of 1.0 mL/min. The elution profile was analyzed by the absorbance at 280 nm.

The purity and aggregation of purified protein were determined using high-performance size exclusion chromatography (SE-HPLC). A Waters HPLC (Alliance 2695) system was used with a Bio SEC-3 column (3 μm, 300 Å, 4.6 × 300 mm, Agilent, Santa Clara, CA, USA) at 0.3 mL/min flow rate (isocratic) using a mobile phase buffer of 20 mM Na-phosphate w/150 mM NaCl, pH 6.8.

4.5. Dynamic Light Scattering (DLS)

DLS was performed using Zetasizer (Malvern, Herrenberg, Germany). After the Z-average of antibody sample was measured at 25 °C, 50 μL of the sample was added to disposable cuvettes (ZEN0040, Malvern, Herrenberg, Germany) and gradually the temperature was increased from 30 °C to 80 °C with 3 °C of temperature interval and a fixed angle of $\theta = 173°$. The Z-average and intensity were calculated using Zetasizer Software version 7.02 (Malvern, Herrenberg, Germany).

4.6. Affinity Determination of Antibodies Using Octet red384 System

The affinity of the antibody was determined using the Octet Red384 system (Sartorius, Goettingen, Germany). Anti-human IgG sensor AHC (ForteBio, Fremont, CA, USA) was firstly soaked in 0.1% PBA for 20 min. The antibody (0.2 mL of 0.5 μg/mL) was captured for 10 min followed by washing with 0.1% PBA for 2 min. hL1-s1 or mL-s1 (25, 12.5, 6.25, 3.125, or 1.5625 nM in 0.1% PBA) was then incubated with the antibody captured on the sensor. Association and dissociation rates were measured for 10 min and 30 min, respectively. For correction of baseline drift, a control sensor was designated as an antibody-captured AHC sensor exposed to running buffer only. All analytes were recalculated by subtraction of the rate of a control sensor. The operating temperature was maintained at 30 °C and agitated at 1000 rpm. Data were analyzed using a 1:1 interaction model (fitting global, R_{max} unlinked by a sensor) with analysis software (ForteBio, ver. 8. 2).

4.7. Capillary Isoelectric Focusing (cIEF) Analysis

cIEF was conducted according to the SCIEX application protocol. All cIEF experiments were performed on SCIEX PA800 plus instrument with a 50 μm i.d. neutral coated capillary (SCIEX P/N 477441) at the length of 30.2 cm. The UV detector was used to detect absorbance at 280 nm wavelength. A cIEF master mix solution was composed of 3 M urea-cIEF gel solution, pharmalyte 3–10 carrier ampholytes, cathodic stabilizer (500 mM arginine), anodic stabilizer (200 mM iminodiacetic acid), and five pI markers (10.0, 9.5, 7.0, 5.5, 4.1). Analytes (5 mg/mL) were also mixed with 10 μL of the master mix solution. All experiments were performed in triplicate. The pI values of the sample were calculated using qualitative analysis of a 32 Karat software.

4.8. In Vivo Antitumor Activities of Ab417 or Ab612

All the animals were housed under a 12/12 h light/dark cycle (light phase, 8:00 A.M. to 8:00 P.M.) with a standard laboratory diet and water ad libitum. All animal handling and experiments were conducted with the approval of the Institutional Animal Care and Use Committee (IACUC) of preclinical CRO Biotoxtech (180678). Nude mice (BALB/cSlc-nu, 5 weeks old) were obtained from Japan SLC, Inc (Shizuoka, Japan). Choi-CK cells (1×10^6) were inoculated into the right flank of each mouse. Constructed Choi-CK tumor tissue ($3 \times 3 \times 3$ mm^3) was subcutaneously inoculated into the back of mice. After tumor volume reached a mean of 100 mm^3 (n = 8 per group), the antibody at a dose of 10 mg/kg was i.v. injected 3 times per week for 3 weeks. Tumor growth was monitored by measuring the length and width of the tumor with a caliper and calculating tumor volume based on the following formula; TV (mm^3) = L (mm) × W2 (mm^2) × 1/2, where L is length and W is width. Body weight was measured twice a week, and tumor tissues were taken out and weighed at the end of the experiment. Tumor growth inhibition rate (IR) was calculated as the following formula; IR (%) = (1 − T/C) × 100. T is the mean tumor weight of the antibody treated group, and C is the mean tumor weight of the mock control group.

Data were validated using SAS (Version 9.3, SAS Institute Inc., Cary, NC, USA). Each point represents the mean ± SD. Statistical comparison between groups were performed by one-way analysis of variance (ANOVA) followed by Dunnett's t-test.

4.9. Production of Ab612 from Research Cell Bank (RCB)

4.9.1. Construction of RCB

RCB was generated by Shanghai OPM Biosciences Co., Ltd. (Shanghai, China). CHO-K1 cells were grown in CD CHO Medium (GIBCO, Thermo Fisher Scientific, Waltham, MA, USA) containing 6 mM L-glutamine (Sigma, St. Louis, MO, USA). Cells were incubated under the condition of 120 rpm, 37 °C, and 8% CO_2. Freshly prepared linearized plasmid was transfected into CHO-K1 cells by electroporation using a Bio-Rad system. For each sample, 1×10^7 cells were transfected with a total of 40 μg of the linear plasmid. At 24 h later, the transfected cells were plated into a 96-well plate with 4000 cells/well. The culture medium was CD CHO Medium containing 50 μM L-Methionine sulfoximine (MSX) (Sigma, St. Louis, MO, USA) and 1 × GS-Supplement (Sigma, St. Louis, MO, USA). Cells were statically cultured in an incubator with 8% CO_2 and 37 °C. The plasmid was transfected into cells twice by electroporation, and then the cells were plated into 20 pieces of a 96-well plate. Mini pool fed-batch assay medium was OPM-CHO CD07 Medium (OPM, China) with 1:200 anti-clumping Agent (ACA, OPM, China). The CDF18 (OPM, China) at 3%, 5%, 6%, 6% and 5% concentration and CDF26 (OPM, China) at 0.3%, 0.5%, 0.6%, 0.6% and 0.5% were fed on day 3, 5, 7, 9, and 11, respectively. The glucose was fed as needed to maintain at 2–6 g/L. The fed-batch was stopped when the viability is about 60% or on day 12.

4.9.2. Stability Study of Research Cell Bank (RCB)

In suspension culture from RCB stock, cells were passaged once every 3 days for 69 days with 0.4×10^6 cells/mL seeding density in OPM-CHO CD07 Medium with 50 μM MSX and 1:200 Anti-Clumping Agent. In a fed-batch assay, cells were incubated at the density of $0.8 \pm 0.1 \times 10^6$ cells/mL with 30 mL culture volume. The medium was OPM-CHO CD07 Medium with 1:200 ACA. The CDF18 was fed on day 3, 5, 7, 9 and 11 at 3%, 5%, 6%, 6% and 5%, respectively, and CDF26 was fed at 0.3%, 0.5%, 0.6%, 0.6% and 0.5%. The glucose was fed as needed to maintain it at 2–8 g/L. The fed-batch was stopped when the viability is about 60% or on 12 days. The culture supernatants were harvested by centrifuging at 3500 rpm for 30 min under 4 °C.

4.9.3. Production and Purification of Antibodies

The HCCF obtained from RCB production was purified using protein A (Repligen, Waltham, MA, USA) packed in XK26/20 column (Cytiva, Marlborough, MA, USA) affinity chromatography. The purified antibody was stored in 10 mM sodium phosphate buffer containing 5% sorbitol and 0.01% tween 20 and dialyzed using HiPrep™ 26/10 Desalting Column (Cytiva, Marlborough, MA, USA). The concentration of purified antibody was determined with a Nanodrop (Thermo fisher scientific, Nanodrop 2000) based on the molar extinction coefficient. The produced Ab612 from RCB was used for analyzing purification by SEC-HPLC and antigen-binding activity by ELISA.

5. Conclusions

In conclusion, we successfully improved the biophysical properties and affinity of Ab417 through antibody engineering based on computational methods, which generated an optimized antibody, Ab612. This antibody exhibited enhanced in vivo anti-tumor efficacy compared to Ab417. Additionally, we successfully generated a highly productive and stable RCB and confirmed the scalability of the production process to a pilot scale. Ab612 is considered a promising candidate antibody for preclinical development.

Supplementary Materials: The following are available online at https://www.mdpi.com/article/10.3390/ijms22136696/s1, Figure S1: Variant combinations of Ab417, Figure S2: pI value of Ab417 and Ab612 using cIEF.

Author Contributions: Conceptualization, H.H. and S.Y.; methodology, H.C., S.C., M.J., K.K., D.C., J.L. (Jaeyoung Lee), J.H. and J.L. (Jiwoo Lee); formal analysis, D.C.; investigation, H.C., S.C., M.J., K.K., D.C., J.L. (Jaeyoung Lee), W.N. and S.Y.; writing—original draft preparation, H.C., D.C., W.N. and H.H.; writing—review and editing, H.H. and S.Y.; Funding acquisition, H.H. and S.Y. All authors have read and agreed to the published version of the manuscript.

Funding: This research was funded by the Korea Drug Development Fund (KDDF) grant (KDDF-201212-12) and the Basic Science Research Program grant (NRF-2018R1D1A1A09084274) to H.J.H. and by the BIG3 Innovative startup package support Program (No. 10449069) & the Technology development Program (No. S3029721) supported by the Ministry of SMEs and Startups to S.Y.

Institutional Review Board Statement: Not applicable.

Informed Consent Statement: Not applicable.

Acknowledgments: We thank Lonza Biologics plc (UK) and Shanghai OPM Biosciences Co. (China) for the excellent services of computational methods and RCB generation, respectively.

Conflicts of Interest: The authors declare no conflict of interest.

References

1. Lu, R.-M.; Hwang, Y.-C.; Liu, I.-J.; Lee, C.-C.; Tsai, H.-Z.; Li, H.-J.; Wu, H.-C. Development of therapeutic antibodies for the treatment of diseases. *J. Biomed. Sci.* **2020**, *27*, 1–30. [CrossRef] [PubMed]
2. Morrison, S.L.; Johnson, M.J.; Herzenberg, L.A.; Oi, V.T. Chimeric human antibody molecules: Mouse antigen-binding domains with human constant region domains. *Proc. Natl. Acad. Sci. USA* **1984**, *81*, 6851–6855. [CrossRef]
3. Jones, P.T.; Dear, P.H.; Foote, J.; Neuberger, M.S.; Winter, G. Replacing the complementarity-determining regions in a human antibody with those from a mouse. *Nature* **1986**, *321*, 522–525. [CrossRef] [PubMed]
4. McCafferty, J.; Griffiths, A.D.; Winter, G.; Chiswell, D.J. Phage antibodies: Filamentous phage displaying antibody variable domains. *Nature* **1990**, *348*, 552–554. [CrossRef]
5. Lonberg, N.; Taylor, L.D.; Harding, F.A.; Trounstine, M.; Higgins, K.M.; Schramm, S.R.; Kuo, C.-C.; Mashayekh, R.; Wymore, K.; McCabe, J.G. Antigen-specific human antibodies from mice comprising four distinct genetic modifications. *Nature* **1994**, *368*, 856–859. [CrossRef]
6. Green, L.; Hardy, M.; Maynard-Currie, C.; Tsuda, H.; Louie, D.; Mendez, M.; Abderrahim, H.; Noguchi, M.; Smith, D.; Zeng, Y. Antigen–specific human monoclonal antibodies from mice engineered with human Ig heavy and light chain YACs. *Nat. Genet.* **1994**, *7*, 13–21. [CrossRef]
7. Derer, S.; Kellner, C.; Berger, S.; Valerius, T.; Peipp, M. Fc engineering: Design, expression, and functional characterization of antibody variants with improved effector function. *Methods Mol. Biol.* **2012**, *907*, 519–536. [PubMed]
8. Drake, P.M.; Rabuka, D. An emerging playbook for antibody–drug conjugates: Lessons from the laboratory and clinic suggest a strategy for improving efficacy and safety. *Curr. Opin. Chem. Biol.* **2015**, *28*, 174–180. [CrossRef]
9. Labrijn, A.F.; Janmaat, M.L.; Reichert, J.M.; Parren, P.W. Bispecific antibodies: A mechanistic review of the pipeline. *Nat. Rev. Drug Discov.* **2019**, *18*, 585–608. [CrossRef]
10. Jones, S.D.; Seymour, P.; Levine, H.L. CMC activities for development of mAbs. *Contract Pharm. Apr.* **2010**, 60–64. Available online: https://www.contractpharma.com/issues/2010-04/view_features/cmc-activities-for-development-of-mabs/ (accessed on 10 June 2021).
11. Chartrain, M.; Chu, L. Development and production of commercial therapeutic monoclonal antibodies in Mammalian cell expression systems: An overview of the current upstream technologies. *Curr. Pharm. Biotechnol.* **2008**, *9*, 447–467. [CrossRef]
12. Liu, H.F.; Ma, J.; Winter, C.; Bayer, R. Recovery and purification process development for monoclonal antibody production. *MAbs* **2010**, *2*, 480–499. [CrossRef]
13. Elgundi, Z.; Reslan, M.; Cruz, E.; Sifniotis, V.; Kayser, V. The state-of-play and future of antibody therapeutics. *Adv. Drug Deliv. Rev.* **2017**, *122*, 2–19. [CrossRef]
14. Joubert, M.K.; Hokom, M.; Eakin, C.; Zhou, L.; Deshpande, M.; Baker, M.P.; Goletz, T.J.; Kerwin, B.A.; Chirmule, N.; Narhi, L.O. Highly aggregated antibody therapeutics can enhance the in vitro innate and late-stage T-cell immune responses. *J. Biol. Chem.* **2012**, *287*, 25266–25279. [CrossRef]
15. Rehder, D.S.; Chelius, D.; McAuley, A.; Dillon, T.M.; Xiao, G.; Crouse-Zeineddini, J.; Vardanyan, L.; Perico, N.; Mukku, V.; Brems, D.N. Isomerization of a single aspartyl residue of anti-epidermal growth factor receptor immunoglobulin $\gamma 2$ antibody highlights the role avidity plays in antibody activity. *Biochemistry* **2008**, *47*, 2518–2530. [CrossRef]
16. Yan, Y.; Wei, H.; Fu, Y.; Jusuf, S.; Zeng, M.; Ludwig, R.; Krystek, S.R., Jr.; Chen, G.; Tao, L.; Das, T.K. Isomerization and oxidation in the complementarity-determining regions of a monoclonal antibody: A study of the modification–structure–function correlations by hydrogen–deuterium exchange mass spectrometry. *Anal. Chem.* **2016**, *88*, 2041–2050. [CrossRef]

17. Ahmadi, M.; Bryson, C.J.; Cloake, E.A.; Welch, K.; Filipe, V.; Romeijn, S.; Hawe, A.; Jiskoot, W.; Baker, M.P.; Fogg, M.H. Small amounts of sub-visible aggregates enhance the immunogenic potential of monoclonal antibody therapeutics. *Pharm. Res.* **2015**, *32*, 1383–1394. [CrossRef]
18. Bessa, J.; Boeckle, S.; Beck, H.; Buckel, T.; Schlicht, S.; Ebeling, M.; Kiialainen, A.; Koulov, A.; Boll, B.; Weiser, T. The immunogenicity of antibody aggregates in a novel transgenic mouse model. *Pharm. Res.* **2015**, *32*, 2344–2359. [CrossRef]
19. Manning, M.C.; Chou, D.K.; Murphy, B.M.; Payne, R.W.; Katayama, D.S. Stability of protein pharmaceuticals: An update. *Pharm. Res.* **2010**, *27*, 544–575. [CrossRef]
20. Sahin, E.; Grillo, A.O.; Perkins, M.D.; Roberts, C.J. Comparative effects of pH and ionic strength on protein–protein interactions, unfolding, and aggregation for IgG1 antibodies. *J. Pharm. Sci.* **2010**, *99*, 4830–4848. [CrossRef]
21. Arosio, P.; Rima, S.; Morbidelli, M. Aggregation mechanism of an IgG2 and two IgG1 monoclonal antibodies at low pH: From oligomers to larger aggregates. *Pharm. Res.* **2013**, *30*, 641–654. [CrossRef]
22. Telikepalli, S.N.; Kumru, O.S.; Kalonia, C.; Esfandiary, R.; Joshi, S.B.; Middaugh, C.R.; Volkin, D.B. Structural characterization of IgG1 mAb aggregates and particles generated under various stress conditions. *J. Pharm. Sci.* **2014**, *103*, 796–809. [CrossRef]
23. Harris, R.J.; Kabakoff, B.; Macchi, F.D.; Shen, F.J.; Kwong, M.; Andya, J.D.; Shire, S.J.; Bjork, N.; Totpal, K.; Chen, A.B. Identification of multiple sources of charge heterogeneity in a recombinant antibody. *J. Chromatogr. B Biomed. Sci. Appl.* **2001**, *752*, 233–245. [CrossRef]
24. Pace, A.L.; Wong, R.L.; Zhang, Y.T.; Kao, Y.-H.; Wang, Y.J. Asparagine deamidation dependence on buffer type, pH, and temperature. *J. Pharm. Sci.* **2013**, *102*, 1712–1723. [CrossRef]
25. Zhang, Y.T.; Hu, J.; Pace, A.L.; Wong, R.; Wang, Y.J.; Kao, Y.-H. Characterization of asparagine 330 deamidation in an Fc-fragment of IgG1 using cation exchange chromatography and peptide mapping. *J. Chromatogr. B* **2014**, *965*, 65–71. [CrossRef] [PubMed]
26. Yi, L.; Beckley, N.; Gikanga, B.; Zhang, J.; Wang, Y.J.; Chih, H.-W.; Sharma, V.K. Isomerization of Asp–Asp motif in model peptides and a monoclonal antibody Fab fragment. *J. Pharm. Sci.* **2013**, *102*, 947–959. [CrossRef]
27. Vlasak, J.; Ionescu, R. Fragmentation of monoclonal antibodies. *MAbs* **2011**, *3*, 253–263. [CrossRef]
28. Chennamsetty, N.; Voynov, V.; Kayser, V.; Helk, B.; Trout, B.L. Design of therapeutic proteins with enhanced stability. *Proc. Natl. Acad. Sci. USA* **2009**, *106*, 11937–11942. [CrossRef]
29. Courtois, F.; Schneider, C.P.; Agrawal, N.J.; Trout, B.L. Rational design of biobetters with enhanced stability. *J. Pharm. Sci.* **2015**, *104*, 2433–2440. [CrossRef]
30. Angarica, V.E.; Sancho, J. Protein dynamics governed by interfaces of high polarity and low packing density. *PLoS ONE* **2012**, *7*, e48212. [CrossRef]
31. Cho, S.; Park, I.; Kim, H.; Jeong, M.S.; Lim, M.; Lee, E.S.; Kim, J.H.; Kim, S.; Hong, H.J. Generation, characterization and preclinical studies of a human anti-L1CAM monoclonal antibody that cross-reacts with rodent L1CAM. *MAbs* **2016**, *8*, 414–425. [CrossRef]
32. Cho, S.; Lee, T.S.; Song, I.H.; Kim, A.-R.; Lee, Y.-J.; Kim, H.; Hwang, H.; Jeong, M.S.; Kang, S.G.; Hong, H.J. Combination of anti-L1 cell adhesion molecule antibody and gemcitabine or cisplatin improves the therapeutic response of intrahepatic cholangiocarcinoma. *PLoS ONE* **2017**, *12*, e0170078. [CrossRef]
33. Jain, T.; Sun, T.; Durand, S.; Hall, A.; Houston, N.R.; Nett, J.H.; Sharkey, B.; Bobrowicz, B.; Caffry, I.; Yu, Y. Biophysical properties of the clinical-stage antibody landscape. *Proc. Natl. Acad. Sci. USA* **2017**, *114*, 944–949. [CrossRef]
34. Katoh, K.; Misawa, K.; Kuma, K.; Miyata, T. MAFFT: A novel method for rapid multiple sequence alignment based on fast Fourier transform. *Nucleic Acids Res.* **2002**, *30*, 3059–3066. [CrossRef] [PubMed]
35. Pawar, A.P.; Dubay, K.F.; Zurdo, J.; Chiti, F.; Vendruscolo, M.; Dobson, C.M. Prediction of "aggregation-prone" and "aggregation-susceptible" regions in proteins associated with neurodegenerative diseases. *J. Mol. Biol.* **2005**, *350*, 379–392. [CrossRef]
36. Laupeze, B.; Fardel, O.; Onno, M.; Bertho, N.; Drenou, B.; Fauchet, R.; Amiot, L. Differential expression of major histocompatibility complex class Ia, Ib, and II molecules on monocytes-derived dendritic and macrophagic cells. *Hum. Immunol.* **1999**, *60*, 591–597. [CrossRef]
37. Ryu, C.J.; Kim, Y.K.; Hur, H.; Kim, H.S.; Oh, J.M.; Kang, Y.J.; Hong, H.J. Mouse monoclonal antibodies to hepatitis B virus preS1 produced after immunization with recombinant preS1 peptide. *Hybridoma* **2000**, *19*, 185–189. [CrossRef] [PubMed]

International Journal of
Molecular Sciences

MDPI

Article

Affinity Maturation of a T-Cell Receptor-Like Antibody Specific for a Cytomegalovirus pp65-Derived Peptide Presented by HLA-A*02:01

Se-Young Lee [1,†], Deok-Han Ko [1,†], Min-Jeong Son [1], Jeong-Ah Kim [1], Keunok Jung [2] and Yong-Sung Kim [1,2,*]

1 Department of Molecular Science and Technology, Ajou University, Suwon 16499, Korea; sylee1117@ajou.ac.kr (S.-Y.L.); kdh701@ajou.ac.kr (D.-H.K.); minjeong96610@ajou.ac.kr (M.-J.S.); rhwjd319@ajou.ac.kr (J.-A.K.)
2 Department of Allergy and Clinical Immunology, Ajou University School of Medicine, Suwon 16499, Korea; jung2767@ajou.ac.kr
* Correspondence: kimys@ajou.ac.kr; Tel.: +82-31-219-2662; Fax: +82-31-219-1610
† These authors have contributed equally to this work.

Abstract: Human cytomegalovirus (CMV) infection is widespread among adults (60–90%) and is usually undetected in healthy individuals without symptoms but can cause severe diseases in immunocompromised hosts. T-cell receptor (TCR)-like antibodies (Abs), which recognize complex antigens (peptide–MHC complex, pMHC) composed of MHC molecules with embedded short peptides derived from intracellular proteins, including pathogenic viral proteins, can serve as diagnostic and/or therapeutic agents. In this study, we aimed to engineer a TCR-like Ab specific for pMHC comprising a CMV pp65 protein-derived peptide (^{495}NLVPMVATV^{503}; hereafter, CMVpp65$_{495\text{-}503}$) in complex with MHC-I molecule human leukocyte antigen (HLA)-A*02:01 (CMVpp65$_{495\text{-}503}$/HLA-A*02:01) to increase affinity by sequential mutagenesis of complementarity-determining regions using yeast surface display technology. Compared with the parental Ab, the final generated Ab (C1-17) showed ~67-fold enhanced binding affinity ($K_D \approx 5.2$ nM) for the soluble pMHC, thereby detecting the cell surface-displayed CMVpp65$_{495\text{-}503}$/HLA-A*02:01 complex with high sensitivity and exquisite specificity. Thus, the new high-affinity TCR-like Ab may be used for the detection and treatment of CMV infection.

Keywords: cytomegalovirus; peptide/major histocompatibility complex class I complex; T-cell-receptor-like antibody; affinity maturation; yeast surface display

Citation: Lee, S.-Y.; Ko, D.-H.; Son, M.-J.; Kim, J.-A.; Jung, K.; Kim, Y.-S. Affinity Maturation of a T-Cell Receptor-Like Antibody Specific for a Cytomegalovirus pp65-Derived Peptide Presented by HLA-A*02:01. *Int. J. Mol. Sci.* **2021**, *22*, 2349. https://doi.org/10.3390/ijms22052349

Academic Editor: Yong-Seok Heo

Received: 1 February 2021
Accepted: 23 February 2021
Published: 26 February 2021

1. Introduction

Human cytomegalovirus (CMV), a β-herpes virus with a double-stranded DNA, infects a wide variety of cells and establishes latency in the host [1]. CMV infection is very common in adults (60-90% of the population), with higher infection rates with age [2], and is usually asymptomatic in healthy subjects but can cause severe diseases in immunocompromised patients with cellular immunosuppression or immunodeficiency, including transplant recipients and fetuses [1,3].

Major histocompatibility complex class I (MHC-I) molecules, also known as human leukocyte antigen I (HLA-I), are cell-surface antigen-presenting proteins displaying peptide fragments (8–10 amino acid residues in length) derived from intracellular cytoplasmic proteins, including self, viral, and tumor antigens, for recognition by CD8$^+$ T cells [4]. In CMV-seropositive hosts, matrix protein pp65 is among the most frequently immunologically recognized CMV antigens [5], accounting for 70–90% of the cytotoxic CD8$^+$ T cells' (CTLs) response to CMV [6]. Among the pp65-derived CTL epitope peptides, the 9-mer peptide ^{495}NLVPMVATV^{503} (residues 495–503; hereafter referred to as CMVpp65$_{495\text{-}503}$ peptide) is the most immunogenic T cell epitope predominantly displayed on HLA-A*02:01, the most common MHC-I allele in the population [6–8]. Hence, detection and targeting of the highly prevalent CMVpp65$_{495\text{-}503}$/HLA-A*02:01 complex on the surface of CMV-infected cells are crucial for the development of detection and/or therapeutic modalities [9,10]. T-cell receptors (TCRs) specifically recognize the peptide–MHC complex (pMHC), but their natural affinity is limited to ~1–100 μM [4]. Alternatively, antibodies (Abs) called TCR-like Abs can be engineered to specifically recognize pMHC with high affinity [9,11].

A number of TCR-like Abs directed toward a particular pMHC derived from a pathogenic viral protein or a tumor-associated antigen have been developed because such Abs have many desirable features of conventional immunoglobulin G (IgG) Abs, including large-scale manufacturing capacity and long serum half-life [11]. However, few of these Abs have reached clinical application, and the optimal specificity and affinity of TCR-like Abs need to be defined. High-affinity TCR-like Abs have several potential biomedical applications and may be valuable research reagents for detecting specific virus-/tumor-associated pMHCs on cell and tissue surfaces [11,12].

Previously, a TCR-like Ab (H9) specific for the CMVpp65$_{495\text{-}503}$/HLA-A*02:01 complex was reported [13]. However, the affinity was relatively weak (K_D = 300 nM), limiting its potential use as a detection or therapeutic reagent. Here, we aimed to engineer H9 to increase its affinity by ~67-fold for pMHC comprising the CMVpp65$_{495\text{-}503}$/HLA-A*02:01 complex by yeast surface display (YSD) technology, thereby enabling highly sensitive and specific detection of the cell surface-displayed pMHC.

2. Results

2.1. Evaluation of Parental H9

The TCR-like H9 antigen-binding fragment (Fab) was previously isolated by screening a large phage-displayed human Fab library against a recombinant CMVpp65$_{495\text{-}503}$/HLA-A*02:01 complex [13]. H9 reformatted into the bivalent IgG form showed binding specificity to soluble pMHC comprising the CMVpp65$_{495\text{-}503}$/HLA-A*02:01 complex with relatively weak binding affinity ($K_D \approx$ 300 nM) [13]. Here, we generated H9 in the mouse IgG2a/κ format and evaluated its binding activity by flow cytometry toward the cell surface-displayed CMVpp65$_{495\text{-}503}$/HLA-A*02:01 complex, generated by external peptide pulsing of cells expressing HLA-A*02:01 at various levels (Figure 1A). Even at 500 nM, H9 manifested very weak binding activity only toward MDA-MB-231 and Malme-3M cells expressing HLA-A*02:01 at relatively high levels (HLA-A*02:01^{++}) but negligible or little binding activity toward HCT116 cells expressing HLA-A*02:01 at moderate levels (HLA-A*02:01^{+}) and toward HLA-A*02:01-negative LoVo cells (Figure 1B). At 100 and 20 nM, H9 binding to peptide-loaded HLA-A*02:01^{++} MDA-MB-231 cells was negligible (Figure 1C). H9 did not react with cells loaded with an off-target peptide of HLA-A*02:01-restricted human papilloma virus (HPV) type 16 E7 protein-derived 9-mer peptide, HPVE7$_{11\text{-}19}$ (^{11}YMLDLQPETV^{19}). These results confirmed the specific binding of H9 to the membrane-bound pMHC comprising the CMVpp65$_{495\text{-}503}$/HLA-A*02:01 complex.

However, the binding strength was too weak to detect the complex on cells expressing HLA-A*02:01 at moderate levels. Thus, we sought to engineer H9 for affinity improvement.

2.2. Affinity Maturation of H9 to Generate C1 Ab

Owing to lack of information regarding specific amino acid residue interactions between H9 and the CMVpp65$_{495\text{-}503}$/HLA-A*02:01 complex, for affinity maturation, we first generated an H9 library by randomization of the third complementarity-determining region (CDR) of variable regions of the heavy chain (VH) and (VL), i.e., VH-CDR3 and VL-CDR3, known to be major contributors to Ab–antigen interaction [14]. Most residues in VH-CDR3 (residues 95–102 in Kabat numbering [15]) and VL-CDR3 (residues 89–97) were randomized with degenerate codons, including the NNK codon encoding all 20 amino acids and one stop codon (Figure 2A). To improve the stability and folding efficiency of the Ab, some highly conserved amino acid residues based on human germline sequences, inferred from the International ImMunoGeneTics information system database [16], were conserved or minimally randomized to maintain the parental amino acid residues at a high frequency. Specifically, in the last three residues of VH-CDR3 (100J, 101, and 102), which are highly conserved with a consensus sequence of 100JPhe/Met/Ile–Asp–Tyr102, only the PheH100J residue was randomized with the degenerate codon WTK (encoding F, I, M, and L) while preserving the other residues, AspH101 and TyrH102. Similarly, for VL-CDR3, the highly conserved residues GlnL89, ProL95, and ThrL97 were retained owing to their high frequency in the human germline sequences. Residues TyrL91, SerL94, and PheL96 were mutated with degenerate codons YHT (encoding F, S, Y, L, P, and H), WHT (encoding F, S, Y, I, T, and N), NNT (encoding F, S, Y, C, L, P, H, R, I, T, N, S, V, A, D, and G), respectively (Figure 2A). The VH-CDR3/VL-CDR3-randomized H9 library was generated by YSD technology in the single-chain Fab (scFab) format, wherein the C-terminus of VL was linked to the N-terminus of VH via a G4S-based 63-amino-acid linker (Figure 2A) [17,18]. The library diversity was ~1.5 × 107, and sequencing of tens of clones confirmed the fidelity of the library diversity.

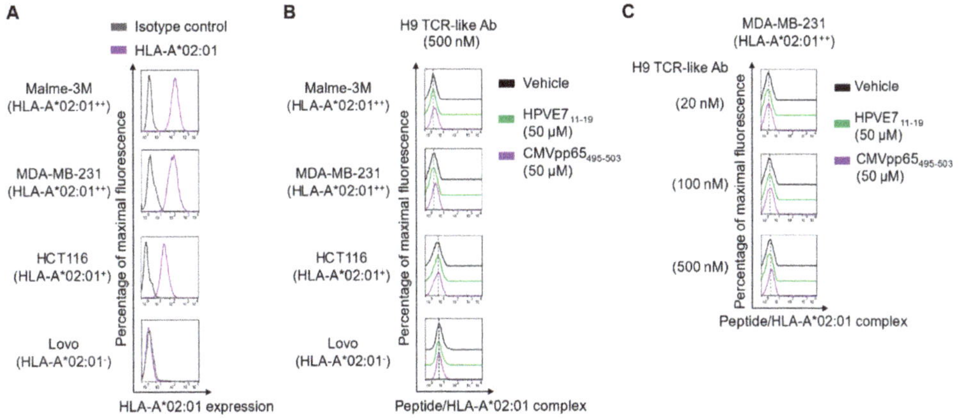

Figure 1. Evaluation of H9 binding to the cell surface-displayed $CMVpp65_{495\text{-}503}$/HLA-A*02:01 complex. (**A**) Flow cytometric analysis of the cell surface expression levels of human leukocyte antigen (HLA)-A*02:01, classified as + + (high level) for both MDA-MB-231 and Malme-3M cells, as + (positive) for HCT116 cells, and as - (negative) for LoVo cells. (**B**,**C**) Flow cytometric analysis of H9 binding at 500 nM (B) to peptide-pulsed cells (B) and at various concentrations to peptide-pulsed MDA-MB-231 cells (**C**). Cells were pulsed with the vehicle, $CMVpp65_{495\text{-}503}$ peptide (50 μM), or the control HLA-A*02:01-restricted $HPVE7_{11\text{-}19}$ (50 μM) peptide for 3 h at 37 °C and incubated with H9 and then the Alexa Fluor 647-conjugated goat anti-mouse immunoglobulin G (IgG)-specific $(Fab')_2$ antibody (Ab) (secondary Ab) prior to flow cytometry. In (A–C), representative histograms from two independent experiments are depicted.

Table 1. Parameters of binding kinetics of TCR-like Abs in relation to the $CMVpp65_{495\text{-}503}$/HLA-A*02:01 SCT protein, as measured using biolayer interferometry.

Abs	K_D (nM)	k_{on} ($M^{-1}s^{-1}$)	k_{off} (s^{-1})	R^2
H9	348 ± 33	$(6.3 \pm 3.3) \times 10^3$	$(2.2 \pm 0.2) \times 10^{-3}$	0.97
C1	12.6 ± 0.3	$(1.8 \pm 0.2) \times 10^5$	$(2.3 \pm 0.4) \times 10^{-3}$	0.97
C38	30.6 ± 0.1	$(1.5 \pm 0.1) \times 10^5$	$(4.7 \pm 0.4) \times 10^{-3}$	0.98
C1-17	5.2 ± 0.1	$(9.3 \pm 0.2) \times 10^5$	$(4.8 \pm 0.1) \times 10^{-3}$	0.99
C1-30	8.7 ± 0.1	$(8.0 \pm 0.2) \times 10^5$	$(7.0 \pm 0.1) \times 10^{-3}$	0.99

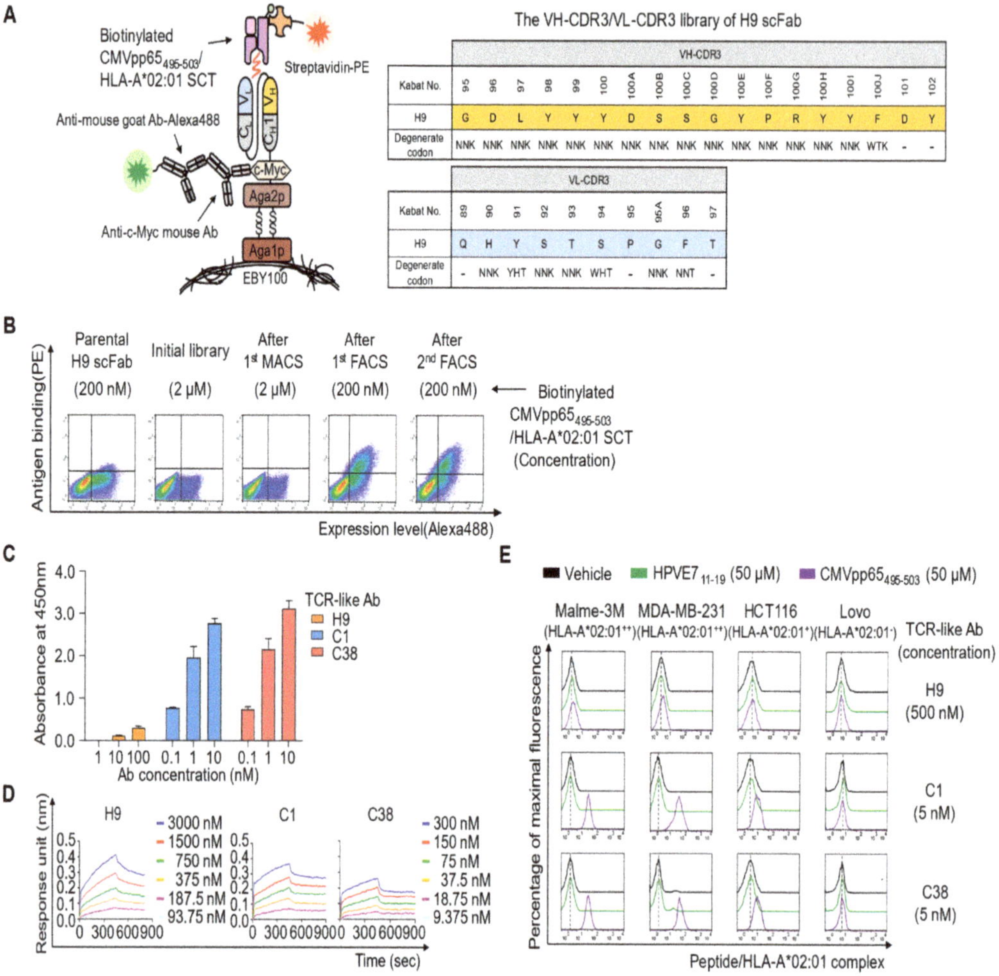

	VH-CDR3																	
Kabat No.	95	96	97	98	99	100	100A	100B	100C	100D	100E	100F	100G	100H	100I	100J	101	102
H9	G	D	L	Y	Y	Y	D	S	S	G	Y	P	R	Y	Y	F	D	Y
Degenerate codon	NNK	NNK	NNK	NNK	NNK	NNK	NNK	NNK	NNK	NNK	NNK	NNK	NNK	NNK	NNK	WTK	-	-

	VL-CDR3									
Kabat No.	89	90	91	92	93	94	95	95A	96	97
H9	Q	H	Y	S	T	S	P	G	F	T
Degenerate codon	-	NNK	YHT	NNK	NNK	WHT	-	NNK	NNT	-

Figure 2. Affinity maturation of H9 and characterization of the isolated clones. (**A**) The scheme of library construction and screening for H9 in the single-chain antigen-binding fragment (scFab) format using YSD technology. The indicated residues in VH-CDR3 and VL-CDR3 were randomized with the indicated degenerate codons. The "-" sign denotes conserved residues.(**B**) Flow cytometric analysis of antigen binding and expression levels of the yeast surface-displayed scFab library pool enriched after each round of screening by magnetically activated cell sorting (MACS) and fluorescence-activated cell sorting (FACS), compared with those of the parental H9 scFab. (**C**) Dose-dependent binding activity of the isolated and purified Abs in mouse IgG2a/κ form toward the microtiter plate coated with peptide–MHC complex (pMHC) comprising CMVpp65$_{495-503}$/HLA-A*02:01 single-chain trimer (SCT) antigen, as determined by ELISA. (**D**) Binding isotherms of the immobilized Abs toward the soluble CMVpp65$_{495-503}$/HLA-A*02:01 SCT antigen, as measured by biolayer interferometry. pMHC concentrations are indicated (colored). The kinetic interaction parameters are listed in Table 1. (**E**) Flow cytometric analysis of the binding of the isolated T-cell receptor (TCR)-like Abs at the indicated concentrations to the peptide-pulsed cells. Peptide pulsing and flow cytometric analysis were performed as described in Figure 1C. Representative histograms from two independent experiments are depicted.

For library screening, we prepared the soluble antigen of CMVpp65$_{495-503}$/HLA-A*02:01 single-chain trimer (SCT) protein with a C-terminal Avi tag (for biotinylation) (Supplementary Figure S1). We engineered the SCT form to have an artificial disulfide bridge between the HLA α1 domain (Tyr108Cys) and linker L1 (position 2 of L1) to maintain stable binding of CMVpp65$_{495-503}$ into the groove of the MHC-I complex (Supplementary Figure S1) [19,20]. The disulfide-bonded SCT format ensured that the TCR-like Ab does not recognize MHC-I alone. As an off-target antigen, the HPVE7$_{11-19}$/HLA-A*02:01 SCT protein was prepared similarly. The pMHC SCT proteins were expressed in cultured HEK293F cells. The purified protein (~49.7 kDa) was site-specifically biotinylated, as confirmed by a streptavidin gel shift assay (Supplementary Figure S1C).

The H9 library was screened by one round of magnetically activated cell sorting (MACS), followed by two rounds of fluorescence-activated cell sorting (FACS) with the biotinylated CMVpp65$_{495-503}$/HLA-A*02:01 SCT antigen in the presence of a 10-fold higher concentration of the non-biotinylated off-target HPVE7$_{11-19}$/HLA-A*02:01 SCT antigen (Figure 2B), thereby yielding two unique good-affinity binders, C1 and C38 scFabs (Supplementary Figure S2). The isolated scFab clones were converted into the mouse IgG2a/κ form and expressed in HEK293F cells. ELISA revealed that purified C1 and C38 bound to the soluble CMVpp65$_{495-503}$/HLA-A*02:01 SCT in proportion to the concentration, thus showing much stronger binding activity than parental H9 (Figure 2C). In a kinetic binding analysis performed by biolayer interferometry, Abs C1 and C38 manifested more than 10-fold stronger affinity ($K_D \approx 13$ and 31 nM, respectively) than that of parental H9 ($K_D \approx 348$ nM; Figure 2D and Table 1). The binding specificity of the affinity-matured TCR-like Abs to the cell surface-displayed CMVpp65$_{495-503}$/HLA-A*02:01 complex was evaluated by flow cytometry using cells pulsed with peptides. Compared with parental H9 at 500 nM, both C1 and C38, even at a 100-fold lower concentration (at 5 nM), exhibited a substantial binding activity toward HLA-A*02:01-positive cells, including HLA-A*02:01$^+$ HCT116 cells (Figure 2E). However, the affinity-matured Abs did not bind at all to the same HLA-A*02:01-positive cells loaded with the off-target HPVE7$_{11-19}$ peptide or to HLA-A*02:01-negative LoVo cells (Figure 2E), thereby confirming their binding specificity to the cell surface-displayed CMVpp65$_{495-503}$/HLA-A*02:01 complex. Thus, both Abs C1 and C38 may exhibit improved affinity while maintaining their specificity.

The association rate constant (k_{on}), dissociation rate constant (k_{off}), and equilibrium dissociation constant (K_D) and an estimate of the goodness of curve fit (R^2) were calculated in the Octet Data Analysis software, v.11.0 (ForteBio).

2.3. *Affinity Maturation of C1 to Generate High-Affinity TCR-Like Abs*

Considering the very low density of specific peptide/HLA complexes on a natural cell surface (≤1000 per cell [21]), successful therapeutic and detection use of a TCR-like Ab requires strong affinity and high specificity [22]. Therefore, we selected C1, which has higher affinity than C38, for the next round of affinity maturation. For affinity maturation of C1, the VH-CDR2 (residues 50–65) and VL-CDR2 (residues 50–56) regions (except for the residues generally conserved in human germline sequences, e.g., IleH51, TyrH59, and AlaH60 in VH-CDR2 and AlaL51 and SerL52 in VL-CDR2) were randomized using degenerate codons (Figure 3A). The library was generated in the scFab format by YSD technology with a diversity of ~1.3×10^7 and was screened by four rounds of FACS against the biotinylated antigen, CMVpp65$_{495-503}$/HLA-A*02:01 SCT, with a gradual decrease in antigen concentration in the presence of a 10-fold higher concentration of the non-biotinylated off-target competitor, HPVE7$_{11-19}$/HLA-A*02:01 SCT (Figure 3B,C). Analysis of more than 50 finally isolated clones yielded two unique clones, C1-17 and C1-30 (Supplementary Figure S2). The isolated clones were reformatted into mouse IgG2a/κ form and purified for further characterization. ELISA indicated improved binding activity of both C1-17 and C1-30 for the soluble CMVpp65$_{495-503}$/HLA-A*02:01 SCT compared with C1 (Figure 3D). Binding kinetics analysis revealed that C1-17 and C1-30 showed single-digit nanomolar affinities (K_D) of ~5.2 and ~8.7 nM, respectively, which were approximately twofold stronger than that of parental C1 ($K_D \approx 13$ nM; Table 1). In all cases, affinity improvement was essentially owing to an increase in the association rate constant k_{on} (Figure 3E and Table 1).

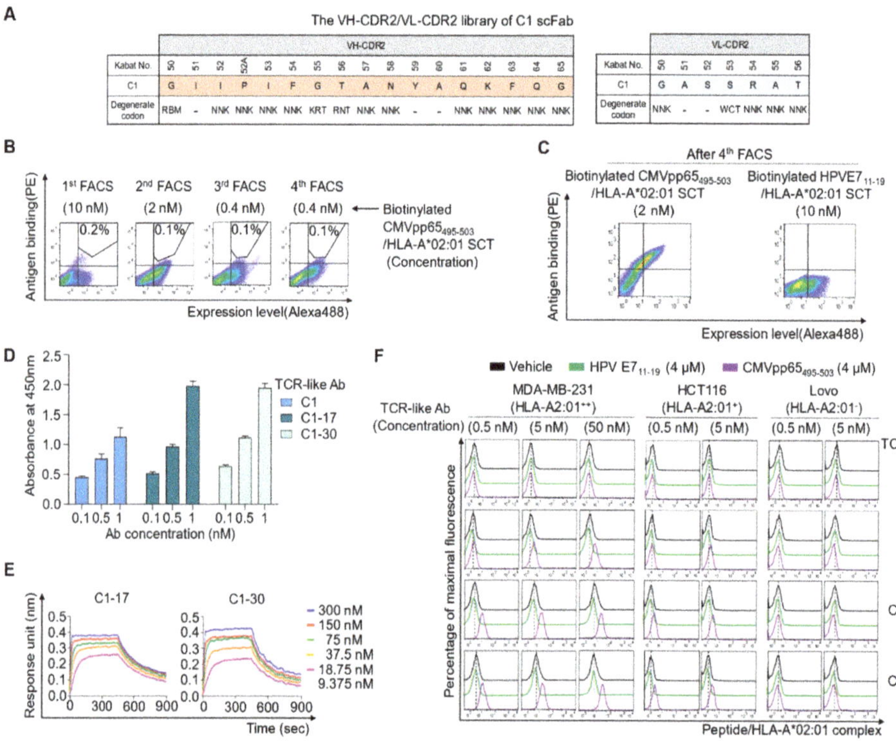

Figure 3. Affinity maturation of C1 Ab to generate high-affinity TCR-like Abs. (**A**) The scheme of yeast scFab library construction for VH-CDR2 and VL-CDR2 of C1 Ab, wherein the indicated residues were randomized with the indicated degenerate codons. The "-" sign indicates conserved residues. (**B**) Flow cytometric sorting gate plots of the yeast surface-displayed scFab library screening in each round of screening by FACS with the indicated concentration of the biotinylated CMVpp65$_{495-503}$/HLA-A*02:01 SCT antigen in the presence of a 10-fold higher concentration of the non-biotinylated off-target HPVE7$_{11-19}$/HLA-A*02:01 SCT protein. (**C**) Flow cytometric analysis of target-specific enrichment for the yeast surface-displayed scFab library pool enriched after four rounds of FACS using the indicated target and off-target antigen. (**D**) Dose-dependent binding activity of the isolated and purified Abs in mouse IgG2a/κ form toward the microtiter plate coated with pMHC comprising CMVpp65$_{495-503}$/HLA-A*02:01 complex antigen, as determined by ELISA. (**E**) Binding isotherms of the immobilized IgG2a/κ Abs toward the soluble CMVpp65$_{495-503}$/HLA-A*02:01 complex antigen, as measured by biolayer interferometry. The concentrations of pMHC are indicated (colored). The kinetic interaction parameters are listed in Table 1. (**F**) Flow cytometric analysis of binding of the TCR-like Abs in IgG2a/κ form at the indicated concentrations to peptide-pulsed cells. Cells were pulsed for 3 h at 37 °C with the vehicle, CMVpp65$_{495-503}$ peptide (4 μM), or the control, HLA-A*02:01-restricted HPVE7$_{11-19}$ (4 μM) peptide, and incubated with the TCR-like Abs at the indicated concentrations and then with the Alexa Fluor 647-conugated goat anti-mouse IgG-specific (Fab')$_2$ Ab (secondary Ab) prior to flow cytometry. Representative histograms from two independent experiments are depicted.

Next, we assessed the specificity and lower detection limits of the affinity-matured Abs toward cells pulsed with the peptide at a low concentration (down to 4 μM) to generate low-density CMVpp65$_{495-503}$/HLA-A*02:01 complex on cells. Both C1-17 and C1-30 strongly stained HLA-A*02:01-positive cells loaded with CMVpp65$_{495-503}$ in proportion to the concentration but did not stain the same cells pulsed with a vehicle or the off-target HPVE7$_{11-19}$ peptide and HLA-A*02:01-negative cells (Figure 3F). Although parental C1 at a low concentration of 0.5 nM failed to detect the membrane-bound CMVpp65$_{495-503}$/HLA-A*02:01 complex, both C1-17 and C1-30 at the same concentration detected it (Figure 3F). Thus, affinity-matured TCR-like Abs C1-17 and C1-30 reliably detected the cell surface-displayed CMVpp65$_{495\text{-}503}$/HLA-A*02:01 complex with high sensitivity and exquisite specificity.

3. Discussion

The low affinity of TCR-like Abs is one of the major hurdles associated with their detection and therapeutic applications. We engineered a TCR-like Ab H9 specific for the CMVpp65$_{495\text{-}503}$/HLA-A*02:01 complex to improve H9's affinity while retaining its specificity. We performed two rounds of affinity maturation by sequential random mutagenesis on the VH-/VL-CDR3 of H9 and then on the VH-/VL-CDR2 of C1 in the scFab format using YSD technology. The finally generated, highest-affinity Ab C1-17 possessed ~67-fold improved affinity ($K_D \approx 5.2$ nM) compared with that of the parental H9 ($K_D \approx 348$ nM). Parental H9 failed to detect the membrane-bound CMVpp65$_{495\text{-}503}$/HLA-A*02:01 complex even on HLA-A*02:01^{++} cells at a concentration below 500 nM. Conversely, both C1-17 and C1-30 with single-digit nanomolar affinities detected the cell surface-displayed CMVpp65$_{495\text{-}503}$/HLA-A*02:01 complex at a 1000-fold lower concentration (0.5 nM) even on HLA-A*02:01^{+} HCT116 cells, thereby showing high sensitivity owing to affinity maturation. They did not bind to HLA-A*02:01-positive cells, unpulsed or pulsed with an off-target peptide, nor to HLA-A*02:01-negative cells, thus confirming their exquisite specificity.

The expression levels of the pMHC complex on the cell surface are relatively low, ranging from tens to hundreds of molecules/cell, compared with other membrane receptors [11]. For example, the CMVpp65$_{495\text{-}503}$/HLA-A*02:01 complex was reported to be ~100 molecules/cell on the surface of CMV-infected fibroblasts [13]. Accordingly, TCRs or TCR-like Abs with high affinity and specificity are necessary for the sensitive detection or targeting of the low copy numbers of pMHC [10,11,22]. Though the H9 Ab detected the CMVpp65$_{495\text{-}503}$/HLA-A*02:01 on the surface of CMV-infected fibroblasts [13], it has not been further developed. The high-affinity TCR-like C1-17 Ab, engineered to have a $K_D \approx$ 5.2 nM in this study, can be developed as a research agent to detect CMVpp65$_{495\text{-}503}$/HLA-A*02:01 presentation on the surface of and inside cells during CMV infection and as a therapeutic agent to eliminate CMV-infected cells.

The full-length TCR-like Ab was generated based on the Fc portion of mouse IgG2a rather than that of human IgG isotype for use as a detection agent for the CMVpp65$_{495\text{-}503}$/HLA-A*02:01 complex on human cells and tissues. The mouse IgG2a isotype also has merits as a primary Ab in detection because it exhibits a detection sensitivity with labeled anti-mouse IgG isotype-specific secondary Abs that is superior to that of the other mouse IgG isotype Abs [23], and the anti-mouse IgG2a-specific secondary Abs are readily available. To be used as a therapeutic Ab, the constant regions of the TCR-like Ab need to be switched into human IgG1 with greater effector functions than the other isotypes [24].

A few antiviral drugs, including ganciclovir and valganciclovir, have been used for treating CMV infection, but viral resistance is a major challenge associated with their use [1]. Another approach is the transfer of donor-derived CMV-specific CTLs, but it remains limited due to the occurrence of graft-versus-host disease (GVHD) in allogeneic recipients [25]. The high-affinity TCR-like Ab C1-17 can be converted into a bispecific T-cell engager [20] and a chimeric antigen receptor (CAR) for CAR-T therapy based on the autologous T-cells to overcome allogeneic immunogenicity [3,26]. Moreover, C1-17 can be developed as a therapeutic Ab to eliminate CMV-infected cells through the effecter functions, such as Ab-dependent cellular cytotoxicity [27,28], or via a targeting agent to deliver cytotoxic payloads, such as potent drugs and toxins [9,29]. Comparative analyses of CTL responses in CMV-seropositive individuals have shown that, among the CMV-derived CTL epitopes, the pp65-derived CMVpp65$_{495\text{-}503}$ and the major immediate-early gene product (IE-1)-derived VLEETSVML peptide (residues 316–324) are the most frequent CTL epitope peptides, with the former being more dominant than the latter [5,6,30]. CMVpp65$_{495\text{-}503}$ is predominantly presented by HLA-A*02:01, one of the most frequent MHC-I alleles in the human population (30~50%, depending on the ethnicity) [27]. Accordingly, C1-17 specific for the CMVpp65$_{495\text{-}503}$/HLA-A*02:01 complex could be used in a maximum of up to

~50% of CMV-infected individuals as a detection or therapeutic agent. Nonetheless, C1-17, restricted to the single HLA-A*02:01 allele, is not suitable for broad applicability due to the three HLA genes and their thousands of polymorphic alleles in humans [9].

This study has some limitations. The engineered TCR-like Abs specific for CMVpp65$_{495\text{-}503}$ -bound HLA-A*02:01 were evaluated only for cells exogenously pulsed with peptides. Thus, the high-affinity TCR-like C1-17 Ab must be further validated as a potential detection and/or therapeutic agent for the pMHC naturally presented on CMV-infected cells, such as fibroblasts, epithelial cells, endothelial cells, neurons, monocytes, and macrophages, which are susceptible to CMV infection [31–33], in comparison with the lower-affinity clones, including the parent H9 Ab [13].

In conclusion, we developed a high-affinity TCR-like Ab (C1-17) specific for the highly prevalent pMHC of CMV infection, i.e., the CMVpp65$_{495\text{-}503}$/HLA-A*02:01 complex, in both soluble and membrane-bound forms. In addition to its value as a study reagent, the high-affinity TCR-like Ab can be utilized as a therapeutic agent against CMV infection.

4. Materials and Methods

4.1. Peptides and Plasmids

Human CMV pp65-derived 9-mer peptide, CMVpp65$_{495\text{-}503}$ (^{495}NLVPMVATV^{503}), and human papilloma virus (HPV) type 16 E7 protein-derived 9-mer peptide, HPVE7$_{11\text{-}19}$ (^{11}YMLDLQPETV^{19}), were synthesized with 95% purity (AnyGen, Gwangju, Korea). DNA fragments encoding the variable regions of the heavy chain (VH) and light chain (VL) of H9 (patent US8361473B2) were synthesized (Bioneer, Daejeon, Korea), and respective VH and VL genes were subcloned into a modified pcDNA 3.4 VH vector (Invitrogen, CA, USA) carrying the mouse IgG2a constant domain and a pcDNA 3.4 VL vector carrying the mouse kappa constant domain, respectively [34,35], to be expressed in mouse IgG2a/κ form. Similarly, engineered H9-derived Abs were subcloned. DNA encoding the full-length HLA-A*02:01 (residues 25–298, GenBank accession #: BC019236) was purchased from SinoBiological (cat. # HG13263-CH, Korea), and the human β2-microglobulin (β2m) gene was prepared by DNA synthesis (Bioneer, Daejeon, Korea). To express the recombinant pMHC protein in the single-chain trimer (SCT) form [19,20], the open-reading frame of the target (CMVpp65$_{495\text{–}503}$) or off-target (HPVE7$_{11\text{–}19}$) peptide-GCGGS(G_4S)$_2$ linker-β2m-(G_4S)$_4$ linker-extracellular domain of the HLA-A*02:01 protein (residues 25–298) with Y108C mutation-GS-Avi tag(GLNDIFEAQKIEWHE)-GS-8×His tag was subcloned in-frame downstream of a secretion signal peptide in the pcDNA3.4 vector to be expressed as the CMVpp65$_{495\text{–}503}$/HLA-A*02:01 or HPVE7$_{11\text{–}19}$/HLA-A*02:01 SCT protein (Supplementary Figure S1).

4.2. Expression and Purification of Abs and Proteins

Plasmids encoding the heavy chain and light chain of Abs were transiently co-transfected in pairs, at equivalent molar ratios, into cultured mammalian human embryonic kidney HEK293F cells in Freestyle 293F medium (Invitrogen, CA, USA, 12338018) following the standard protocol [34,35]. Culture supernatants were collected after 6 days by centrifugation and filtration (0.22 μm, polyethersulfone; Corning). Abs were purified from the culture supernatants using a CaptivA™ Protein A-agarose chromatographic column (Repligen, MA, USA) and were extensively dialyzed to achieve the final composition of phosphate-buffered saline (PBS; pH 7.4). Likewise, the plasmid encoding the pMHC SCT protein was transfected into HEK293F cells. The pMHC protein was purified from the culture supernatant using Ni-NTA resin (GE Healthcare, IL, USA). Protein concentrations were determined using a bicinchoninic acid kit (Thermo Fisher Scientific, Waltham, MA, USA). To prepare an Ab-screening antigen, the purified pMHC SCT proteins were biotinylated using a BirA500 kit (Avidity LLC, Colorado, USA) following the manufacturer's instructions [35].

4.3. Enzyme-Linked Immunosorbent Assay (ELISA)

Binding activity and specificity of Abs to the purified $CMVpp65_{495\text{-}503}$/HLA-A*02:01 SCT protein were determined by ELISA, as described previously [17].

4.4. Cell Cultures

HLA-A*02:01-expressing cell lines Malme-3M, MDA-MB-231, and HCT116 and an HLA-A*02:01-negative LoVo cell line were purchased from the Korean Cell Line Bank and maintained and cultured in an RPMI-1640 medium (HyClone, Busan, Korea) supplemented with 10% heat-inactivated fetal bovine serum (FBS) (HyClone, Busan, Korea), penicillin (100 U/mL), streptomycin (100 μg/mL), and amphotericin B (0.25 μg/mL; HyClone) [35,36]. All cell lines were maintained at 37 °C in a humidified 5% CO_2 incubator and routinely screened for *Mycoplasma* contamination (CellSafe, Yongin-si, Korea).

4.5. Flow Cytometry

To determine the expression levels of HLA-A*02:01, cells (2.0×10^5 cells/mL) were incubated for 30 min with a PE-conjugated mouse anti-HLA-A2 monoclonal Ab (cat. # sc-32236 PE, Santa Cruz Biotechnology, diluted 1:100). After washing with 1 mL ice-cold PBS, cells were analyzed on a FACSCalibur flow cytometer (Becton-Dickinson, Franklin lakes, New Jersey, USA). All staining procedures were performed at 4°C.

To detect pMHC on cell surfaces, cells (3.0×10^5 cells/mL) were pulsed with the vehicle, $CMVpp65_{495\text{-}503}$, or $HPVE7_{11\text{-}19}$ peptide at the indicated concentration for 3 h at 37 °C, washed with fluorescence-activated cell sorting (FACS) buffer (1% FBS in PBS, pH 7.4), and resuspended at 1.5×10^5 cells/sample. All staining procedures were performed at 4 °C. Cells were incubated for 1 h with the TCR-like Ab at the indicated concentration, washed with 1 mL FACS buffer, and incubated with an Alexa Fluor 647-conjugated goat anti-mouse IgG-specific $F(ab')_2$ polyclonal Ab (cat. # 115-606-008, Jackson ImmunoResearch, diluted 1:600) for 30 min. After washing with 1 mL ice-cold PBS, cells were analyzed on the FACSCalibur flow cytometer. Data were analyzed using FlowJo V10 software (Tree Star).

4.6. Affinity Maturation of Abs

The yeast strains and media compositions have been previously described in detail [34,35]. Library generation of Abs by complementarity-determining region (CDR) mutagenesis was performed in the scFab format involving a G_4S-based 63-amino-acid linker between VL and VH, using YSD technology as described previously [17]. The yeast library was screened using magnetically activated cell sorting (MACS) and an FACS Aria III instrument (BD Biosciences) against biotinylated $CMVpp65_{495\text{-}503}$/HLA-A*02:01 SCT protein (with a gradual decrease in concentration from 2 μM to 0.4 nM) in the presence of a 10-fold higher concentration of non-biotinylated $HPVE7_{11\text{-}19}$/HLA-A*02:01 SCT protein as a competitor, as specified in the text. In FACS, cell surface expression and antigen binding levels of the scFab library were monitored by indirect double immunofluorescence labeling of the CH1 C-terminal c-myc tag (anti-c-myc mouse Ab [9E10], diluted 1:100) with an Alexa 488-labeled goat anti-mouse IgG Ab (Invitrogen, diluted 1:600) and streptavidin-conjugated R-phycoerythrin (Invitrogen, diluted 1:600). Typically, the top 0.1–0.2% of target-binding cells were sorted. The final sorted yeast cells were plated on a selective medium, and individual clones were isolated and further analyzed. DNA from the screened yeast cells was recovered using a Zymoprep kit (Zymo Research, CA, USA) as previously described [34,35].

4.7. Biolayer Interferometry

Kinetic binding interactions of TCR-like Abs with $CMVpp65_{495\text{-}503}$/HLA-A*02:01 SCT protein were monitored at pH 7.4 using an Octet QKe System (ForteBio, California, USA), as described previously [17,35]. All data were globally fitted via the 1:1 Langmuir binding model, and association and dissociation rate constants were calculated using Octet Data Analysis Software, version 11.0 (ForteBio, Fremont, CA, USA).

5. Patents

Patents resulting from the work reported in this manuscript have been filed in the Republic of Korea (Application number: KR 10-2020-0138273) and PCT (application number: PCT/KR2020/017067).

Supplementary Materials: The following are available online at https://www.mdpi.com/1422-0067/22/5/2349/s1.

Author Contributions: Conceptualization, Y.-S.K. and S.-Y.L.; methodology, S.-Y.L. and J.-A.K.; validation, D.-H.K. and M.-J.S.; investigation, S.-Y.L., D.-H.K., M.-J.S., J.-A.K., and K.J.; writing—original draft preparation, S.-Y.L. and Y.-S.K.; writing—review and editing, K.J. and Y.-S.K.; supervision, Y.-S.K.; project administration, Y.-S.K.; funding acquisition, Y.-S.K. All authors have read and agreed to the published version of the manuscript.

Funding: This research was funded by Samsung Future Technology Center (grant number SRFC-MA1802-09).

Institutional Review Board Statement: Not applicable.

Informed Consent Statement: Not applicable.

Data Availability Statement: All data in this study are available within the article or from the authors on request.

Conflicts of Interest: Y.S.K. and S.Y.L. are listed as inventors on the patent application (KR 10-2020-0138273; PCT/KR2020/017067) related to the technology described in this work. The other authors declare no conflicts of interest. The funders had no role in the design of the study; in the collection, analyses, or interpretation of data; in the writing of the manuscript, or in the decision to publish the results.

References

1. Limaye, A.P.; Babu, T.M.; Boeckh, M. Progress and Challenges in the Prevention, Diagnosis, and Management of Cytomegalovirus Infection in Transplantation. *Clin. Microbiol. Rev.* **2021**, *34*. [CrossRef]
2. Cannon, M.J.; Schmid, D.S.; Hyde, T.B. Review of cytomegalovirus seroprevalence and demographic characteristics associated with infection. *Rev. Med. Virol.* **2010**, *20*, 202–213. [CrossRef]
3. Lerias, J.R.; Paraschoudi, G.; Silva, I.; Martins, J.; de Sousa, E.; Condeco, C.; Figueiredo, N.; Carvalho, C.; Dodoo, E.; Jager, E.; et al. Clinically Relevant Immune Responses against Cytomegalovirus: Implications for Precision Medicine. *Int. J. Mol. Sci.* **2019**, *20*, 1986. [CrossRef]
4. Van der Merwe, P.A.; Davis, S.J. Molecular interactions mediating T cell antigen recognition. *Annu. Rev. Immunol.* **2003**, *21*, 659–684. [CrossRef] [PubMed]
5. Sylwester, A.W.; Mitchell, B.L.; Edgar, J.B.; Taormina, C.; Pelte, C.; Ruchti, F.; Sleath, P.R.; Grabstein, K.H.; Hosken, N.A.; Kern, F.; et al. Broadly targeted human cytomegalovirus-specific CD4+ and CD8+ T cells dominate the memory compartments of exposed subjects. *J. Exp. Med.* **2005**, *202*, 673–685. [CrossRef] [PubMed]
6. Wills, M.R.; Carmichael, A.J.; Mynard, K.; Jin, X.; Weekes, M.P.; Plachter, B.; Sissons, J.G. The human cytotoxic T-lymphocyte (CTL) response to cytomegalovirus is dominated by structural protein pp65: Frequency, specificity, and T-cell receptor usage of pp65-specific CTL. *J. Virol.* **1996**, *70*, 7569–7579. [CrossRef]
7. Weekes, M.P.; Wills, M.R.; Mynard, K.; Carmichael, A.J.; Sissons, J.G. The memory cytotoxic T-lymphocyte (CTL) response to human cytomegalovirus infection contains individual peptide-specific CTL clones that have undergone extensive expansion in vivo. *J. Virol.* **1999**, *73*, 2099–2108. [CrossRef] [PubMed]
8. Reiser, J.B.; Legoux, F.; Machillot, P.; Debeaupuis, E.; Le Moullac-Vaydie, B.; Chouquet, A.; Saulquin, X.; Bonneville, M.; Housset, D. Crystallization and preliminary X-ray crystallographic characterization of a public CMV-specific TCR in complex with its cognate antigen. *Acta Cryst. Sect. F Struct. Biol. Cryst. Commun.* **2009**, *65*, 1157–1161. [CrossRef]
9. Bewarder, M.; Held, G.; Thurner, L.; Stilgenbauer, S.; Smola, S.; Preuss, K.D.; Carbon, G.; Bette, B.; Christofyllakis, K.; Bittenbring, J.T.; et al. Characterization of an HLA-restricted and human cytomegalovirus-specific antibody repertoire with therapeutic potential. *Cancer Immunol. Immunother.* **2020**, *69*, 1535–1548. [CrossRef]

10. Wagner, E.K.; Qerqez, A.N.; Stevens, C.A.; Nguyen, A.W.; Delidakis, G.; Maynard, J.A. Human cytomegalovirus-specific T-cell receptor engineered for high affinity and soluble expression using mammalian cell display. *J. Biol. Chem.* **2019**, *294*, 5790–5804. [CrossRef] [PubMed]
11. Hoydahl, L.S.; Frick, R.; Sandlie, I.; Loset, G.A. Targeting the MHC Ligandome by Use of TCR-Like Antibodies. *Antibodies* **2019**, *8*, 32. [CrossRef] [PubMed]
12. He, Q.; Liu, Z.; Liu, Z.; Lai, Y.; Zhou, X.; Weng, J. TCR-like antibodies in cancer immunotherapy. *J. Hematol. Oncol.* **2019**, *12*, 99. [CrossRef] [PubMed]
13. Makler, O.; Oved, K.; Netzer, N.; Wolf, D.; Reiter, Y. Direct visualization of the dynamics of antigen presentation in human cells infected with cytomegalovirus revealed by antibodies mimicking TCR specificity. *Eur. J. Immunol.* **2010**, *40*, 1552–1565. [CrossRef]
14. Lefranc, M.P.; Lefranc, G. Immunoglobulins or Antibodies: IMGT((R)) Bridging Genes, Structures and Functions. *Biomedicines* **2020**, *8*, 319. [CrossRef]
15. Dunbar, J.; Deane, C.M. ANARCI: Antigen receptor numbering and receptor classification. *Bioinformatics* **2016**, *32*, 298–300. [CrossRef] [PubMed]
16. Lefranc, M.P.; Giudicelli, V.; Duroux, P.; Jabado-Michaloud, J.; Folch, G.; Aouinti, S.; Carillon, E.; Duvergey, H.; Houles, A.; Paysan-Lafosse, T.; et al. IMGT(R), The international ImMunoGeneTics information system(R) 25 years on. *Nucleic Acid. Res.* **2015**, *43*. [CrossRef] [PubMed]
17. Kim, J.E.; Jung, K.; Kim, J.A.; Kim, S.H.; Park, H.S.; Kim, Y.S. Engineering of anti-human interleukin-4 receptor alpha antibodies with potent antagonistic activity. *Sci. Rep.* **2019**, *9*, 7772. [CrossRef] [PubMed]
18. Kim, J.E.; Lee, D.H.; Jung, K.; Kim, E.J.; Choi, Y.; Park, H.S.; Kim, Y.S. Engineering of Humanized Antibodies Against Human Interleukin 5 Receptor Alpha Subunit That Cause Potent Antibody-Dependent Cell-Mediated Cytotoxicity. *Front. Immunol.* **2021**, *11*, 593748. [CrossRef] [PubMed]
19. Truscott, S.M.; Lybarger, L.; Martinko, J.M.; Mitaksov, V.E.; Kranz, D.M.; Connolly, J.M.; Fremont, D.H.; Hansen, T.H. Disulfide bond engineering to trap peptides in the MHC class I binding groove. *J. Immunol.* **2007**, *178*, 6280–6289. [CrossRef]
20. Schmittnaegel, M.; Hoffmann, E.; Imhof-Jung, S.; Fischer, C.; Drabner, G.; Georges, G.; Klein, C.; Knoetgen, H. A New Class of Bifunctional Major Histocompatibility Class I Antibody Fusion Molecules to Redirect CD8 T Cells. *Mol. Cancer. Ther.* **2016**, *15*, 2130–2142. [CrossRef]
21. Schirle, M.; Keilholz, W.; Weber, B.; Gouttefangeas, C.; Dumrese, T.; Becker, H.D.; Stevanovic, S.; Rammensee, H.G. Identification of tumor-associated MHC class I ligands by a novel T cell-independent approach. *Eur. J. Immunol.* **2000**, *30*, 2216–2225. [CrossRef]
22. Li, Y.; Moysey, R.; Molloy, P.E.; Vuidepot, A.L.; Mahon, T.; Baston, E.; Dunn, S.; Liddy, N.; Jacob, J.; Jakobsen, B.K.; et al. Directed evolution of human T-cell receptors with picomolar affinities by phage display. *Nat. Biotechnol.* **2005**, *23*, 349–354. [CrossRef]
23. Manning, C.F.; Bundros, A.M.; Trimmer, J.S. Benefits and pitfalls of secondary antibodies: Why choosing the right secondary is of primary importance. *PLoS ONE* **2012**, *7*. [CrossRef]
24. Vidarsson, G.; Dekkers, G.; Rispens, T. IgG subclasses and allotypes: From structure to effector functions. *Front. Immunol.* **2014**, *5*, 520. [CrossRef]
25. Kim, N.; Nam, Y.S.; Im, K.I.; Lim, J.Y.; Jeon, Y.W.; Song, Y.; Lee, J.W.; Cho, S.G. Robust Production of Cytomegalovirus pp65-Specific T Cells Using a Fully Automated IFN-gamma Cytokine Capture System. *Transfus. Med. Hemother.* **2018**, *45*, 13–22. [CrossRef]
26. Akatsuka, Y. TCR-Like CAR-T Cells Targeting MHC-Bound Minor Histocompatibility Antigens. *Front. Immunol.* **2020**, *11*, 257. [CrossRef]
27. Lai, J.; Choo, J.A.L.; Tan, W.J.; Too, C.T.; Oo, M.Z.; Suter, M.A.; Mustafa, F.B.; Srinivasan, N.; Chan, C.E.Z.; Lim, A.G.X.; et al. TCR-like antibodies mediate complement and antibody-dependent cellular cytotoxicity against Epstein-Barr virus-transformed B lymphoblastoid cells expressing different HLA-A*02 microvariants. *Sci. Rep.* **2017**, *7*, 9923. [CrossRef] [PubMed]
28. Zhao, Q.; Ahmed, M.; Tassev, D.V.; Hasan, A.; Kuo, T.Y.; Guo, H.F.; O'Reilly, R.J.; Cheung, N.K. Affinity maturation of T-cell receptor-like antibodies for Wilms tumor 1 peptide greatly enhances therapeutic potential. *Leukemia* **2015**, *29*, 2238–2247. [CrossRef] [PubMed]
29. Lowe, D.B.; Bivens, C.K.; Mobley, A.S.; Herrera, C.E.; McCormick, A.L.; Wichner, T.; Sabnani, M.K.; Wood, L.M.; Weidanz, J.A. TCR-like antibody drug conjugates mediate killing of tumor cells with low peptide/HLA targets. *mAbs* **2017**, *9*, 603–614. [CrossRef]
30. Khan, N.; Cobbold, M.; Keenan, R.; Moss, P.A. Comparative analysis of CD8+ T cell responses against human cytomegalovirus proteins pp65 and immediate early 1 shows similarities in precursor frequency, oligoclonality, and phenotype. *J. Infect. Dis.* **2002**, *185*, 1025–1034. [CrossRef] [PubMed]
31. Gerna, G.; Kabanova, A.; Lilleri, D. Human Cytomegalovirus Cell Tropism and Host Cell Receptors. *Vaccines* **2019**, *7*, 70. [CrossRef] [PubMed]
32. Plachter, B.; Sinzger, C.; Jahn, G. Cell types involved in replication and distribution of human cytomegalovirus. *Adv. Virus Res.* **1996**, *46*, 195–261. [CrossRef] [PubMed]
33. Stern-Ginossar, N.; Weisburd, B.; Michalski, A.; Le, V.T.; Hein, M.Y.; Huang, S.X.; Ma, M.; Shen, B.; Qian, S.B.; Hengel, H.; et al. Decoding human cytomegalovirus. *Science* **2012**, *338*, 1088–1093. [CrossRef] [PubMed]

34. Shin, S.M.; Choi, D.K.; Jung, K.; Bae, J.; Kim, J.S.; Park, S.W.; Song, K.H.; Kim, Y.S. Antibody targeting intracellular oncogenic Ras mutants exerts anti-tumour effects after systemic administration. *Nat. Commun.* **2017**, *8*, 15090. [CrossRef] [PubMed]
35. Shin, S.M.; Kim, J.S.; Park, S.W.; Jun, S.Y.; Kweon, H.J.; Choi, D.K.; Lee, D.; Cho, Y.B.; Kim, Y.S. Direct targeting of oncogenic RAS mutants with a tumor-specific cytosol-penetrating antibody inhibits RAS mutant-driven tumor growth. *Sci. Adv.* **2020**, *6*. [CrossRef] [PubMed]
36. Jung, K.; Kim, J.A.; Kim, Y.J.; Lee, H.W.; Kim, C.H.; Haam, S.; Kim, Y.S. A Neuropilin-1 Antagonist Exerts Antitumor Immunity by Inhibiting the Suppressive Function of Intratumoral Regulatory T Cells. *Cancer Immunol. Res.* **2020**, *8*, 46–56. [CrossRef] [PubMed]

International Journal of
Molecular Sciences

MDPI

Article

Neutralizing Human Antibodies against Severe Acute Respiratory Syndrome Coronavirus 2 Isolated from a Human Synthetic Fab Phage Display Library

Yu Jung Kim, Min Ho Lee, Se-Ra Lee, Hyo-Young Chung, Kwangmin Kim, Tae Gyu Lee and Dae Young Kim *,†

New Drug Development Center, Osong Medical Innovation Foundation, Cheongju-si, Chungcheongbuk-do 28160, Korea; yjkim@kbiohealth.kr (Y.J.K.); hpimh3@kbiohealth.kr (M.H.L.); srlee@kbiohealth.kr (S.-R.L.); hchung@kbiohealth.kr (H.-Y.C.); kwangmin.kim@kbiohealth.kr (K.K.); tglee17@gmail.com (T.G.L.)
* Correspondence: kdypsh99@gmail.com; Tel.: +82-10-2460-4630
† Current address: PnP Biopharm Ltd., #1304, Acetechno Tower 8 cha, 11, Digital-ro 33 gil, Guro-gu, Seoul 08380, Korea.

Abstract: Since it was first reported in Wuhan, China, in 2019, the severe acute respiratory syndrome coronavirus 2 (SARS-CoV-2) has caused a pandemic outbreak resulting in a tremendous global threat due to its unprecedented rapid spread and an absence of a prophylactic vaccine or therapeutic drugs treating the virus. The receptor-binding domain (RBD) of the SARS-CoV-2 spike protein is a key player in the viral entry into cells through its interaction with the angiotensin-converting enzyme 2 (ACE2) receptor protein, and the RBD has therefore been crucial as a drug target. In this study, we used phage display to develop human monoclonal antibodies (mAbs) that neutralize SARS-CoV-2. A human synthetic Fab phage display library was panned against the RBD of the SARS-CoV-2 spike protein (SARS-2 RBD), yielding ten unique Fabs with moderate apparent affinities (EC_{50} = 19–663 nM) for the SARS-2 RBD. All of the Fabs showed no cross-reactivity to the MERS-CoV spike protein, while three Fabs cross-reacted with the SARS-CoV spike protein. Five Fabs showed neutralizing activities in in vitro assays based on the Fabs' activities antagonizing the interaction between the SARS-2 RBD and ACE2. Reformatting the five Fabs into immunoglobulin Gs (IgGs) greatly increased their apparent affinities (K_D = 0.08–1.0 nM), presumably due to the effects of avidity, without compromising their non-aggregating properties and thermal stability. Furthermore, two of the mAbs (D12 and C2) significantly showed neutralizing activities on pseudo-typed and authentic SARS-CoV-2. Given their desirable properties and neutralizing activities, we anticipate that these human anti-SARS-CoV-2 mAbs would be suitable reagents to be further developed as antibody therapeutics to treat COVID-19, as well as for diagnostics and research tools.

Keywords: SARS-CoV-2; spike protein; receptor-binding domain; phage display; monoclonal antibody

Citation: Kim, Y.J.; Lee, M.H.; Lee, S.-R.; Chung, H.-Y.; Kim, K.; Lee, T.G.; Kim, D.Y. Neutralizing Human Antibodies against Severe Acute Respiratory Syndrome Coronavirus 2 Isolated from a Human Synthetic Fab Phage Display Library. *Int. J. Mol. Sci.* **2021**, *22*, 1913. https://doi.org/10.3390/ijms22041913

Academic Editor: Philippe Rondard
Received: 18 January 2021
Accepted: 12 February 2021
Published: 15 February 2021

1. Introduction

Since the pandemic outbreak of the severe acute respiratory syndrome coronavirus 2 (SARS-CoV-2), first discovered in Wuhan, China, in 2019, the rapidly growing number of infected people and casualties has posed a serious global threat [1]. SARS-CoV-2 causes severe respiratory symptoms that are accompanied by high fever, cough, and severe pneumonia [2], and although the mortality rate has been reported to be lower than that of severe acute respiratory syndrome coronavirus (SARS-CoV) or Middle East respiratory syndrome coronavirus (MERS-CoV), the overall risk remains highly significant, and thus novel prophylactic agents such as therapeutic drugs and vaccines are urgently in need.

Among the four coronavirus genera (α, β, γ, and δ), SARS-CoV-2 belongs to the β-coronaviruses and is an enveloped, positive-sense single-stranded RNA (or (+) ssRNA) virus, the RNA genome of which encodes structural proteins including the spike (S)

protein [3,4]. SARS-CoV-2 shares similarities in its genome sequences with those of SARS-CoV and MERS-CoV, which are respectively about 79.5% and 50% similar, indicating homologous structures and similar infectious pathways to SARS-CoV [5].

As in all coronaviruses, the S protein is present on the surface of the virus and plays a critical role in the viral entry to host cells [6,7]. The S protein consists of two subunits, S1 and S2, which are non-covalently associated as a homotrimeric form that comprises a prefusion state. The receptor-binding domain (RBD, residues 387–516) of the S1 subunit consists of a core domain and a receptor-binding motif (RBM, residues 438–505), and this motif directly engages with the host receptor, known as angiotensin-converting enzyme 2 (ACE2) [8]. Upon entry of the virus into cells, the RBD of the S1 subunit recognizes ACE2 on the surface of host cells as a receptor, while the S2 subunit has a role in viral fusion with host cell membranes and is primed by the S protein cleavage at the S1/S2 and S2′ sites on the S2 subunit through intracellular proteases such as TMPRSS2, triggering the conformational change of the S protein to the postfusion state [8–13].

Due to the urgent situation in which no drugs or vaccines are available, researchers and medical doctors have worked in close cooperation to develop a variety of therapeutic approaches, mostly repurposed from existing drugs, including nucleoside analogs such as remdesivir [14–16], antiparasitics such as chloroquine [17], protease inhibitors such as lopinavir and ritonavir [18], indole-derivate molecules such as arbidol [19], plasma therapy from convalescent patients who recovered from the infection [20], and, lastly, antibodies that treat the viral infection by blocking the S protein or pro-inflammatory cytokines, such as IL-6, TNF-α, GM-CSF, and IFN-γ [21,22].

Monoclonal antibodies (mAbs) have been recognized as significant biologics in therapeutic fields and are now rapidly taking a position as an alternative treatment that complements vaccines in working against newly emerging pathogenic viruses, such as SARS-CoV-2 [22–25]. Since viral neutralization by targeting the S protein has previously been shown to correlate with therapeutic efficacy in animal models [26], tremendous efforts have been made, based on the structural information of the S protein and its critical role in viral entry, to discover neutralizing mAbs that block the RBD of the S1 subunit through a variety of approaches, such as phage display library selection [27–30]; antibody selection through immunization of animals, such as humanized mice, dromedary camels, or sharks [31–34]; and antibody isolation from memory or plasma B cells of naturally infected human donors [31,35–39]. At the time of writing, 198 antibodies programs are in discovery and development phases globally, among which 66 are going through clinical trials (phase 1/2/3). In particular, 122 antibodies programs (~62%) are known to target the S protein of SARS-CoV-2, highlighting the importance of the S protein as a target. Last November, the United States Food and Drug Administration (US FDA) approved two antibodies targeting the S protein (REGN-COV2 (REGN10933 + REGN10987) and Bamlanivimab from Regeneron and Eli Lilly, respectively) for the treatment of COVID-19 patients [21].

However, the mAb approach, mainly based on the immunoglobulin G (IgG) format, has a drawback in that it relies on mammalian cell lines for the production of antibodies, which is costly and time-consuming. Moreover, viruses can easily evolve to generate RBD variants with mutations avoiding immune responses [39]. Therefore, in order to protect against the immune escapers, it would be useful to identify a selection of mAbs broadly acting on different epitopes that could contribute to a therapeutic antibody cocktail that might induce resistance to mutations in the RBD variants [29,40,41].

In this study, we panned a human Fab synthetic phage display library on the RBD of the SARS-CoV-2 S protein and obtained human mAbs with desirable properties that successfully neutralized the viral entry upon SARS-CoV-2 infection. We anticipate that these mAbs can be further developed as a promising antibody therapy against the pathogenic virus and as tools for diagnosis.

2. Results

2.1. Selection of Human Anti-SARS-2 RBD Fabs

To isolate a specific SARS-CoV-2 antibody, the KFab-I library [42,43] was panned against a recombinant SARS-2 RBD immobilized on magnetic beads (Figure 1a). After five rounds of panning, the phage ELISA was performed on immobilized SARS-2 RBD surfaces, using each panning library to monitor the enrichment (Figure 1b). Ninety-five monoclonal phages were randomly picked from the third and fourth rounds, and the binding on the SARS-2 RBD was evaluated by ELISA (Figure S1). Of the 190 individual clones from the third and fourth rounds, 70 clones showed higher absorbances at 450 nm (A450 nm) than those of the negative control (no immobilized SARS-2 RBD control) in the ELISA read-out. The 70 clones were sequenced: 55 were confirmed to be complete and the remaining clones had mutations, such as frame-shifts and stop codons. By analyzing the CDR sequences of the 55 clones, ten unique Fab clones were identified in total and, of these, D12 (Fab) was dominantly selected (60% of sequenced clones (33 out of the 55)), while the other clones showed selection frequencies of about 11% (G3 (Fab)), 9% (E10 (Fab)), 7% (E4 (Fab)), 4% (F7 (Fab)), and 2% (C2 (Fab), C12 (Fab), G9 (Fab), H1 (Fab), and H3 (Fab)) (Figure 1c). In addition, it was observed that nine out of the ten Fabs had CDR3 lengths greater than 12 amino acid residues (70% and 20% for 12 and 14 amino acid residues, respectively), while 10% of the Fabs had shorter CDR3 lengths, such as eight amino acid residues (Figure 1c). In order to confirm that the ten selected clones bound to the SARS-2 RBD and SARS-2 S1 proteins as well, a binding assay was performed, revealing that all of the antibody clones bound to the RBD and the S1 proteins (Figure 1d). In parallel, a binding analysis for RBD variants was also performed using the ten selected clones (Figure S2). This showed that all the phage clones bound to each RBD variant. Two of them (G9 and E4) bound weakly to one RBD variant (N354D; D364Y).

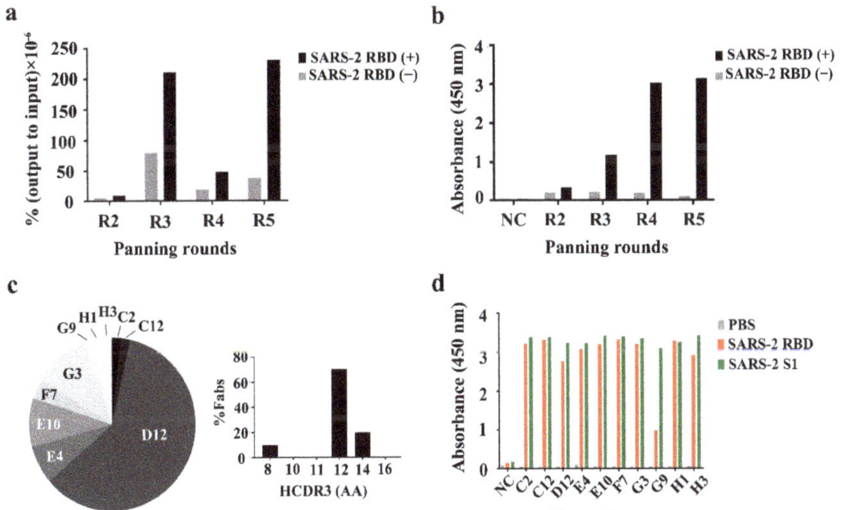

Figure 1. Panning of the phage-displayed synthetic Fab library on an immobilized SARS-2 receptor-binding domain (RBD). (**a**) Monitoring of the phage titers over four rounds (R2–R5) of panning. Black and gray bars indicate the ratio of the phage output to the input titers, presented as a percentage (%), from panning on immobilized SARS-2 RBD (black, SARS-2 RBD (+)) and non-immobilized SARS-2 RBD (gray, SARS-2 RBD (−)) surfaces. The ratio of the output to the input (%) = (phage output titer ÷ phage input titer) × 100. (**b**) Phage ELISA performed on the immobilized SARS-2 RBD surfaces using each panning library phage. (**c**) Frequency of ten Fab phage clones selected in the third and fourth rounds (left) and the distribution of HCDR3 lengths (right). The selection frequency of a unique clone (%) = (number of unique clones ÷ total number of phage ELISA positives) × 100. (**d**) Monoclonal ELISA of ten Fab phage clones against the SARS-2 RBD (red) and SARS-2 S1 protein (green). AA: amino acid residue; NC: negative control.

2.2. Production and Characterization of Human Anti-SARS-2 RBD Fabs

To order to produce and characterize the selected clones as Fab proteins, clones were cloned into an in-house *E. coli* expression vector (pKFAB). The Fab proteins were expressed and purified as described in the Section 4. The protein yields of these Fab clones were 11 mg/L, 6.5 mg/L, 106 mg/L, 15.5 mg/L, 12.5 mg/L, 125.5 mg/L, 8.5 mg/L, 17.5 mg/L, 9.5 mg/L, and 40 mg/L for C2 (Fab), C12 (Fab), D12 (Fab), F7 (Fab), H1 (Fab), E4 (Fab), E10 (Fab), G3 (Fab), G9 (Fab), and H3 (Fab), respectively (Figure S3 and Table 1).

Table 1. Physicochemical properties of human anti-SARS-2 RBD antibodies.

Clones	Yield (mg/L Culture)	T_m1/T_m2 (°C)	Monomericity (Mon./Agg.)	EC_{50} (nM)	K_D (nM)	$IC_{50}{}^P$ (μg/mL)	$IC_{50}{}^A$ (mg/mL)
C2 (Fab)	11	80.2	n.d.	121	n.d.	n.d.	n.d.
C12 (Fab)	6.5	76.7/83.2	n.d.	83	n.d.	n.d.	n.d.
D12 (Fab)	106	76.2/83.0	n.d.	19	n.d.	n.d.	n.d.
F7 (Fab)	15.5	76.4	n.d.	125	n.d.	n.d.	n.d.
H1 (Fab)	12.5	76.8	n.d.	126	n.d.	n.d.	n.d.
E4 (Fab)	125.5	n.d.	n.d.	663	n.d.	n.d.	n.d.
E10 (Fab)	8.5	n.d.	n.d.	62	n.d.	n.d.	n.d.
G3 (Fab)	17.5	n.d.	n.d.	67	n.d.	n.d.	n.d.
G9 (Fab)	9.5	n.d.	n.d.	112	n.d.	n.d.	n.d.
H3 (Fab)	40	n.d.	n.d.	174	n.d.	n.d.	n.d.
C2 (IgG)	9.6	70.3/89.6	Mon.	0.07	0.134	0.015	0.018
C12 (IgG)	12.9	70.3/86.5	Mon.	1.0	n.d.	0.263	0.232
D12 (IgG)	13.5	70.5/91.9	Mon.	0.2	0.57	0.035	0.036
F7 (IgG)	13.2	70.2/81.1	Mon.	0.5	n.d.	0.219	0.151
H1 (IgG)	12.5	70.3/80.1	Mon.	0.16	n.d.	0.042	0.102

Fab: antigen-binding fragment; IgG: immunoglobulin G; n.d.: not determined; T_m: melting temperature. T_m1 and T_m2 are the first and second apparent melting temperatures determined by differential scanning fluorimetry (DSF), respectively; EC_{50}: half maximal effective concentration; K_D: equilibrium dissociation constant; IC_{50}: half maximal inhibitory concentration; Mon.: monomer; Agg.: aggregate; $IC_{50}{}^P$ and $IC_{50}{}^A$: IC_{50} determined by a pseudo-typed virus (D614 spike) and authentic SARS-CoV-2 virus, respectively.

The apparent affinities of the ten Fabs for the SARS-2 RBD were assessed using an ELISA (EC_{50}, nM) (Figure 2a and Table 1). While six Fabs (G9 (Fab), C2 (Fab), F7 (Fab), H1 (Fab), H3 (Fab), and E4 (Fab)) had low to intermediate apparent affinities for the SARS-2 RBD (EC_{50} = 112–663 nM), the remaining four Fabs—D12 (Fab), E10 (Fab), G3 (Fab), and C12 (Fab)—showed relatively higher apparent affinities (19 nM, 62 nM, 67 nM, and 83 nM, respectively) (Figure 2a).

To examine the potential neutralizing ability of the selected Fabs, we conducted a competitive binding assay between the SARS-2 RBD and ACE2 protein or ACE2-overexpressed cells (Figure 2b). It was found that five Fabs (C2 (Fab), C12 (Fab), D12 (Fab), F7 (Fab), and H1 (Fab)) significantly antagonized the interaction between the SARS-2 RBD and biotinylated ACE2 protein (Figure 2c). The same five Fabs seemed to block the interaction between SARS-2 RBD-mFc protein and ACE2-overexpressed cells in a flow cytometry analysis as well (Figure 2d and Figure S4).

Next, in order to determine whether the ten Fabs could cross-react with the S1 proteins from other coronaviruses, such as SARS-CoV and MERS-CoV, an ELISA was conducted. This showed that three of the Fabs (E4 (Fab), E10 (Fab), and G3 (Fab)) indeed cross-reacted with the SARS-CoV S1, whereas no Fabs bound with the MERS-CoV S1 (Figure S5).

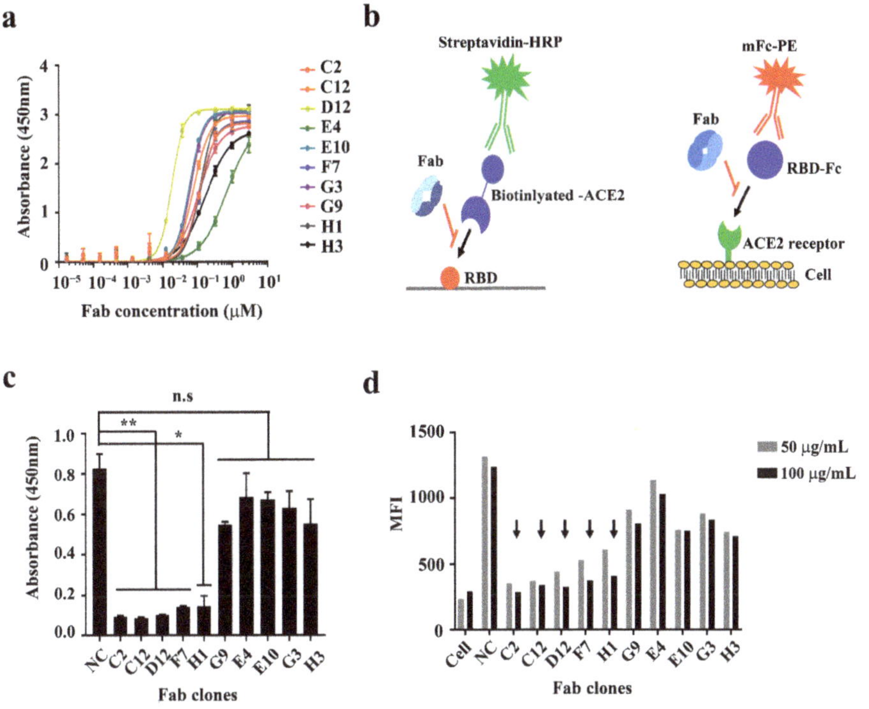

Figure 2. Characterization of human anti-SARS-2 RBD Fabs. (**a**) Soluble ELISA of ten serially diluted human anti-SARS-2 RBD Fabs on immobilized SARS-2 RBD surfaces to measure their apparent affinities (EC_{50}, nM). (**b**) Schematic drawings of a competitive ELISA of human anti-SARS-2 RBD Fabs between the SARS-2 RBD and ACE2 protein (left) or ACE2-overexpressed cells (right). (**c**) Competitive ELISA of human anti-SARS-2 RBD Fabs antagonizing the interaction between ACE2 and the SARS-CoV-2 RBD. (**d**) Competitive flow cytometry analysis of human anti-SARS-2 RBD Fabs antagonizing the interaction between ACE2 on cells and the SARS-CoV-2 RBD (tagged with mouse Fc (mFc)). Arrows indicate potentially neutralizing clones. mFc-PE: anti-mouse PE (phycoerythrin) conjugate; MFI: mean fluorescence intensity; n.s: not significant ($p > 0.05$); NC: negative control. * and **: $p < 0.05$ and $p < 0.01$, respectively.

2.3. Production and Characterization of Human Anti-SARS-2 RBD IgGs

To produce and characterize the five anti-SARS-2 RBD antibodies that seemed to have neutralizing activities in IgG forms, the five Fabs were individually reformatted to IgG forms. That is, the individual VH and VL sequences from each of the Fabs were cloned into heavy- (IgG1 Fc) and light-chain (Ck1) expression vectors, respectively. The five IgGs were transiently expressed in HEK293 cells and subsequently purified as described in the Section 4. The resulting IgGs were highly pure and their protein yields were 9.6 mg/L, 12.9 mg/L, 13.5 mg/L, 13.2 mg/L, and 12.5 mg/L for C2 (IgG), C12 (IgG), D12 (IgG), F7 (IgG), and H1 (IgG), respectively (Figure S6 and Table 1).

In order to confirm whether the purified IgGs could bind to the SARS-2 RBD and its variants—and also whether they could cross-react with other coronavirus S1 proteins, as observed with the Fabs—an ELISA binding assay was conducted, revealing that all the IgGs bound to the SARS-2 RBD and SARS-2 S1, as well as the RBD variants, whereas all of them did not bind to the MERS-CoV S1 (Figure 3a). In particular, one clone, H1 (IgG), was found to cross-react with the SARS-CoV S1 and three IgGs (C2 (IgG), D12 (IgG), and F7 (IgG)) seemed to bind with the SARS-CoV S1 but the binding was too weak to confirm their cross-reactivity.

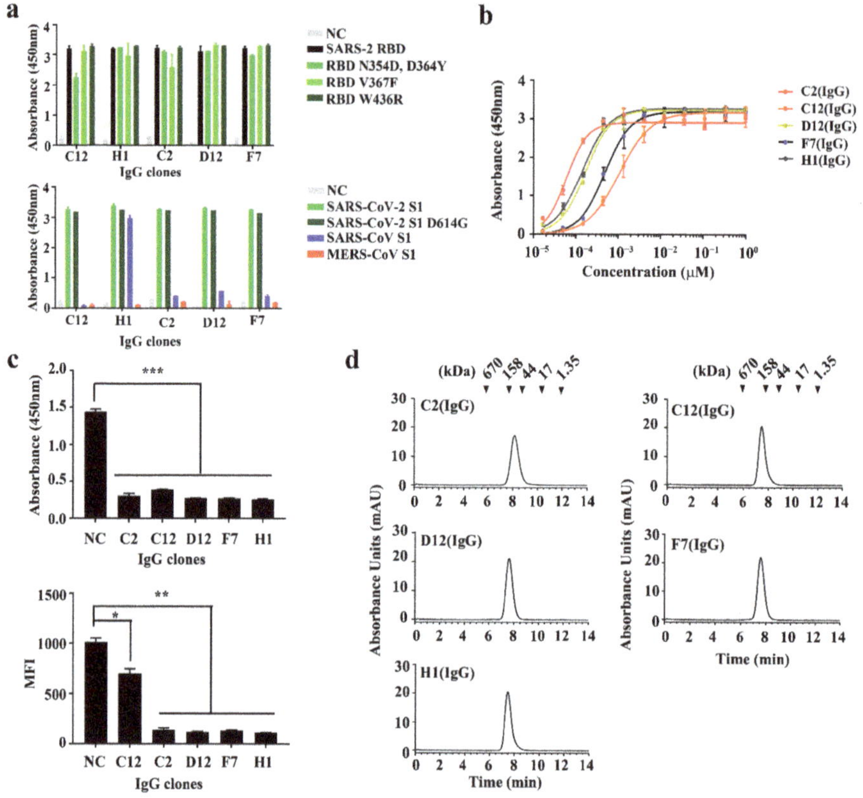

Figure 3. Characterization of anti-SARS-2 RBD immunoglobulin Gs (IgGs). (**a**) Binding analysis of five human anti-SARS-2 RBD IgGs—C12 (IgG), H1 (IgG), C2 (IgG), D12 (IgG), and F7 (IgG)—to the SARS-2 RBD and its variants (top) and the SARS-CoV-2 S1 (D614G) and other coronavirus S1 proteins (bottom), respectively. (**b**) Soluble ELISA of five serially diluted human anti-SARS-2 RBD IgGs on immobilized SARS-2 RBD surfaces to measure their apparent affinities (EC_{50}, nM). (**c**) ELISA detection for five human anti-SARS-2 RBD IgGs blocking the binding of the ACE2 protein with the SARS-CoV-2 RBD (top) and analysis of the flow cytometry for the blocking effect between the SARS-CoV-2 RBD and an ACE2-overexpressed cell (bottom). (**d**) Size-exclusion chromatography analysis of five human anti-SARS-2 RBD IgGs. The positions of the molecular mass markers, shown as kDa, on the retention time *x*-axis are indicated above the peaks. The data are presented as the mean ± standard error (SEM). MFI: mean fluorescence intensity; NC: negative control; *, **, and ***: $p < 0.05$, $p < 0.01$, and $p < 0.001$, respectively.

To determine whether the apparent affinities of the anti-SARS-2 RBD IgGs were altered by reformatting the Fabs into the IgGs, the apparent affinities of the IgGs were examined using ELISA (EC_{50}, nM). As shown in Figure 3b, the five clones (C2 (IgG), C12 (IgG), D12 (IgG), F7 (IgG), and H1 (IgG)) increased their apparent affinities approximately 100- to 1800-fold compared to their Fab formats (Figure 3b and Table 1), which might have been due to an avidity effect [42,43]. Next, a size-exclusion chromatography analysis was performed to assess their non-aggregation properties, revealing that the IgGs were monomeric without forming high molecular weight (HMW) aggregates (Figure 3d and Table 1). The five IgGs were further analyzed using a protein thermal shift (PTS) assay to determine their thermal stabilities; the assay showed that all the IgGs had T_m over 70.0 °C, confirming that they were thermally stable (Figure S7 and Table 1). To determine whether the thermal stability of the IgGs was due to the intrinsically high stability of the Fabs, the five Fabs were analyzed with the same PTS assay and the results showed that all of the Fabs had T_m values over

76.0 °C, indicating that the high thermal stability of the IgGs was derived from the intrinsic properties of the Fabs (Figure S8).

Next, to determine whether the neutralizing activities of the SARS-2 RBD IgGs remained after reformatting the Fabs into IgGs, we performed a competitive binding assay demonstrating the IgGs' antagonizing activities in the interaction between the SARS-2 RBD and ACE2 protein or ACE2-expressed cells (Figure 3c). All the IgGs significantly antagonized the interaction between the RBD and biotinylated ACE2 protein (Figure 3c top) and also inhibited the interaction between the SARS-2 RBD-mFc protein and ACE2-overexpressed cells in a flow cytometry analysis, although C12 (IgG) showed a slightly reduced inhibition compared to the other IgGs (Figure 3c bottom and Figure S9).

2.4. Neutralization Assay against SARS-CoV-2 Pseudovirus and Authentic SARS-CoV-2

To evaluate the neutralization potency of the five human SARS-CoV-2 RBD IgGs, we carried out a pseudo-typed virus neutralization assay using a lentiviral HIV-1 pseudo-typing system [44]. The five IgGs were found to display strong neutralizing activity against the SARS-CoV-2 pseudo-typed virus, among which C2 (IgG) and D12 (IgG) showed the most potent activity. The IC_{50} values of C2 (IgG) and D12 (IgG) in the pseudo-typed virus neutralization were 0.015 and 0.035 μg/mL, respectively (Figure 4a and Table 1).

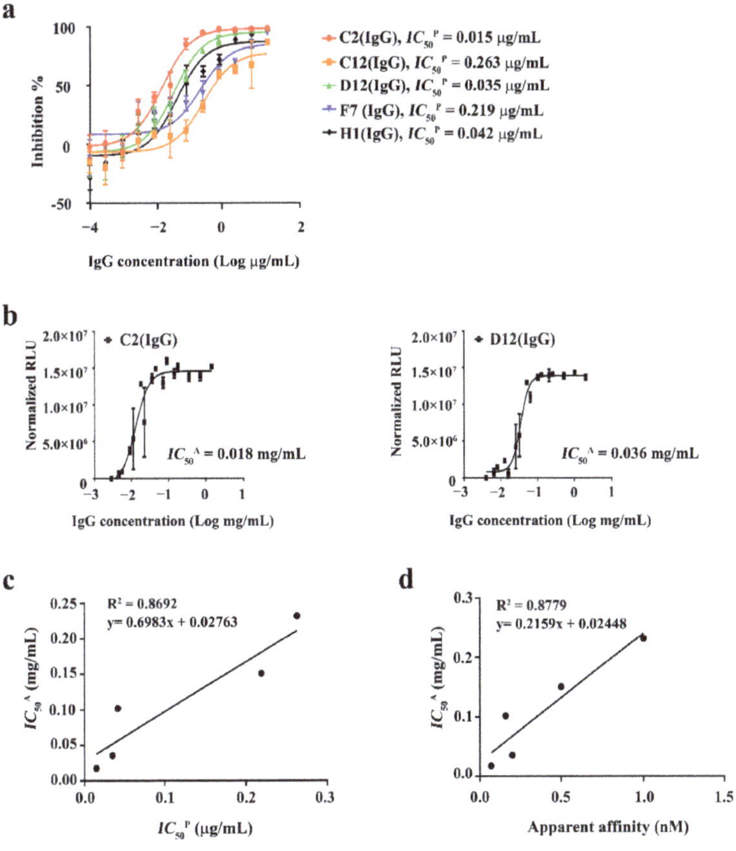

Figure 4. In vitro neutralization assay of human anti-SARS-2 RBD IgGs. Pseudo-typed virus-based neutralization (**a**) and a neutralization assay using authentic SARS-CoV-2 (**b**). (**c**) Correlation in neutralization potencies between pseudo-typed virus- and authentic virus-based assays. (**d**) Correlation between affinities of anti-SARS-2 RBD IgGs and their neutralization potencies for the authentic virus. The data are showed as the mean ± standard error (SEM).

Based on our previous competitive binding assays, we examined the five IgGs in order to evaluate their neutralizing effects on authentic SARS-CoV-2. The observations of luminescent signals showed that two of the IgGs, C2 (IgG) and D12 (IgG), exhibited high protection upon SARS-CoV-2 exposure for three days. The IC_{50} values of C2 (IgG) and D12 (IgG) in the authentic SARS-CoV-2 neutralization were 0.018 and 0.036 mg/mL, respectively (Figure 4b, Figure S10, and Table 1). The rest of the IgGs showed less neutralization compared to the two IgGs: 0.102 mg/mL, 0.151 mg/mL, and 0.232 mg/mL for H1 (IgG), F7 (IgG), and C12 (IgG), respectively (Table 1). In order to know whether there was any correlation present between the neutralization potencies from the pseudo-typed virus and the authentic virus, we compared and plotted the values from the assays and found that a strong correlation was indeed present between the neutralization potencies from the two different neutralization assays (Figure 4c). In addition, we also found that there was a strong correlation between the affinity and the neutralization potency of the anti-SARS-2 RBD IgGs as well (Figure 4d).

The two human anti-SARS-2 RBD IgGs, C2 and D12, were further characterized by BLI (Octet) in order to determine their affinities with the SARS-2 RBD, and it was found that C2 (IgG) and D12 (IgG) had binding affinities of 0.13 nM and 0.57 nM, respectively (Figure S11). This confirmed that some avidity effects were reflected in the apparent affinities from the previous ELISA (Figure 3b and Table 1), which was performed with an immobilized SARS-2 RBD, unlike the BLI (Octet), which was undertaken with the human IgGs immobilized on the sensor.

3. Discussion

We here report on the selection of human mAbs specific to the SARS-CoV-2 RBD (SARS-2 RBD) using a human synthetic Fab phage display library. Phage display is a powerful tool that has been used for both discovery and therapeutic applications against various malignancies, including infectious diseases [45–49]. In particular, phage display has been demonstrated to be highly effective for the selection of human antibodies against SARS-CoV-2 in both synthetic and immune phage display libraries built with immune repertoires of memory or plasma B cells from convalescent patients who recovered from the viral infection [27–30]. In our phage display panning, we employed two in-house human synthetic Fab phage display libraries: KFab-I and KFab-II. The KFab-I library was built on V_H3 and V_k1 frameworks by randomizing their complementarity-determining regions (CDRs) and yielded ten human anti-SARS-2 RBD mAb clones, whereas no binder was yielded by panning with the KFab-II library, another in-house human synthetic Fab phage display library built on V_H1 and V_k1 frameworks. Due to the same CDR randomization design being applied to the two libraries, we reasoned that the framework could have made a difference in the panning outcome. The human V_H3 family has been shown to have the highest stability and soluble protein yield, and its germline usage out of 51 germline genes is about 43%, which is considerably higher than that of other families of human V_H [43,50]. Indeed, for various antibody libraries, such as the Griffiths and the HuCAL libraries, it has been shown that a considerable number of antibodies selected from the libraries belonged to the human V_H3 family (74% and 36% for the Griffiths and HuCAL libraries, respectively) [51,52], indicating that the human V_H3 framework may be inevitably favored in the phage display selection due to its desirable properties. Moreover, our previous phage display panning against human YKL-40, which was also performed with the two Fab libraries, showed a similar outcome in that, unlike the KFab-I library, the KFab-II yielded no binders with desirable properties [43]. However, it is believed that a panning with a mixture of both V_H3 and V_H1 frameworks from KFab-I and KFab-II libraries might result in a different outcome from the previous panning performed separately with each Fab library.

Our study revealed that only one anti-SARS-2 RBD IgG clone (H1) cross-reacted with the S protein of SARS-CoV and the rest of the anti-SARS-2 RBD IgGs reacted specifically with the S protein of SARS-CoV-2, while no anti-SARS-2 RBD IgGs cross-reacted with the

S protein of MERS-CoV, as expected based on the low protein sequence identity between SARS-CoV-2 and MERS-CoV [5,53]. The difference in the cross-reactivity of the antibodies between SARS-CoV and SARS-CoV-2 could be related to whether the epitopes recognized by antibodies are located on regions that are conserved between SARS-CoV-2 and SARS-CoV. The amino acid sequence identity of the RBD (residues 387–516) between SARS-CoV-2 and SARS-CoV is quite high (86.3%), whereas the sequence identity of the receptor-binding motif (RBM; residues 438–505) is substantially lower (46.7%) [8,22,32]. This suggests that our antibodies likely recognize epitopes on the RBM of each virus, not on the conserved regions of the RBD. In addition, the RBM is known to have a loop structure and is thus likely subjected to the conformational variation, which may further reduce the structural homology between SARS-CoV-2 and SARS-CoV [8,22]. In addition, we also observed that all of the anti-SARS-2 RBD IgGs cross-reacted with the SARS-2 RBD variants tested, indicating that the antibody epitopes might not have overlapped with the regions of the RBD in which mutations occurred or that the anti-SARS-2 RBD IgGs might have been tolerable enough to bind to the RBD variants, although the antibody epitopes overlapped with regions where mutations occurred. Due to the limited numbers of the variants tested, it is hard to tell how tolerable our antibodies are to the genetic variations. More information on the antibody epitopes and antibody binding against increased numbers of the RBD variants will surely elucidate this.

Although in general human mAbs targeting the RBD of the S1 subunit have higher neutralizing potencies than those targeting other regions of the S protein, such as the S2 subunit and other regions of the S1 (e.g., the N-terminal domain (NTD)), it is still necessary to combine human mAbs that recognize different neutralizing epitopes due to the emergence of viruses carrying RBD mutations. Indeed, this was nicely demonstrated by the Regeneron antibodies (REGN10933 + REGN10987): an antibody cocktail consisting of these two antibodies, which recognize distinct, non-overlapping epitopes on the RBD, helped to avoid escape mutants after treatment thanks to the unlikely occurrence of simultaneous mutations on two distinct genetic sites [40]. By the same rationale, the neutralizing antibody (4A8 mAb) targeting the NTD of the S1 subunit could also be a good candidate for antibody cocktail therapy [35]. We are currently working to figure out whether our neutralizing antibodies (C2 and D12) can compete with other neutralizing antibodies, such as REGN-COV2, by charactering their antibody epitopes and by using a competitive enzyme-linked immunosorbent assay (ELISA) or bio-layer interferometry (BLI).

In order to identify potential neutralizing antibody candidates out of the ten Fab clones from the panning, we used in vitro competitive assays, namely an ELISA and an ACE2-overexpressed cell-based assay, to enable the Fab clones to compete with either a biotinylated ACE2 or the SARS-2 RBD, respectively. The two assays led to the identification of five Fabs as potential neutralizing antibodies, with the five candidate Fab clones behaving similarly in both assays. When the same assays were performed with the same five candidate antibodies that were reformatted from Fabs to IgGs, the two assays confirmed the five IgG antibodies as competitors, although the clone C12 (IgG) showed slightly less competition, albeit still significant, in both assays, especially in the ACE2-overexpressed cell-based assay. Although the two in vitro assays we adopted were not sensitive enough to discern their subtle differences and the antibodies could therefore not be ranked, it was strongly demonstrated that they could still be useful to handle many clones when screening potential candidates prior to a virus-mediated neutralization assay for either a pseudo-typed or authentic virus.

In the characterization of the antibodies in terms of affinity and neutralization, we also noticed that the affinity of the antibodies seemed to correlate with the neutralization potency. That is, the order of the affinity, C2 > D12 > H1 > F7 > C12, strongly correlated with the order of the neutralization potency, C2 > D12 > H1 > F7 > C12. This observed correlation is strongly supported by previous studies: (1) in a study of the mAb IIB4 recognizing influenza A virus haemagglutinin (HA), a strong positive correlation between its affinity and viral neutralization was found [54]; (2) in a study with potential SARS-

CoV-2 neutralizing antibodies from convalescent human patients, RBD binding and viral neutralization were well correlated [55].This therefore suggests that further maturation of the affinity of the mAbs may somehow enhance their neutralization potency accordingly; studies are underway to explore this. Moreover, the neutralization potencies determined by an in vitro neutralization assay for pseudo-typed and authentic SARS-CoV-2 also correlated with each other: the order of neutralization potency from the pseudo-typed virus, C2 > D12 > H1 > F7 > C12, nicely correlated with the order of potency from the authentic virus, C2 > D12 > F7 > H1 > C12, indicating that a neutralization assay for a pseudo-typed virus can be reliably applied to assess the neutralization potency of clones prior to the authentic virus-based assay, which, unlike the pseudo-typed viral assay, must be done under Biosafety Level 3 (BSL3) conditions. Consistent with the antibody binding against the D614G S1 variant, the order of neutralization potency for the pseudo-typed virus (carrying the D614G S1 variant) remained the same as the order for the pseudo-typed virus (carrying the D614 wildtype S1), with C2 (IgG) and C12 (IgG) showing the highest and the lowest neutralizations, respectively, thus confirming that the antibodies were tolerable to the D614G variation on the S1. This result highlights that current vaccinations relying on the neutralization of antibodies targeting the wildtype S protein of SARS-CoV-2 in vivo may somehow also be effective in coping with the new SARS-CoV-2 variants, including the D614G variant [56].

In conclusion, we selected human anti-SARS-2 RBD mAbs from a human synthetic Fab phage display library. We characterized the resulting Fabs and IgGs in order to observe their desirable biophysical properties, such as their affinity, non-aggregation, and thermal stability. We conducted in vitro assays to assess their neutralizing activities against pseudo-typed and authentic SARS-CoV-2 and identified two clones, C2 and D12, which demonstrated an exceptional ability to block the viral entry into cells. Further refinement of the mAbs should allow for the development of promising anti-SARS-CoV-2 therapeutics, as well as reagents for diagnosis.

4. Materials and Methods

4.1. A Phage Library Display Panning

Human synthetic Fab phage display libraries produced in-house (KFab-I and KFab-II, respectively built on human VH3/Vk1 and human VH1/Vk1 germline-based scaffolds, with randomized complementarity-determining regions) were used for the selection of specific binders against a SARS-CoV-2 spike protein (SARS-2 RBD) (Sino Biological, Cat. 40592-V08H, Beijing, China). The SARS-2 RBD was coupled to beads following the protocol for dynabeads (Thermofisher Scientific, Cat. 14301, Waltham, MA, USA). After removing the supernatant on the beads, the coated beads were blocked with 5% skimmed milk (BD, Cat. 232100, Franklin Lakes, NJ, USA) in PBS for 1 h at room temperature. At the same time, the phage library was incubated in 2% skimmed milk in PBS for 1 h at room temperature. The blocked phages were transferred to the beads coated with SARS-2 RBD and incubated for 2 h at room temperature. After separating the beads from the supernatant, the beads bound with phages were washed three times with PBST (PBS containing 0.05% Tween 20) and bound phages were eluted from the beads with 100 mM triethylamine (Sigma-Aldrich, Cat. 90335, St. Louis, MO, USA) for 10 min at room temperature, followed by neutralization with 1 M Tris-HCl (pH 7.4) (Biosesang, Cat. T2016-7.5, Seongnam, Korea). The eluted phages were used to infect *E. coli* TG1 cells at OD_{600} 0.6~0.8. Phage particles were prepared for subsequent rounds of panning by amplification and rescue using VCSM13 helper phages (provided by Dr. Hong from Kangwon National University, Chuncheon, Gangwon-do, Korea) according to standard procedures. The amplified phage was used for the next round of panning, and so forth.

4.2. Polyclonal Phage ELISA

A polyclonal phage ELISA was performed using pools of purified phage from each library stock. A 96-Well Half-Area Microplate (Corning, Cat. 3690, New York, NY, USA) was coated overnight at 4 °C, with 30 µL per well of 1 µg/mL SARS-2 RBD (Sino Biological, Cat. 40592-V08H, Beijing, China), and each well was blocked with 5% skimmed milk in PBS (MPBS) for 1 h at room temperature. Phage pools (~10^{12} phage particles) were also blocked in MPBS for 1 h at room temperature and then blocked phage pools were added to the SARS-2 RBD-coated plate and incubated for 1 h at 37 °C. After washing four times with PBST, the horseradish peroxidase (HRP)-conjugated anti-M13 antibody (1:5000, Sino Biological, Cat. 11973-MM05, Beijing, China) was incubated for 1 h at 37 °C. After washing four times with PBST, a TMB substrate solution (Sigma-Aldrich, Cat. T0440, St. Louis, MO, USA) was added for 8 min, and the reaction was stopped with 1 N sulfuric acid (Merck, Cat. 100731, Darmstadt, Germany). The absorbance was measured at 450 nm using a SpectraMax 190 Microplate Reader (Molecular Devices, Sunnydale, CA, USA).

4.3. Monoclonal Phage ELISA

Individual phage clones from either the third or fourth round were tested for binding to the SARS-2 RBD-coated plate. Several 96-Well Half-Area Microplates (Corning, Cat. 3690, New York, NY, USA) were coated overnight at 4 °C, with 30 µL per well of 1 µg/mL SARS-2 RBD, and each well was blocked with 5% skimmed milk in PBS for 1 h at room temperature. The amplified phages of individual clones from the third or fourth rounds of panning were added and incubated for 1 h at 37 °C. After washing four times with PBST, the horseradish peroxidase-conjugated anti-M13 antibody (1:5000, Sino Biological, Cat. 11973-MM05, Beijing, China) was incubated for 1 h at 37 °C. After washing four times with PBST, a TMB substrate solution (Sigma-Aldrich, Cat. T0440, St. Louis, MO, USA) was added for 8 min, and the reaction was stopped with 1 N sulfuric acid (Merck, Cat. 100731, Darmstadt, Germany). The absorbance was measured at 450 nm using a SpectraMax 190 Microplate Reader (Molecular Devices, Sunnydale, CA, USA).

4.4. Production of Fab Proteins

An in-house bacterial expression vector (pKFAB) was used to construct the Fab expression vectors. The Fab fragments and pKFAB vector were amplified by a polymerase chain reaction (PCR) for each primer set. The PCR products were treated with DpnI (New England Biolabs, Cat. R0176L, Ipswich, MA, USA) for 1 h at 37 °C, separated on a 1.2% agarose gel, and the single band was purified using a Wizard SV Gel and PCR Clean-Up System (New England Biolabs, Cat. A9282, Ipswich, MA, USA). The fragments were assembled following the Gibson assembly protocol (New England Biolabs, Cat. E2611, Ipswich, MA, USA). The assembled products were used to transform *E. coli* DH5α competent cells (Enzynomics, Cat. CP010, Daejeon, Korea). The individual colonies of the transformed cells were isolated and the sequences of the isolated clones were verified.

Top10F′ Competent Cells (Invitrogen, Cat. C303003, Carlsbad, CA, USA) were transformed with the Fab expression vectors and the transformants were grown in 200 mL of TB (Terrific Broth) (Thermofisher Scientific, Cat. 22711022, Waltham, MA, USA) media supplemented with 100 µg/mL ampicillin at 37 °C until the OD_{600} reached 0.5. The log-phase cultures were then induced with 0.5 mM isopropyl β-D-1-thiogalactopyranoside (IPTG) (DAWINBIO, Cat. I0355-005, Hanam, Gyeonggi, Seoul) and incubated overnight at 30 °C. The cells were collected and resuspended in 16 mL of 1× TES (50 mM Tris-HCl, 1 mM EDTA, 20% Sucrose, pH 8.0). After incubation for 30 min on ice, 24 mL of 0.2× TES was added and incubated for 1 h on ice. The periplasmic fractions were collected after centrifugation at 12,000 rpm for 30 min and filtered through a 0.22 µm filter (Milipore, Cat. SCGP00525, Carrigtwohill, Co., Cork, Ireland). The periplasmic extracts were loaded on a column packed with 0.5 mL of ProL (rProtein L) Agarose resin (Amicogen, Cat. 3010125, Jinju, Gyeongnam-do, Korea). The column was washed with 10 column volumes (CVs) of PBS and eluted with 30 CVs of Buffer W (100 mM Glycine, pH 2.5). The eluted proteins were neutralized with 1M Tris-HCl (pH 9.0) (Biosesang, Cat. TR2016-050-90, Seongnam, Gyeonggi, Korea). The eluted protein was concentrated and buffer-exchanged with PBS using Amicon Ultra-15 Centrifuge Filter Units (Milipore, Cat. UFC903024, Carrigtwohill, Co., Cork, Ireland).

4.5. Determination of Apparent Affinity by ELISA

Several 96-Well Half-Area Microplates (Corning, Cat. 3690, New York, NY, USA) were coated overnight at 4 °C, with 30 μL per well of 2 μg/mL SARS-2 RBD. After rinsing them twice with tap water, the wells were blocked with 5% skimmed milk in PBS for 1 h at room temperature. Serially diluted anti-SARS-2 RBD Fabs or IgGs were added and incubated for 1 h at 37 °C. After washing the plates four times with PBST, the HRP-conjugated human kappa light-chain antibody (1:5000, Bethyl laboratories, Cat. A80-115P, Montgomery, TX, USA) or HRP-conjugated human IgG Fc (1:5000, Abcam, Cat. ab97225, Cambridge, USA) were added to the plates and incubated at 37 °C for 1 h. After washing the plates four times with PBST, a TMB substrate solution was incubated for 8 min, and the reaction was stopped with 1 N sulfuric acid. The absorbance was measured at 450 nm using a SpectraMax 190 Microplate Reader. A plot was created using a nonlinear regression with Graphpad Prism 7 (GraphPad Software, San Diego, CA, USA), and half-maximal effective concentration (EC_{50}) values were determined accordingly.

4.6. ELISA-Based Neutralizing Assay

A 96-Well Half-Area Microplate (Corning, Cat. 3690, New York, NY, USA) was coated overnight at 4 °C, with 30 μL per well of 2 μg/mL SARS-2 RBD. After rinsing them twice with tap water, the wells were blocked with 5% skimmed milk in PBS for 1 h at room temperature. Both anti-SARS-2 RBD Fabs or IgGs and biotinylated human ACE2 (Acrobiosystems, Cat. AC2-H82E6, Newark, NJ, USA) were added and incubated for 1 h at 37 °C. After washing the plates four times with PBST, High Sensitivity Streptavidin-HRP (1:5000, Thermofisher, Cat. 21130, Waltham, MA, USA) was added to the plates and incubated for 1 h at 37 °C. After washing the plates four times with PBST, a TMB substrate solution was incubated for 8 min, and the reaction was stopped with 1 N sulfuric acid. The absorbance was measured at 450 nm using a SpectraMax 190 Microplate Reader. Graphpad Prism 7 (GraphPad Software, San Diego, CA, USA) was used to plot data using a two-way ANOVA algorithm.

4.7. Flow Cytometry-Based Neutralizing Assay

Calu-3 cells were obtained from the American Type Culture Collection (Manassas, VA, USA). Calu-3 cells were seeded in a 96-well plate (Corning, Cat. 3894, New York, NY, USA) at a density 1×10^6 cells per well. Afterward, 50 μg/mL, 100 μg/mL Fabs, or 50 μg/mL IgGs were mixed with 5 μg/mL SARS-2 RBD-mFc (mouse IgG2a Fc-tagged SARS-2 RBD) (Acrobiosystems, Cat. SPD-C5259, Newark, NJ, USA), and the mixture was then incubated with cells for 1 h at 4 °C. After washing, the cell was labeled with the PE anti-mouse IgG2a antibody (Biolegend, Cat. 407108, San Diego, CA, USA) and incubated for 1 h at 4 °C. The cells were analyzed by FACS canto II (BD Biosciences, San Jose, CA, USA). Data were analyzed by FlowJo (downloadable at https://www.flowjo.com/solutions/flowjo/downloads (accessed on 1 January 2021)).

4.8. Conversion to IgG and Production of IgG Proteins

The light- and heavy-chain vectors (pcDNA3.4) were used as the backbone vectors. The VL and VH genes were individually amplified by polymerase chain reaction (PCR) from each Fab. The PCR products (VL and VH) were purified with an Expin PCR SV Mini Kit (Geneall, Cat. 103-102, Seoul, Korea) and digested with the following restriction enzymes (New England Biolabs, Ipswich, MA, USA): for VH, EcoRI (Cat. R3101S) and NheI (Cat. R3131S); for VL, XhoI (Cat. R0146S) and BsiWI (Cat. R3553S). The digestion products were separated on a 1.2% agarose gel, and the single band was purified with an Expin Gel SV Kit (Geneall, Cat. 102-102, Seoul, Korea). The fragments were ligated with the same restriction enzyme-digested vector using T4 DNA ligase (Promega, Cat. M1801,

Madison, WI, USA). The ligation mixtures were used to transform *E. coli* DH5α Competent Cells (Enzynomics, Cat. CP010, Daejeon, Korea). Individual colonies of the transformed cells were isolated and the sequences of selected clones were confirmed by sequencing.

Freestyle 293 cells were cultured in Freestyle 293 Expression Medium (Thermofisher Scientific, Cat. 12338018, Waltham, MA, USA) in a humidified 8% CO_2 incubator at 37 °C and 125 rpm. On the day of transfection, Freestyle 293 cell density was approximately 2.0×10^6 cells/mL. Cells were transfected with plasmid DNA and these were mixed by DNA/PEI (polyethylenimine, Sigma-Aldrich, Cat. 913375, St. Louis, MO, USA) in a 1:2 ratio in the medium. Culture supernatants were collected after five days by centrifugation and filtration (0.22 μm, Polyethersulfone, Milipore, Cat. SLGPR33RB, Burlington, MA, USA).

Antibodies were purified from the culture supernatants using HiTrap MabSelect SuRe (GE Healthcare, Cat. 11-0034-94, Chicago, IL, USA) columns. Briefly, equilibration was carried out using Buffer A (1xPBS). The sample was loaded onto the equilibrated column. Following the sample loading, the column was washed with Buffer A until a stable baseline was established. Following the wash step, the protein was eluted with Buffer B (IgG elution buffer or 100 mM citrate buffer, pH 3.0). Following the elution, the IgG was brought to neutral pH with 1 M Tris base, pH 9.0, and dialyzed into a final buffer composition of PBS (pH 7.4) (Thermofisher Scientific, Cat. 10010023, Waltham, MA, USA). Each antibody was separated on 4–12% Bis-Tris gels (Thermofisher Scientific, Cat. NP0321, Waltham, MA, USA) with reducing or non-reducing conditions and stained with Sun-Gel Staining Solution (LPS Solution, Cat. SGS01, Daejeon, Korea).

4.9. Size-Exclusion Chromatography

The separation of the IgGs using size-exclusion chromatography (SEC) was performed using a Waters Alliance 2695 (Waters, Milford, MA, USA) connected to a Biosuite high-resolution SEC column (7.5 mm × 300 mm, 10 μm particle size, Waters, Milford, MA, USA). The separation was conducted using an isocratic elution with PBS, pH 7.4, at a flow rate of 1 mL/min. The effluent detection was conducted using a UV/Vis detector 2489 at 280 nm.

4.10. Determination of Melting Temperature by a Protein Thermal Shift (PTS) Assay

To each well of a MicroAmp Fast Optical 96-Well Reaction Plate (Applied Biosystems, Cat. 4346906, Foster City, CA, USA), 12.5 μL of anti-SARS-2 RBD Fabs or anti-SARS-2 RBD IgGs, 5 μL of Protein Thermal Shift Buffer and 2.5 μL of Protein Thermal Shift Dye (10×, Applied Biosystems, Cat. 4461146, Foster City, CA, USA) were mixed. As a negative control, PBS was mixed with the Protein Thermal Shift Dye. The plate was sealed with a MicroAmp Optical Adhesive Film (Applied Biosystems, Cat. 4306311, Foster City, CA, USA) and centrifuged at 1000 rpm for 1 min. The measurement was conducted using a real-time PCR instrument (ViiA 7 Real-Time PCR System, Thermofisher Scientific, Waltham, MA, USA). The instrument was set up according to the manufacturer's instructions. All the experiments were performed at least in triplicate.

4.11. Production of SARS-CoV-2 Spike pseudovirus

Plasmids encoding the SARS-CoV-2 spike protein (D614) were purchased from Sino Biological (pCMV3-SARS-CoV-2 Spike, Cat. VG40589-UT, Beijing, China). The SARS-CoV-2 spike protein (D614G) was made by site-directed mutagenesis. The mutation was confirmed by full-length spike gene sequencing. The SARS-CoV-2 pseudoviruses were produced by co-transfection HEK-293T cells with pMDLg/pRRE (Addgene plasmid, 12251), pRSV-Rev (Addgene plasmid, 12253), pCDH-CMV-Nluc-copGFP-Puro (Addgene plasmid, 73037), and plasmids encoding either SARS-CoV-2 spike (D614) or SARS-CoV-2 spike (D614G) by using polyetherimide. Sixty hours post-infection, SARS-CoV-2 spike pseudoviruses containing culture supernatants were harvested, filtered (0.45 μm pore size, Millipore, Cat. S2HVU01RE, Burlington, MA, USA), and stored at −80 °C in 1 mL aliquots until use.

4.12. Pseudovirus Neutralization Assay

Derivatives of HEK-293T cells expressing ACE2 were generated by transducing HEK-293T cells with ACE2 (Addgene plasmid, 145839). Cells were used as single cell clones derived by limiting dilution from the bulk populations. The HEK-293T cells expressing ACE2 were seeded at a density of 1.5×10^4 cells/well in 96-well luminometer-compatible tissue culture plates (Corning, Cat. 3610, New York, NY, USA) 24 h before infection. For the neutralization assay, 30 uL of pseudoviruses (~1×10^6 RLU) was incubated with serial dilutions of the test antibody (12 dilutions in a threefold stepwise manner) for 1 h at 37 °C, together with the virus control, and then added to the 96-well 293T-ACE2 cells. After 24 h of incubation, the inoculum was replaced with fresh medium. Luciferase activity was measured 72 h after infection. Briefly, cells were washed twice, carefully, with PBS and lysed with 40 µL/well of a Passive Lysis buffer (Promega, Cat. E1941, Madison, WI, USA). Luciferase activity in lysates was measured using the Nano-Glo Luciferase Assay System (Promega, Cat. N1130, Madison, WI, USA). Specifically, 40 µL of the substrate in a Nano-Glo buffer was mixed with 40 µL of cell lysate and incubated for 3 min at RT. NanoLuc luciferase activity was measured using a Filter max F5 (Molecular Devices, San Jose, CA, USA) with an integration time of 1000 ms. The IC_{50} values were calculated with nonlinear regression using GraphPad Prism 7 (GraphPad Software, Inc., San Diego, CA, USA).

4.13. Authentic Virus Neutralization Assay

The SARS-CoV-2 virus (NCCP43326) for this study was provided by the National Culture Collection for Pathogens (Osong Health Technology Administration Complex, Cheongju, Chungbuk-do, Korea). Vero cells were seeded in a 96-well plate (Greiner Bio-One, Cat. 655180, Kremsmünster, Austria) at a density of 1×10^4 cells per well. Serially, twofold-diluted mAbs and $100TCID_{50}$ (median tissue culture infectious dose) SARS-CoV-2 virus were incubated at RT for 0.5 h. mAb–virus mixtures were added to the Vero cells and incubated at 37 °C for 72 h. After 72 h of incubation, the supernatant was replaced with 100 µL of CellTiter-Glo® 2.0 Reagent (Promega, Cat. G9241, Madison, WI, USA) and incubated at RT for 10 min. Luciferase activity in lysates was measured using the CellTiter-Glo® 2.0 Assay (Promega, Cat. G9241, Madison, WI, USA). The luminescent signal was measured using a GloMax® Discover Microplate Reader (Promega, Cat. GM3000, Madison, WI, USA) and the IC_{50} values were calculated by nonlinear regression using GraphPad Prism 7 (GraphPad Software, Inc., San Diego, CA, USA). This experiment was conducted at Chungbuk National University in a BSL3 facility (KCDC (Korea Center for Disease Control)-14-3-07).

4.14. Measurements of Affinity Using Bio-Layer Interferometry

Affinity measurement was performed by BLI using an Octet QK384 (ForteBio, Menlo Park, CA, USA) instrument. The anti-SARS-2 RBD human antibody was immobilized at 15 µg/mL in 10× Kinetic Buffer (KB) (ForteBio, Cat. 18-1105, Menlo Park, CA, USA). SARS-2 RBD protein was prepared in six different concentrations (100~0 nM, in twofold serial dilutions) in 10× KB for baseline stabilization. Before the binding measurements, the Anti-Human IgG Fc Capture (AHC; Cat. 18-5060) (ForteBio, Menlo Park, CA, USA) sensor tips were washed with 10× KB for 60 s and incubated in a binding buffer for 300 s (loading step). After a 180 s baseline dip in the same buffer, the binding kinetics were measured by dipping each human IgG (C2 and D12)-coated sensor into a well containing SARS-CoV-2 RBD protein at the above six concentrations. The binding interactions were monitored over a 300 s association step, followed by a 500 s dissociation step, in which the sensors were dipped into new wells containing 10× KB only. Non-specific binding was assessed using sensor tips without human IgGs. Data analysis was performed using Octet Data Analysis Software v6.4 (ForteBio, Menlo Park, CA, USA). Data were fitted to a 1:1 binding model to determine an association rate (K_{on}, $M^{-1}s^{-1}$) and a dissociation rate (K_{off}, s^{-1}), and the equilibrium dissociation constant (K_D) was calculated using the kinetic constants as follows: equilibrium dissociation constant (K_D, M) = $K_{off} \div K_{on}$.

4.15. Statistical Analysis

Statistical analysis was carried out using GraphPad Prism version 7.0 (GraphPad Software, San Diego, CA, USA). All error bars reported are the standard error of the mean (± SEM), unless otherwise indicated. Pairwise comparisons were conducted using an unpaired *t*-test. Differences between groups were considered significant at *p*-values below 0.05 (* $p < 0.05$; ** $p < 0.01$; *** $p < 0.001$).

5. Conclusions

We selected human anti-SARS-2 RBD mAbs from human synthetic Fab phage display libraries. We characterized the resulting Fabs and IgGs to observe their desirable biophysical properties, such as their high affinity, non-aggregation, and thermal stability. We conducted in vitro assays to assess their neutralizing activities against pseudo-typed and authentic SARS-CoV-2 and identified two clones, C2 and D12, which demonstrated an exceptional ability to block the viral entry into cells. Further refinement of the mAbs should allow for the development of promising human anti-SARS-CoV-2 therapeutic and diagnostic reagents.

6. Patents

We are in the process of obtaining a patent for the data on the human anti-SARS-2 RBD Fabs and IgGs in Korea (patent application number 10-2020-0161180; application date 26th November 2020).

Supplementary Materials: Supplementary materials can be found at https://www.mdpi.com/1422-0067/22/4/1913/s1.

Author Contributions: Conceptualization and experiment design, Y.J.K. and D.Y.K.; investigation, Y.J.K., S.-R.L., M.H.L., H.-Y.C., and K.K.; supervision, D.Y.K.; project administration, D.Y.K. and T.G.L.; writing—original draft preparation, Y.J.K. and D.Y.K.; writing—review and editing, Y.J.K. and D.Y.K.; funding acquisition, T.G.L. All authors have read and agreed to the published version of the manuscript.

Funding: This research was funded by the Osong Medical Innovation Foundation and Chungcheongbuk-do (no grant numbers issued).

Institutional Review Board Statement: Not applicable.

Informed Consent Statement: Not applicable.

Data Availability Statement: Data sharing is not applicable due to patent-pending and tech-transfer issue.

Acknowledgments: We thank Hyo Jeong Hong (Kangwon National University, Gangwon-do, Korea) for her work in constructing the human Fab synthetic phage display library. We also thank Min-Seok Song for his support in the neutralization assay on authentic SARS-CoV-2. Lastly, we are grateful to Gu-Sun Park, the Chairman of the Osong Medical Innovation Foundation, for his support throughout the research.

Conflicts of Interest: Y.J.K. and D.Y.K. are inventors with the Korean patent application number 10-2020-0161180 (application date 26th November 2020). The authors declare no other conflicts of interest.

Abbreviations

mAb	Monoclonal antibody
SARS-CoV	Severe acute respiratory syndrome coronavirus
SARS-CoV-2	Severe acute respiratory syndrome coronavirus 2
MERS-CoV	Middle East respiratory syndrome coronavirus
ACE2	Angiotensin-converting enzyme 2
RBD	Receptor-binding domain
RBM	Receptor-binding motif
SARS-2 RBD	Receptor binding domain of severe acute respiratory syndrome coronavirus 2

ELISA	Enzyme-linked immunosorbent assay
HRP	Horseradish peroxidase
EC_{50}	Half maximal effective concentration
IgG	Immunoglobulin G
Fab	Antigen-binding fragment
SEC	Size-exclusion chromatography
PTS	Protein thermal shift
T_m	Melting temperature
K_D	Equilibrium dissociation constant
K_{on}	Association constant
K_{off}	Dissociation constant
IPTG	Isopropyl β-D-1-thiogalactopyranoside
PBS	Phosphate-buffered saline
SDS-PAGE	Sodium dodecyl sulfate-polyacrylamide gel electrophoresis
CDR	Complementarity-determining region
FR	Framework
VH	Heavy-chain variable domain
VL	Light-chain variable domain
CL	Light-chain constant domain
BLI	Bio-layer Interferometry
IC_{50}	Half maximal inhibitory concentration
$TCID_{50}$	Median tissue culture infectious dose
RLU	Relative luminescence unit
MFI	Mean fluorescence intensity

References

1. Zhu, N.; Zhang, D.; Wang, W.; Li, X.; Yang, B.; Song, J.; Xiang , Z.; Baoying , H.; Weifeng , S.; Roujian , L.; et al. A Novel Coronavirus from Patients with Pneumonia in China, 2019. *N. Engl. J. Med.* **2020**, *38*, 727–733. [CrossRef]
2. Wang, C.; Horby, P.W.; Hayden, F.G.; Gao, G.F. A novel coronavirus outbreak of global health concern. *Lancet* **2020**, *395*, 470–473. [CrossRef]
3. Van Boheemen, S.; de Graaf, M.; Lauber, C.; Bestebroer, T.M.; Raj, V.S.; Zaki, A.M.; Osterhaus, A.D.M.E.; Haagmans, B.L.; Gorbalenya, A.E.; Snijder, E.J.; et al. Genomic characterization of a newly discovered coronavirus associated with acute respiratory distress syndrome in humans. *mBio.* **2012**, *3*, e00473–e12. [CrossRef] [PubMed]
4. Rossi, G.A.; Sacco, O.; Mancino, E.; Cristiani, L.; Midulla, F. Differences and similarities between SARS-CoV and SARS-CoV-2: Spike receptor-binding domain recognition and host cell infection with support of cellular serine proteases. *Infection* **2020**, *48*, 665–669. [CrossRef]
5. Zhu, Z.; Lian, X.; Su, X.; Wu, W.; Marraro, G.A.; Zeng, Y. From SARS and MERS to COVID-19: A brief summary and comparison of severe acute respiratory infections caused by three highly pathogenic human coronaviruses. *Respir. Res.* **2020**, *21*, 224–237. [CrossRef]
6. Li, F. Evidence for a common evolutionary origin of coronavirus spike protein receptor-binding subunits. *J. Virol.* **2012**, *86*, 2856–2858. [CrossRef] [PubMed]
7. Li, F. Structure, function, and evolution of coronavirus spike proteins. *Annu. Rev. Virol.* **2016**, *3*, 237–261. [CrossRef]
8. Lan, J.; Ge, J.; Yu, J.; Shan, S.; Zhou, H.; Fan, S.; Zhang, Q.; Shi, X.; Wang, Q.; Zhang, L.; et al. Structure of the SARS-CoV-2 spike receptor-binding domain bound to the ACE2 receptor. *Nature* **2020**, *581*, 215–220. [CrossRef]
9. Kirchdoerfer, R.N.; Cottrell, C.A.; Wang, N.; Pallesen, J.; Yassine, H.M.; Turner, H.L.; Corbett, K.S.; Graham, B.S.; McLellan, J.S.; Ward, A.B. Prefusion structure of a human coronavirus spike protein. *Nature* **2016**, *531*, 118–121. [CrossRef]
10. Barnes, C.O.; Jette, C.A.; Abernathy, M.E.; Dam, K.A.; Esswein, S.R.; Gristick, H.B.; Malyutin, A.G.; Sharaf, N.G.; Huey-Tubman, K.E.; Lee, Y.E.; et al. SARS-CoV-2 neutralizing antibody structures inform therapeutic strategies. *Nature* **2020**, *588*, 682–687. [CrossRef]
11. Gui, M.; Song, W.; Zhou, H.; Xu, J.; Chen, S.; Xiang, Y.; Wang, X. Cryo-electron microscopy structures of the SARS-CoV spike glycoprotein reveal a prerequisite conformational state for receptor binding. *Cell Res.* **2017**, *27*, 119–129. [CrossRef]
12. Wrapp, D.; Wang, N.; Corbett, K.S.; Goldsmith, J.A.; Hsieh, C.L.; Abiona, O.; Graham, B.S.; McLellan, J.S. Cryo-EM structure of the SARS-CoV-2 spike in the prefusion conformation. *Science* **2020**, 1260–1263. [CrossRef]
13. Wang, L.; Xiang, Y. Spike Glycoprotein-Mediated Entry of SARS Coronaviruses. *Viruses* **2020**, *12*, 1289. [CrossRef]
14. De Clercq, E. New Nucleoside Analogues for the Treatment of Hemorrhagic Fever Virus Infections. *Chem. Asian J.* **2019**, *14*, 3962–3968. [CrossRef] [PubMed]
15. Wang, M.; Cao, R.; Zhang, L.; Yang, X.; Liu, J.; Xu, M.; Shi, Z.; Hu, Z.; Zhong, W.; Xiao, G. Remdesivir and chloroquine effectively inhibit the recently emerged novel coronavirus (2019-nCoV) in vitro. *Cell Res.* **2020**, *30*, 269–271. [CrossRef] [PubMed]
16. Zumla, A.; Chan, J.F.; Azhar, E.I.; Hui, D.S.; Yuen, K.Y. Coronaviruses—Drug discovery and therapeutic options. *Nat. Rev. Drug Discov.* **2016**, *15*, 327–347. [CrossRef]
17. Vincent, M.J.; Bergeron, E.; Benjannet, S.; Erickson, B.R.; Rollin, P.E.; Ksiazek, T.G.; Seidah, N.G.; Nichol, S.T. Chloroquine is a potent inhibitor of SARS coronavirus infection and spread. *Virol. J.* **2005**, *2*, 69–78. [CrossRef] [PubMed]
18. Chu, C.M.; Cheng, V.C.; Hung, I.F.; Wong, M.M.; Chan, K.H.; Chan, K.S.; Kao, R.Y.; Poon, L.L.; Wong, C.L.; Guan, Y.; et al. Role of lopinavir/ritonavir in the treatment of SARS: Initial virological and clinical findings. *Thorax* **2004**, *59*, 252–256. [CrossRef]

19. Boriskin, Y.S.; Leneva, I.A.; Pecheur, E.I.; Polyak, S.J. Arbidol: A broad-spectrum antiviral compound that blocks viral fusion. *Curr. Med. Chem.* **2008**, *15*, 997–1005. [CrossRef]
20. Duan, K.; Liu, B.; Li, C.; Zhang, H.; Yu, T.; Qu, J.; Zhou, M.; Chen, L.; Meng, S.; Hu, Y.; et al. Effectiveness of convalescent plasma therapy in severe COVID-19 patients. *Proc. Natl. Acad. Sci. USA* **2020**, *117*, 9490–9496. [CrossRef]
21. Yang, L.; Liu, W.; Yu, X.; Wu, M.; Reichert, J.M.; Ho, M. COVID-19 Antibody Therapeutics Tracker: A Global Online Database of Antibody Therapeutics for the Prevention and Treatment of COVID-19. *Antibody Therapeutics* **2020**, *3*, 205–212. [CrossRef]
22. Renn, A.; Fu, Y.; Hu, X.; Hall, M.D.; Simeonov, A. Fruitful Neutralizing Antibody Pipeline Brings Hope To Defeat SARS-Cov-2. *Trends Pharmacol. Sci.* **2020**, *41*, 815–829. [CrossRef] [PubMed]
23. Jin, Y.; Lei, C.; Hu, D.; Dimitrov, D.S.; Ying, T. Human monoclonal antibodies as candidate therapeutics against emerging viruses. *Front. Med.* **2017**, *11*, 462–470. [PubMed]
24. Zhou, G.; Zhao, Q. Perspectives on therapeutic neutralizing antibodies against the Novel Coronavirus SARS-CoV-2. *Int. J. Biol. Sci.* **2020**, *16*, 1718–1723. [CrossRef]
25. Jiang, S.; Hillyer, C.; Du, L. Neutralizing Antibodies against SARS-CoV-2 and Other Human Coronaviruses. *Trends Immunol.* **2020**, *41*, 355–359. [CrossRef] [PubMed]
26. Pascal, K.E.; Coleman, C.M.; Mujica, A.O.; Kamat, V.; Badithe, A.; Fairhurst, J.; Hunt, C.; Strein, J.; Berrebi, A.; Sisk, J.M.; et al. Pre- and post-exposure efficacy of fully human antibodies against Spike protein in a novel humanized mouse model of MERS-CoV infection. *Proc. Natl. Aca. Sci. USA* **2015**, *112*, 8738–8743. [CrossRef]
27. Li, W.; Chen, C.; Drelich, A.; Martinez, D.R.; Gralinski, L.E.; Sun, Z.; Schäfer, A.; Kulkarni, S.S.; Liu, X.; Leist, S.R.; et al. Rapid identification of a human antibody with high prophylactic and therapeutic efficacy in three animal models of SARS-CoV-2 infection. *Proc. Natl. Acad. Sci. USA* **2020**, *117*, 29832–29838. [CrossRef] [PubMed]
28. Sun, Z.; Chen, C.; Li, W.; Martinez, D.R.; Drelich, A.; Baek, D.S.; Liu, X.; Mellors, J.W.; Tseng, C.T.; Baric, R.S.; et al. Potent neutralization of SARS-CoV-2 by human antibody heavy-chain variable domains isolated from a large library with a new stable scaffold. *mAbs* **2020**, *12*, 1–6.
29. Noy-Porat, T.; Makdasi, E.; Alcalay, R.; Mechaly, A.; Levy, Y.; Bercovich-Kinori, A.; Zauberman, A.; Tamir, H.; Yahalom-Ronen, Y.; Israeli, M.; et al. A panel of human neutralizing mAbs targeting SARS-CoV-2 spike at multiple epitopes. *Nature Commun.* **2020**, *11*, 4303–4309. [CrossRef]
30. Zeng, X.; Li, L.; Lin, J.; Li, X.; Liu, B.; Kong, Y.; Zeng, S.; Du, J.; Xiao, H.; Zhang, T.; et al. Isolation of a human monoclonal antibody specific for the receptor binding domain of SARS-CoV-2 using a competitive phage biopanning strategy. *Antibody Therapeutics* **2020**, *3*, 95–100. [CrossRef]
31. Hansen, J.; Baum, A.; Pascal, K.E.; Russo, V.; Giordano, S.; Wloga, E.; Fulton, B.O.; Yan, Y.; Koon, K.; Patel, K.; et al. Studies in humanized mice and convalescent humans yield a SARS-CoV-2 antibody cocktail. *Science* **2020**, *369*, 1010–1014. [CrossRef]
32. Wang, C.; Li, W.; Drabek, D.; Okba, N.; van Haperen, R.; Osterhaus, A.; van Kuppeveld, F.; Haagmans, B.L.; Grosveld, F.; Bosch, B.J. A human monoclonal antibody blocking SARS-CoV-2 infection. *Nature Commun.* **2020**, *11*, 2251–2256. [CrossRef]
33. Esparza, T.J.; Martin, N.P.; Anderson, G.P.; Goldman, E.R.; Brody, D.L. High affinity nanobodies block SARS-CoV-2 spike receptor binding domain interaction with human angiotensin converting enzyme. *Sci. Rep.* **2020**, *10*, 22370–22382. [CrossRef] [PubMed]
34. Cheong, W.S.; Leow, C.Y.; Abdul Majeed, A.B.; Leow, C.H. Diagnostic and therapeutic potential of shark variable new antigen receptor (VNAR) single domain antibody. *Int. J. Biol. Macromol.* **2020**, *147*, 369–375. [CrossRef]
35. Chi, X.; Yan, R.; Zhang, J.; Zhang, G.; Zhang, Y.; Hao, M.; Zhang, Z.; Fan, P.; Dong, Y.; Yang, Y.; et al. A neutralizing human antibody binds to the N-terminal domain of the Spike protein of SARS-CoV-2. *Science* **2020**, *369*, 650–655. [CrossRef]
36. Pinto, D.; Park, Y.J.; Beltramello, M.; Walls, A.C.; Tortorici, M.A.; Bianchi, S.; Jaconi, S.; Culap, K.; Zatta, F.; De Marco, A.; et al. Cross-neutralization of SARS-CoV-2 by a human monoclonal SARS-CoV antibody. *Nature* **2020**, *583*, 290–295. [CrossRef]
37. Cao, Y.; Su, B.; Guo, X.; Sun, W.; Deng, Y.; Bao, L.; Zhu, Q.; Zhang, X.; Zheng, Y.; Geng, C.; et al. Potent Neutralizing Antibodies against SARS-CoV-2 Identified by High-Throughput Single-Cell Sequencing of Convalescent Patients' B Cells. *Cell* **2020**, *182*, 73–84. [CrossRef] [PubMed]
38. Chen, X.; Li, R.; Pan, Z.; Qian, C.; Yang, Y.; You, R.; Zhao, J.; Liu, P.; Gao, L.; Li, Z.; et al. Human monoclonal antibodies block the binding of SARS-CoV-2 spike protein to angiotensin converting enzyme 2 receptor. *Cell. Mol. Immunol.* **2020**, *17*, 647–649.
39. Zost, S.J.; Gilchuk, P.; Chen, R.E.; Case, J.B.; Reidy, J.X.; Trivette, A.; Nargi, R.S.; Sutton, R.E.; Suryadevara, N.; Chen, E.C.; et al. Rapid isolation and profiling of a diverse panel of human monoclonal antibodies targeting the SARS-CoV-2 spike protein. *Nature Med.* **2020**, *26*, 1422–1427. [CrossRef] [PubMed]
40. Baum, A.; Fulton, B.O.; Wloga, E.; Copin, R.; Pascal, K.E.; Russo, V.; Giordano, S.; Lanza, K.; Negron, N.; Ni, M.; et al. Antibody cocktail to SARS-CoV-2 spike protein prevents rapid mutational escape seen with individual antibodies. *Science* **2020**, *369*, 1014–1018. [CrossRef]
41. Wang, L.; Shi, W.; Chappell, J.D.; Joyce, M.G.; Zhang, Y.; Kanekiyo, M.; Becker, M.M.; van Doremalen, N.; Fischer, R.; Wang, N.; et al. Importance of neutralizing monoclonal antibodies targeting multiple antigenic sites on MERS-CoV Spike to avoid neutralization escape. *J. Virol.* **2018**, *92*, e02002–e02017. [CrossRef]
42. Kim, Y.; Lee, H.; Park, K.; Park, S.; Lim, J.-H.; So, M.K.; Woo, H.-M.; Ko, H.; Lee, J.-M.; Lim, S.H.; et al. Selection and characterization of monoclonal antibodies targeting Middle East respiratory syndrome coronavirus through a human synthetic Fab phage display library panning. *Antibodies* **2019**, *8*, 42. [CrossRef]

43. Kang, K.; Kim, K.; Lee, S.R.; Kim, Y.; Lee, J.E.; Lee, Y.S.; Lim, J.H.; Lim, C.S.; Kim, Y.J.; Baek, S.I.; et al. Selection and Characterization of YKL-40-Targeting Monoclonal Antibodies from Human Synthetic Fab Phage Display Libraries. *Int. J. Mol. Sci.* **2020**, *21*, 6354–6370.
44. Crawford, K.H.D.; Eguia, R.; Dingens, A.S.; Loes, A.N.; Malone, K.D.; Wolf, C.R.; Chu, H.Y.; Tortorici, M.A.; Veesler, D.; Murphy, M.; et al. Protocol and Reagents for Pseudotyping Lentiviral Particles with SARS-CoV-2 Spike Protein for Neutralization Assays. *Viruses* **2020**, *12*, 513. [CrossRef]
45. Smith, G.P. Filamentous Fusion Phage: Novel Expression Vectors That Display Cloned Antigens on the Virion Surface. *Science* **1985**, *228*, 1315–1317. [CrossRef]
46. Hoogenboom, H.R. Selecting and screening recombinant antibody libraries. *Nat. Biotechnol.* **2005**, *23*, 1105–1116. [CrossRef]
47. Winter, G.; Griffiths, A.D.; Hawkins, R.E.; Hoogenboom, H.R. Making antibodies by phage display technology. *Ann. Rev. Immunol.* **1994**, *12*, 433–455. [CrossRef] [PubMed]
48. Bradbury, A.R.M.; Sidhu, S.; Dübel, S.; McCafferty, J. Beyond natural antibodies: The power of in vitro display technologies. *Nat. Biotechnol.* **2011**, *29*, 245–254. [PubMed]
49. Huang, J.X.; Bishop-Hurley, S.L.; Cooper, M.A. Development of anti-infectives using phage display: Biological agents against bacteria, viruses, and parasites. *Antimicrob. Agents Chemother.* **2012**, *56*, 4569–4582. [CrossRef] [PubMed]
50. Ewert, S.; Huber, T.; Honegger, A.; Pluckthün, A. Biophysical properties of human antibody variable domains. *J. Mol. Biol.* **2003**, *325*, 531–553. [CrossRef]
51. Griffiths, A.D.; Williams, S.C.; Hartley, O.; Tomlinson, I.M.; Waterhouse, P.; Crosby, W.L.; Kontermann, R.E.; Jones, P.T.; Low, N.M.; Allison, T.J. Isolation of high affinity human antibodies directly from large synthetic repertoires. *EMBO J.* **1994**, *13*, 3245–3260. [CrossRef]
52. Knappik, A.; Ge, L.; Honegger, A.; Pack, P.; Fischer, M.; Wellnhofer, G.; Hoess, A.; Wolle, J.; Pluckthün, A.; Virnekas, B. Fully synthetic human combinatorial antibody libraries (HuCAL) based on modular consensus frameworks and CDRs randomized with trinucleotides. *J. Mol. Biol.* **2000**, *296*, 57–86. [CrossRef]
53. Tai, W.; He, L.; Zhang, X.; Pu, J.; Voronin, D.; Jiang, S.; Zhou, Y.; Du, L. Characterization of the receptor-binding domain (RBD) of 2019 novel coronavirus: Implication for development of RBD protein as a viral attachment inhibitor and vaccine. *Cell Mol. Immunol.* **2020**, *17*, 613–620. [CrossRef] [PubMed]
54. Kostolanský, F.; Varecková, E.; Betáková, T.; Mucha, V.; Russ, G.; Wharton, S.A. The strong positive correlation between effective affinity and infectivity neutralization of highly cross-reactive monoclonal antibody IIB4, which recognizes antigenic site B on influenza A virus haemagglutinin. *J. Gen. Virol.* **2000**, *81*, 1727–1735. [CrossRef] [PubMed]
55. Rogers, T.F.; Zhao, F.; Huang, D.; Beutler, N.; Burns, A.; He, W.T.; Limbo, O.; Smith, C.; Song, G.; Woehl, J.; et al. Isolation of potent SARS-CoV-2 neutralizing antibodies and protection from disease in a small animal model. *Science* **2020**, *369*, 956–963. [CrossRef]
56. Hou, Y.J.; Chiba, S.; Halfmann, P.; Ehre, C.; Kuroda, M.; Dinnon, K.H., 3rd; Leist, S.R.; Schäfer, A.; Nakajima, N.; Takahashi, K.; et al. SARS-CoV-2 D614G variant exhibits efficient replication ex vivo and transmission in vivo. *Science* **2020**, *370*, 1464–1468. [PubMed]

International Journal of
Molecular Sciences

MDPI

Article

ABL001, a Bispecific Antibody Targeting VEGF and DLL4, with Chemotherapy, Synergistically Inhibits Tumor Progression in Xenograft Models

Dong-Hoon Yeom [1,2], Yo-Seob Lee [1], Ilhwan Ryu [1], Sunju Lee [1], Byungje Sung [1], Han-Byul Lee [1], Dongin Kim [1], Jin-Hyung Ahn [1], Eunsin Ha [1], Yong-Soo Choi [2], Sang Hoon Lee [1] and Weon-Kyoo You [1,*]

1 R&D Center, ABL Bio Inc., 2F, 16 Daewangpangyo-ro, 712 beon-gil, Bundang-gu, Seongnam-si, Gyeonggi-do 13488, Korea; donghoon.yeom@ablbio.com (D.-H.Y.); yoseob.lee@ablbio.com (Y.-S.L.); ilhwan.ryu@ablbio.com (I.R.); sunju.lee@ablbio.com (S.L.); byungje.sung@ablbio.com (B.S.); hanbyul.lee@ablbio.com (H.-B.L.); dongin.kim@ablbio.com (D.K.); jinhyung.ahn@ablbio.com (J.-H.A.); eunsin.ha@ablbio.com (E.H.); sang.lee@ablbio.com (S.H.L.)

2 Department of Biotechnology, CHA University, Pangyo-ro 335, Bundang-gu, Seongnam-si, Gyeonggi-do 13488, Korea; yschoi@cha.ac.kr

* Correspondence: weonkyoo.you@ablbio.com; Tel.: +82-31-8018-9803; Fax: +82-31-8018-9836

Abstract: Delta-like-ligand 4 (DLL4) is a promising target to augment the effects of VEGF inhibitors. A simultaneous blockade of VEGF/VEGFR and DLL4/Notch signaling pathways leads to more potent anti-cancer effects by synergistic anti-angiogenic mechanisms in xenograft models. A bispecific antibody targeting VEGF and DLL4 (ABL001/NOV1501/TR009) demonstrates more potent in vitro and in vivo biological activity compared to VEGF or DLL4 targeting monoclonal antibodies alone and is currently being evaluated in a phase 1 clinical study of heavy chemotherapy or targeted therapy pre-treated cancer patients (ClinicalTrials.gov Identifier: NCT03292783). However, the effects of a combination of ABL001 and chemotherapy on tumor vessels and tumors are not known. Hence, the effects of ABL001, with or without paclitaxel and irinotecan were evaluated in human gastric or colon cancer xenograft models. The combination treatment synergistically inhibited tumor progression compared to each monotherapy. More tumor vessel regression and apoptotic tumor cell induction were observed in tumors treated with the combination therapy, which might be due to tumor vessel normalization. Overall, these findings suggest that the combination therapy of ABL001 with paclitaxel or irinotecan would be a better clinical strategy for the treatment of cancer patients.

Keywords: anti-angiogenesis; delta-like ligand; irinotecan; paclitaxel; therapeutic antibody; VEGF

Citation: Yeom, D.-H.; Lee, Y.-S.; Ryu, I.; Lee, S.; Sung, B.; Lee, H.-B.; Kim, D.; Ahn, J.-H.; Ha, E.; Choi, Y.-S.; et al. ABL001, a Bispecific Antibody Targeting VEGF and DLL4, with Chemotherapy, Synergistically Inhibits Tumor Progression in Xenograft Models. *Int. J. Mol. Sci.* **2021**, *22*, 241. https://doi.org/10.3390/ijms22010241

Received: 7 December 2020
Accepted: 25 December 2020
Published: 29 December 2020

Publisher's Note: MDPI stays neutral with regard to jurisdictional claims in published maps and institutional affiliations.

1. Introduction

Tumor angiogenesis, the formation of new blood vessels in solid tumors, plays an important role in tumor cell survival, growth, and metastasis [1]. A major driving force of tumor angiogenesis is the signaling pathway involving vascular endothelial growth factor (VEGF) and its receptors (VEGFRs) [2]. Several angiogenesis inhibitors, including antibodies and small molecule compounds targeting the VEGF/VEGFR signaling pathway, have been approved by the Food and Drug Administration (FDA), and used for the treatment of many different types of cancers [3]. Besides cancer treatment, VEGF/VEGFR inhibitors, including antibody fragments, aptamers, and VEGF-Traps were also approved and used for the treatment of ocular diseases caused by pathological angiogenesis [4–8]. VEGF/VEGFR blockade can inhibit VEGF-driven tumor angiogenesis, and the regression of tumor vessels is dependent on the VEGF signaling pathway. However, VEGF inhibitors alone are not capable of destroying all tumor blood vessels. In addition, preclinical studies indicate that VEGF inhibitors alone resulted in an increasingly aggressive and invasive pattern of tumors [9]. Some cancer patients are eventually refractory to anti-VEGF therapy, hence, next-generation angiogenesis inhibitors are being sought to augment the effects of VEGF inhibitors [10–12].

The DLL4/Notch signaling pathway can be a promising target of the next angiogenesis inhibitors, as this pathway regulates tumor angiogenesis with a different mechanism of action compared to that of the VEGF inhibitors [13–15]. Several preclinical xenograft studies have demonstrated that DLL4/Notch blockade inhibited tumor progression by promoting hyperproliferation of endothelial cells, which resulted in an increase in vascular density and a decrease in functional tumor vasculature [14–20]. DLL4/Notch inhibition is also known to reduce the number of cancer stem cells (CSCs), which are an important cancer cell population responsible for malignancy [21]. ABL001 is a bispecific antibody that simultaneously targets both DLL4 and VEGF, by linking each C-terminal of an anti-VEGF antibody (bevacizumab-similar) with a DLL4-binding single-chain Fv (scFv) [22,23]. In previous studies, ABL001 has demonstrated anti-cancer effects with higher potency in several human cancer xenograft models compared to that shown by the VEGF-targeting antibody (bevacizumab-similar) and the DLL4-targeting monoclonal antibody alone [23,24].

The safety and tolerability of ABL001 in cancer patients are now being evaluated in a phase 1 dose escalation study. The study was designed in a classical 3+3 dose-escalation schema where ABL001 is administered by IV across nine dose cohorts ranging from 0.3, 1, 2.5, 5, 7.5, 10, 12.5, 15, to 17.5 mg/kg biweekly [25]. No dose-limiting toxicity (DLT) was observed during the final cohort dose (17.5 mg/kg), and the maximum tolerated dose (MTD) was not reached. The most common treatment-related adverse events (AEs) (including all dose levels and all grades) were hypertension, anemia, anorexia, general weakness, and headache. However, they were well managed for all cohorts. Although the current phase 1 trial of monotherapy of ABL001 is ongoing, further clinical studies should be performed in combination with chemotherapy after the selection of optimal anti-cancer agents and cancer types. Since angiogenesis inhibitors target tumor endothelial cells, most VEGF/VEGFR blocking agents demonstrate clinical benefits for cancer patients when combined with chemotherapy [3]. Two different mechanisms of action of the combination therapy could provide synergistic anti-cancer efficacy for cancer patients. First, the combination therapy can destroy two separate components of tumors, tumor cells and tumor endothelial cells [26,27]. Second, the tumor vessel normalization by angiogenesis inhibitors enhances the delivery of cytotoxic anti-cancer agents [28,29]. However, the effects of a combination of ABL001 with chemotherapy on tumors and tumor blood vessels have not been fully studied. In this report, the in vivo anti-cancer effects of ABL001 with chemotherapy were evaluated in human gastric and colon cancer xenograft models and were compared to each monotherapy alone.

2. Results

2.1. Suppression of Tumor Progression in Various Cancer Xenograft Models by ABL001

To confirm the effects of ABL001 on tumor progression and to select the appropriate xenograft models for testing a combination treatment of ABL001 with chemotherapy, we evaluated the anti-cancer effects of ABL001 using several human gastric cancer (NUGC-3, MKN45, and SNU16 for mABL001, and GAPF006 for ABL001) xenograft models (Figure 1A), and human colon cancer (Colo205, WiDr, SW48, and SW620 for mABL001) xenograft models (Figure 1B). In the case of general xenograft models using human cancer cell lines, we used the mouse surrogate version of ABL001 (mABL001: binding to human VEGF and mouse DLL4) for the studies, as DLL4 is expressed by mouse endothelial cells involving tumor angiogenesis in tumor xenografts [23]. However, we used ABL001 in a patient-derived xenograft (PDX) model using GAPF006, which mimics the human tumor microenvironment from patients. Both bispecific antibodies, mABL001 and ABL001, inhibited tumor progression in the tested xenograft models at doses ranging from 1 to 6.5 mg/kg (Figure 1). The anti-cancer effects of mABL001 or ABL001 monotherapy were calculated as %TGI ranging from 27.4% to 57.2%, depending on the doses of mABL001 or ABL001 and cancer cell lines in xenograft models (Table 1). We focused on the dose level of ABL001 showing %TGI_{50} (50% tumor growth inhibition ratio) in each xenograft model because the dose of ABL001 and the xenograft model would be used for the combination therapy with paclitaxel or irinotecan. Based on the results from the dose range-finding studies, we selected GAPF006 gastric PDX, and SW48 or SW620 colon cancer xenograft models to address the efficacy of the combination treatment.

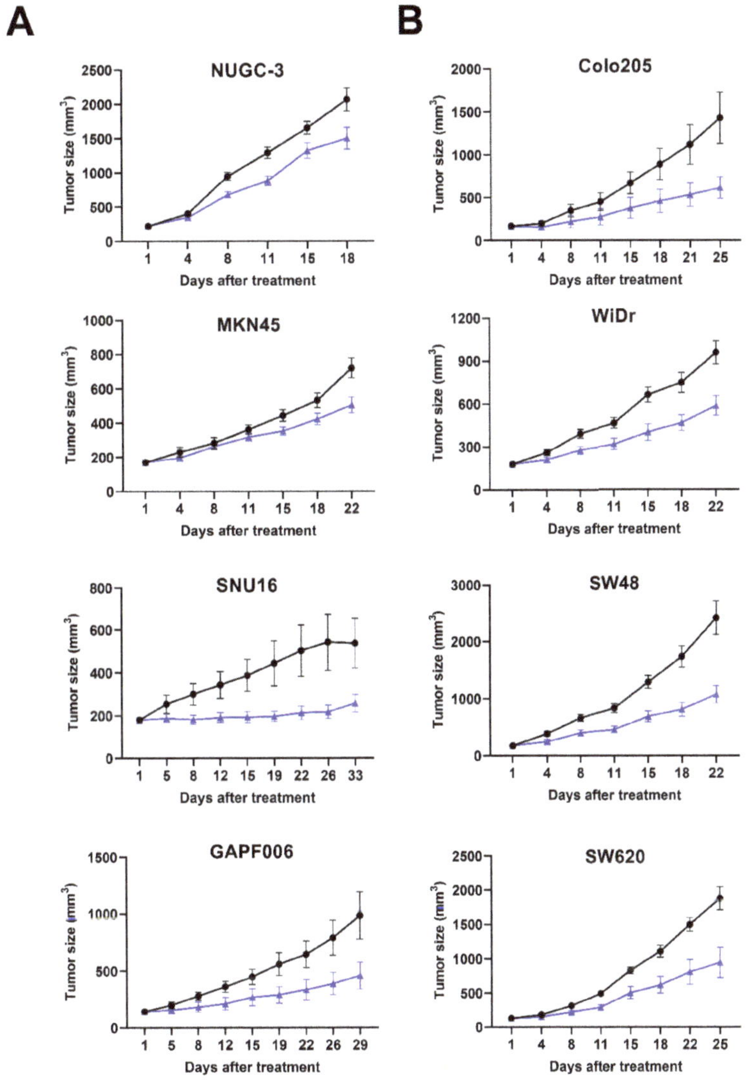

Figure 1. ABL001 strongly inhibited tumor progression of various human gastric and colon cancer xenograft models. Tumor size was measured twice per week and compared between vehicle (closed circle) and ABL001 (closed triangle) in human gastric cancer (NUGC-3, MKN45, SNU16 for mABL001, and human patient-derived gastric cancer GAPF006 for ABL001) xenograft model (**A**) and human colon cancer (Colo205, WiDr, SW48, SW620 for mABL001) xenograft model (**B**). ABL001 treatment significantly delayed tumor progression in different cancer xenograft models compared to control group of vehicle treatment. Error bars: mean ± SEM.

Table 1. Summarized information of animal studies using human gastric and colon cancer xenograft models.

Cancer Type	Cancer Cell Line	Dose (mg/kg)	Treatment Schedule	Animal Number (*n*/Group)	%TGI	*p* Value
Gastric	NUGC-3	1	Biweekly	11	27.4	0.0275
	MKN45	1.25		10	30.0	0.0378
	SNU16	3.25		12	52.2	0.0010
	GAPF006	6.5		10	53.3	0.0051
Colon	SW48	1.25	Biweekly	10	55.5	0.0264
	SW620	2		6	49.7	0.0224
	Colo205	3.25		8	57.2	0.0177
	WiDr	6.5		9	38.8	0.0131

GAPF006, gastric patient-derived xenograft model, %TGI = tumor growth inhibition, *p* value: Student's *t*-test.

2.2. Synergistic Suppression on Tumor Progression by Combination Therapy

To determine whether the combination treatment of ABL001 with chemotherapy suppressed tumor progression with a higher strength as compared to that of each monotherapy, we evaluated the anti-cancer effects of the combination therapy using xenograft models compared to ABL001 or chemotherapy alone (Figure 2). In this study, we tested paclitaxel as chemotherapy in combination with ABL001 in gastric GAPF006 PDX (human gastric origin) xenograft, and irinotecan with mABL001 in SW48 or SW620 human colon tumor xenografts. In the gastric PDX model, the combination of paclitaxel and ABL001 demonstrated the most potent inhibition of tumor progression (74.75% TGI compared to 40.33% TGI in the paclitaxel-treated group and 46.20% TGI in the ABL001-treated group) (Figure 2A). Similarly, the combination of irinotecan with mABL001 suppressed tumor progression of SW48 and SW620 human colon cancer xenografts more potently compared to that by irinotecan or mABL001 alone (Figure 2B,C). At the endpoint of the SW48 xenograft study, the combination of irinotecan and mABL001 demonstrated 77.7% TGI, which was significantly different from the %TGI of the vehicle ($p < 0.0001$) group and irinotecan ($p < 0.005$) or mABL001 alone ($p < 0.05$) (Figure 2B). In the case of the SW620 xenograft model (human colon cancer), the combination treatment of irinotecan and mABL001 also exhibited the most potent anti-cancer effect (94.47% TGI) on tumor progression in the SW620 xenograft (Figure 2C).

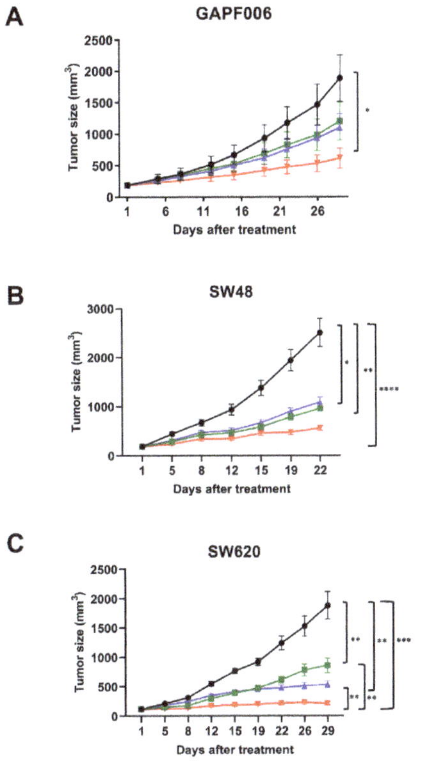

Figure 2. ABL001 in combination with chemotherapy with paclitaxel or irinotecan synergistically inhibited tumor progression in human gastric PDX and colon cancer xenograft models. In GAPF006 human gastric PDX model (**A**), mice were treated with vehicle (closed circle, black), paclitaxel alone (closed rectangle, green), ABL001 (closed triangle, blue), or a combination of ABL001 and paclitaxel (closed reverse triangle, red). Compared to vehicle, each treatment group inhibited tumor progression (40.33% TGI in paclitaxel, 46.20% TGI in ABL001, and 74.75% TGI in the combination treatment). In the studies using SW48 (**B**) and SW620 (**C**) colon cancer xenograft models, mice were treated with vehicle (closed circle, black), irinotecan alone (closed rectangle, green), mABL001 (closed triangle, blue), or a combination of mABL001 and irinotecan (closed reverse triangle, red). In the case of both colon cancer xenograft models, the combination treatment of mABL001 and irinotecan showed the most potent effects on tumor progression (77.7% TGI in SW48 and 94.47% TGI in SW620 xenograft models). Each line represents the average tumor size (mm^3) of each treatment group ± SEM. * $p < 0.05$, ** $p < 0.01$, *** $p < 0.001$, **** $p < 0.0001$ by Tukey's test.

2.3. More Potent Regression of Tumor Vessels by Combination Therapy

In order to evaluate the effects of the combination therapy on tumor blood vessels in xenograft models, the tumor vessels of SW620 tumor sections were analyzed using immunohistochemical staining for CD31 and VEGFR-2. Fluorescence microscopy images revealed that CD31-positive staining was localized in the vascular endothelial cells in the tumors (Figure 3A). The tumor vessel densities positive for CD31 in SW620 tumors treated with vehicle, irinotecan, mABL001, and combination were 0.71 ± 0.05%, 0.48 ± 0.03%, 0.36 ± 0.03%, and 0.18 ± 0.01%, respectively (Figure 3B). The percentage of positive area for CD31 in the combination was significantly lower than that of irinotecan or mABL001 alone. The area density of CD31-positive vessels in irinotecan-treated tumors was decreased by 32.4% and the density in mABL001-treated tumors was decreased by 49.3%, compared to the vehicle-treated group. However, the density of CD31-positive tumor vessels in the combination treatment decreased by 74.6% compared to the vehicle group (Figure 3B). VEGFR-2 was also strongly expressed on the endothelial cell membrane and cytoplasm in SW620 tumors (Figure 3A). The area densities of VEGFR-2-positive tumor vessels in the four groups were 0.65 ± 0.06%, 0.43 ± 0.04%, 0.23 ± 0.02%, and 0.13 ± 0.02%, respectively (Figure 3C). Compared to the vehicle-treated group, VEGFR-2-positive tumor vessels were reduced by 33.8% in the irinotecan-treated group, by 64.6% in the mABL001-treated group, and by 80% in the combination treatment group (Figure 3C). Based on the comparison of relative reduced levels between CD31-positive vessels with VEGFR-2-positive vessels in each tumor, VEGFR-2 expression was more reduced in tumor blood vessels compared to CD31 expression after VEGF blockade, mABL001 treatment, or the combination treatment (Figure 3B,C).

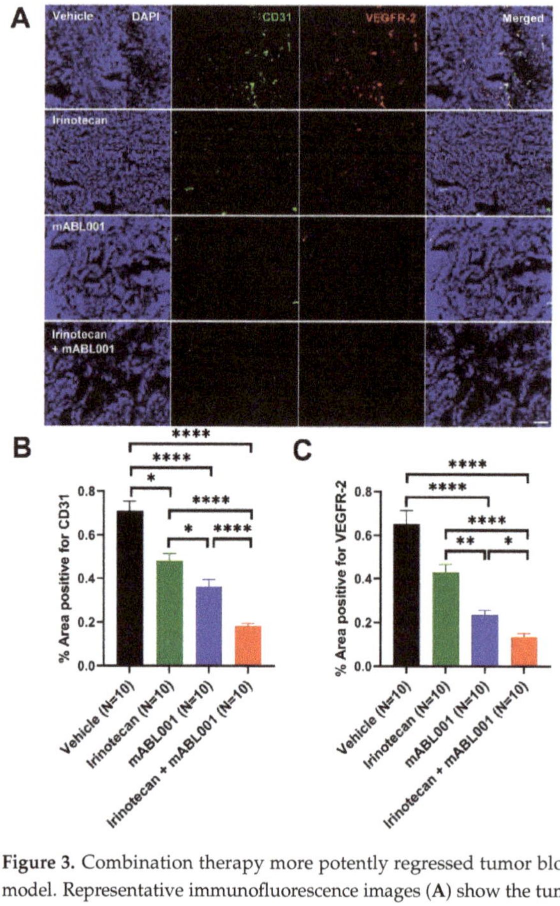

Figure 3. Combination therapy more potently regressed tumor blood vessels in SW620 xenograft model. Representative immunofluorescence images (**A**) show the tumor vasculature in SW620 tumor tissues stained for CD31, a generally conserved endothelial cell marker (green) and VEGFR-2 (red) with DAPI (blue). Most tumor blood vessels in vehicle group were stained and colocalized with both markers, CD31 and VEGFR-2. The area densities of CD31 (**B**) and VEGFR-2 (**C**) positive vessels were measured in each group. After irinotecan treatment, CD31 or VEGFR-2 positive tumor blood vessels were slightly regressed compared to vehicle treatment. However, after mABL001 or the combination treatment of mABL001 and irinotecan, CD31 and VEGFR-2 positive tumor vessels were significantly reduced (**B**,**C**). VEGFR-2 expression reduced more rapidly on tumor vessels. Scale bar indicates 200 μm. Error bars: mean ± SEM. * $p < 0.05$, ** $p < 0.01$, **** $p < 0.0001$ by Kruskal–Wallis test.

2.4. Decrease of DLL4 Expression on Tumor Vessels by Combination Therapy

DLL4 is expressed by tumor endothelial cells to regulate tumor angiogenesis, and by some tumor cells to maintain cancer stemness [14,15,21]. To address whether treatment with irinotecan, mABL001, or their combination affects DLL4 expression in tumors of xenograft models, DLL4 expression was examined using immunohistochemical staining using SW620 tumor sections from each group (Figure 4). DLL4 was mainly expressed on tumor blood vessels rather than tumor cells in this xenograft tumor and colocalized with CD31-positive tumor vessels (Figure 4A). The area densities of DLL4-positive tumor vessels were 0.40 ± 0.03% in vehicle, 0.24 ± 0.03% in irinotecan, 0.11 ± 0.02% in mABL001, and 0.05 ± 0.01% in the combination treatment group, respectively (Figure 4B). DLL4-positive tumor vessels were significantly reduced in the combination group compared to other groups. Compared to the vehicle group, DLL4-positive tumor vessels were reduced by 40% in the irinotecan group, by 72.5% in the mABL001 group, and by 87.5% in the combination group (Figure 4B). Similar to VEGFR-2 expression in tumor vessels, DLL4 expression was markedly reduced in tumor vessels compared to CD31 after treatment with mABL001 or the combination, rather than treatment with irinotecan alone (Figure 4B). Such a rapid reduction of DLL4 expression after mABL001 caused some tumor vessels to be stained only by CD31 but not by DLL4 (arrows in Figure 4A).

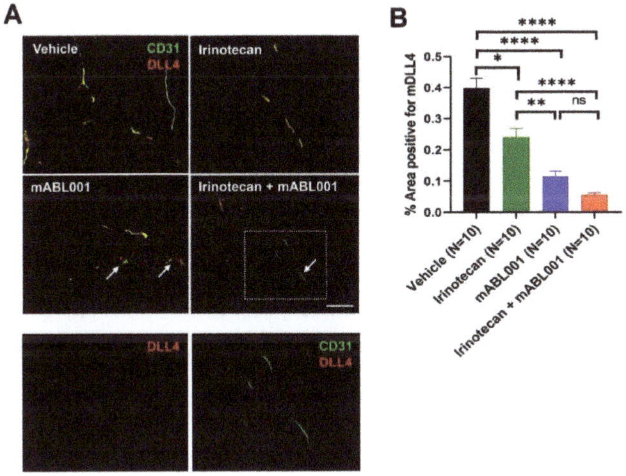

Figure 4. ABL001 significantly reduced DLL4 expression in tumor blood vessels. Representative immunofluorescence images (**A**) indicate the tumor vasculature in SW620 tumor tissues stained for CD31 (green) and DLL4 (red). The bottom figures (**A**) are magnified images of the dotted region of the combination treatment of mABL001 and irinotecan. The left image was shown only by red channel, whereas the right one was shown by merged channels (red and green). Similar to VEGFR-2, DLL4 was stained and colocalized on CD31 positive tumor blood vessels. The area density of DLL4 (**B**) positive vessels was measured in tumors of each group. Compared to vehicle or irinotecan treatment, DLL4 positive tumor vessels were significantly reduced in tumors after mABL001 or the combination treatment. Some tumor vessels were stained only for CD31 but not for DLL4, after mABL001 or the combination treatment group (arrows and dotted box in A). Scale bar indicates 50 μm in the bottom two images and 100 μm in the other images. Error bars: mean ± SEM. * $p < 0.05$, ** $p < 0.01$, **** $p < 0.0001$ by Kruskal–Wallis test.

2.5. Increase of Tumor Apoptosis by Combination Therapy

Since the combination treatment of mABL001 with irinotecan showed more potent anti-cancer effects on tumor progression and anti-angiogenic effects on tumor vessels, the effects of the combination therapy on tumor cells were analyzed by immunohistochemical staining for activated caspase-3, an apoptotic cell marker. Immunofluorescence imaging revealed that activated caspase-3 was largely stained in the tumor cell nuclei rather than in the tumor endothelial cell nuclei in the tumor sections (Figure 5A). The area densities of activated caspase-3/DAPI positive cells were 5.16 ± 0.74% in the vehicle-treated group, 7.92 ± 1.05% in the irinotecan-treated group, 8.92 ± 1.65% in mABL001-treated group, and 10.87 ± 1.78% in the combination group (Figure 5B). The level of apoptotic tumor cells was significantly increased in the tumor sections after the combination treatment compared with the other groups. Such a potent increase in tumor cell apoptosis by the combination treatment might be due to direct cytotoxic effects of irinotecan against highly proliferating tumor cells together with the anti-angiogenic effects of mABL001, a bispecific antibody binding against dual antigens, VEGF, and mouse DLL4. The results suggest that the combination treatment of ABL001 with chemotherapy might provide better clinical benefits for cancer patients in clinical trials than ABL001 monotherapy.

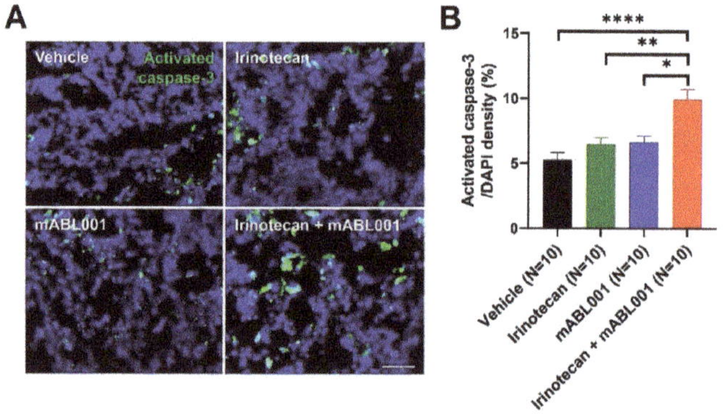

Figure 5. Combination therapy markedly increased apoptotic tumor cells in SW620 xenograft model. Representative immunofluorescence images (**A**) reveal apoptotic cells stained for activated caspase-3 (green) with DAPI (blue) in SW620 tumor tissues. The area densities of activated caspase-3-positive apoptotic cells were measured in each group (**B**). Apoptotic cells in tumors were marginally increased after irinotecan or mABL001 treatment, but the increase was not significant compared to vehicle treatment. However, the combination treatment of mABL001 and irinotecan markedly increased the apoptotic cell population in tumors. Scale bar indicates 50 μm. Error bars: mean ± SEM. * $p < 0.05$, ** $p < 0.01$, **** $p < 0.0001$ by Kruskal–Wallis test.

3. Discussion

ABL001 (NOV1501/TR009), a bispecific antibody targeting VEGF and DLL4, is being developed as an anti-angiogenic cancer therapeutic that strengthens the effects of VEGF inhibitors and eventually overcomes resistance to anti-VEGF therapy [16,19,20,23]. ABL001 demonstrated more potent anti-angiogenic and anti-cancer effects in vitro and in vivo, as compared to the VEGF-targeting or the DLL4-targeting monoclonal antibodies alone, in various assay systems [23,24]. Based on the overall results of preclinical studies, the safety and tolerability of ABL001 are currently being tested with cancer patients previously treated heavily with chemotherapy or targeted therapy [25]. Other approved anti-angiogenic antibody therapeutics including bevacizumab, an antagonist of the VEGF ligand (VEGF-A: Avastin®), and ramucirumab, an antagonist of the VEGF receptor (VEGFR-2: Cyramza®), are generally used in a combination regimen with chemotherapy to treat cancer patients, providing more efficacious therapeutic options for cancer patients [3,30]. Anti-VEGF therapy is known to normalize tumor blood vessels, leading to a more efficient delivery of cytotoxic anti-cancer agents into tumor tissues [28,29], hence, most anti-VEGF therapy are used in the clinic in combination with chemotherapy [3,30]. Based upon the rationale mentioned above, newly developing VEGF/VEGFR inhibitors of monoclonal or bispecific antibodies, small molecule compounds, aptamers, and VEGF-Traps, have been evaluated synergistic anti-cancer effects with chemotherapy in various preclinical models before entering clinical trials [27,31,32].

Not only VEGF but DLL4 is also known to impair efficient delivery of anti-cancer drugs and to enhance chemoresistance in pancreatic cancer model due to induction of defective tumor angiogenesis [33]. However, little is known about the effects of a combination of ABL001, targeting dual antigens VEGF and DLL4, and chemotherapy on tumor vessels and tumor cells in xenograft models compared to each monotherapy alone. In this study, we evaluated the anti-angiogenic and anti-cancer effects of the combination treatment of ABL001 with paclitaxel or irinotecan in human gastric and colon cancer xenograft models.

The combination treatment of ABL001 with paclitaxel or irinotecan demonstrated more potent inhibition of tumor progression in these xenograft models, which is consistent with the previous report of the study collaborator [24]. Such potent anti-cancer effects of the combination therapy might be related to more significantly regressed tumor blood vessels, as compared to monotherapy with ABL001 or chemotherapy alone. Eventually, these anti-angiogenic and anti-cancer effects increased the apoptotic tumor status in the tumors post the combination treatment of ABL001 and chemotherapy. The underlying molecular mechanisms of action of the potent anti-cancer effects of ABL001 with chemotherapy might be due to the optimal combination effects of cytotoxic activity on tumor cells by paclitaxel or irinotecan together with more potent anti-angiogenic activity on tumor endothelial cells by ABL001, a VEGF, and DLL4 dual inhibitor. Moreover, because the VEGF-binding part of ABL001 is composed of the same IgG backbone and sequence as bevacizumab, ABL001 may have similar activity and function as bevacizumab in tumor vessels, resulting in a more effective delivery of anti-cancer agents, such as paclitaxel or irinotecan.

Based on the results of immunohistochemical analysis of tumor blood vessels, the expression levels of VEGFR-2 and DLL4, dual targets of ABL001, were markedly reduced in tumor endothelial cells after ABL001 treatment compared to that of CD31, a conventional endothelial cell marker. These findings are consistent with the previous results that VEGF blockade downregulates the levels of its receptor, VEGFR-2, and of DLL4 on endothelial cells [34,35]. Therefore, these results strongly support that the VEGF/VEGFR signaling pathway interacts with the DLL4/Notch signaling pathway in the tumor vasculature [35].

In addition to the cytotoxic anti-cancer agents, tumor vessel normalization by anti-VEGF therapy is also able to provide a better infiltration of immune cells, including cytotoxic T cells, into tumor tissues [36]. These reports suggest that anti-VEGF therapy can be the best option for combination therapy with immune checkpoint inhibitors for non-responsive cancer patients due to the lack of immune cells in the tumors, which are so-called 'cold tumors' or 'non-inflamed tumors'. Indeed, a number of clinical studies for combination trials using anti-VEGF therapy with immune checkpoint inhibitors are ongoing for various cancer types [37]. During the past two years, 114 new combination regimens of VEGF and immune checkpoint inhibitors entered into clinical studies [38,39]. Among a large number of clinical studies, the FDA has approved several combination regimens of VEGF and immune checkpoint inhibitors, such as atezolizumab (an antagonist of PD-L1, Tecentriq®) plus bevacizumab with carboplatin and paclitaxel for the treatment of non-small cell lung cancer (NSCLC), avelumab (an antagonist of PD-L1, Bavencio®) plus axitinib (AG013736, a small molecule inhibitor of VEGFR tyrosine kinase, Inlyta®), and pembrolizumab (an antagonist of PD-1, Keytruda®) plus axitinib for the treatment of advanced renal carcinoma [40–42]. Recently, another combination regimen of atezolizumab plus bevacizumab was approved for the treatment hepatocellular carcinoma (HCC) as a first-line therapeutic option [43]. In this point of view, the results obtained in the current study imply that ABL001 may be another promising partner for combination therapy with immune checkpoint inhibitors, through the facilitation of immune cell infiltration via dual blockade of VEGF and DLL4 [28,29,33].

Currently, ABL001 is being tested for its safety, tolerability, and efficacy in phase 1 clinical studies with heavily pre-treated metastatic cancer patients. ABL001 has been well tolerated and no DLT is observed during dose escalation up to the final cohort, with manageable adverse effects generally exhibited by anti-cancer antibody therapeutics [25]. After the current dose escalation study of ABL001, further clinical development is scheduled to evaluate the efficacy of ABL001 in combination with chemotherapy. In conclusion, the results of this study provide important information for the clinical study design and plan for the combination treatment of ABL001 with chemotherapy.

4. Materials and Methods

4.1. Antibodies and Compounds

A human version of ABL001 bispecific antibody (ABL001) was produced under Good Manufacturing Practices (GMP) regulation by Bi-Nex (Incheon, Korea), and a mouse version of ABL001 bispecific antibody (mABL001) was produced by ABL Bio Inc., R&D Center (Gyeonggi-do, Seongnam-si, Korea), as described in a previous report [23]. Paclitaxel and irinotecan HCl were purchased from Hanmi Pharmaceutical Co. Ltd. (Seoul, Korea).

4.2. Cancer Cell Lines and Culture

Human gastric cancer cell lines, MKN45 (KCLB No.80103) and SNU16 (KCLB No.00016), were purchased from KCLB (Korea Cell Line Bank, Seoul, Korea), and NUGC-3 (JCRB0822) was obtained from JCRB (JCRB Cell Bank, Ibaraki, Japan). Human colon cancer cell lines, Colo205 (CCL-222), WiDr (CCL-218), and SW48 (CCL-231) were purchased from ATCC (American Type Culture Collection, Manassas, VA, USA). GAPF006 gastric cancer patient-derived tissues and SW620 human colon cancer cell line (LIDE, Shanghai, China) were also used for in vivo mouse xenograft studies. DMEM/F12, RPMI-1640, Leibovitz's L-15, PBS, fetal bovine serum, 0.05% trypsin-EDTA, and antibiotic-antimycotic were purchased from Gibco (Carlsbad, CA, USA). Colo205, MKN45, SNU16, and NUGC-3 cells were cultured in RPMI-1640 culture medium containing 10% fetal bovine serum and antibiotic-antimycotic (1X). SW48 cells were cultured in DMEM/F12 culture medium containing 10% fetal bovine serum and antibiotic-antimycotic (1X). Colo205, MKN45, SNU16, NUGC-3, and SW48 cells were cultured in an incubator at 37 °C in a humidified atmosphere with 5% CO_2 and 95% air. SW620 cells were cultured in Leibovitz's L-15 medium containing 10% fetal bovine serum in an incubator at 37 °C in free gas exchange with atmospheric air.

4.3. Animals

Eight-week-old female BALB/c nu/nu mice (Orient Bio Inc., Gyeonggi-do, Korea) were used for the efficacy tests in Colo205, WiDr, MKN45, and SNU16 xenograft models, eight-week-old female CB17 SCID (Envigo, Indianapolis, IN, USA) were used for the efficacy tests in the SW48 xenograft model, and eight-week-old female BALB/c nu/nu mice (Beijing Vital River Laboratory Animal Technology Co., Ltd, Beijing, China) were used for the efficacy tests in the SW620 xenograft model and human gastric PDX (Patient-Derived Xenograft) model (LIDE). All animal experiments were approved by the Institutional Animal Care and Use Committee (IACUC), approval number: IACUC180067, approval date: 17 April 2018. Mice were maintained in a controlled environment (12 h light-dark cycle; temperature, 20–22 °C; 50–60% humidity), and ad libitum access to food and water.

4.4. Animal Studies

To evaluate the in vivo efficacy of mABL001, MKN45, SNU16, and NUGC-3 human gastric cancer cells (5×10^6 cells/head) or Colo205, SW48, and WiDr human colon cancer cells (5×10^6 cells/head) were implanted in the flank of BALB/c nu/nu mice or CB17 SCID mice. When the tumors had grown to an average volume of 150–200 mm^3, the mice were divided into homogenous groups (6–12 mice/group), and treated with an intraperitoneal injection mABL001 (1.25, 2, 3.25, or 6.5 mg/kg), or ABL001 (GAPF006 PDX model, 6.5 mg/kg) twice per week. To evaluate the in vivo efficacy of mABL001 with chemotherapy, tumor growth was measured after treatment with the mouse version, mABL001 in SW48 or SW620 human colorectal cancer xenograft models, with or without irinotecan

(20 or 40 mg/kg), respectively. BALB/c nu/nu mice were injected subcutaneously in the flank region with SW620 cells (5 $\times$ 10^6 cells/head) in 0.1 mL of HBSS or GAPF006 tumor tissue fragments (9 mm^3, approximately 50–90 mg), and CB17 SCID mice were injected subcutaneously in the flank region with SW48 cells (5 $\times$ 10^6 cells/head). When the tumors had grown to an average volume of 150–200 mm^3, the mice were divided into homogenous groups (7–10 mice/group). GAPF006 PDX model treated ABL001 (3.25 mg/kg) twice per week, and paclitaxel (15 mg/kg) was administered with an intraperitoneal injection once a week for three weeks. SW620 xenograft model treated mABL001 (2 mg/kg) twice per week, and irinotecan (40 mg/kg) were administered with an intraperitoneal injection once a week for three weeks.

Tumor size was measured twice per week using a caliper and then calculated using the formula, (length) $\times$ $(\text{width})^2$ $\times$ 0.5. When the average tumor size of the control group reached 2000 mm^3, the treatment was stopped, and the mice were sacrificed to measure the tumor weight, and immunofluorescence analysis was performed (SW620 xenograft model). The efficacy was expressed as tumor growth inhibition [%TGI (mean volume of treated tumors/mean volume of control tumors) $\times$ 100]. Some mice were perfused with 4% paraformaldehyde in PBS for further immunofluorescence analysis of tumors.

4.5. Immunofluorescence Staining Analysis

To investigate whether mABL001 affects tumor angiogenesis and tumor cell survival, SW620 tumor sections were analyzed by immunofluorescence staining. For immunofluorescence staining analysis, SW620 tumors were removed from mice after cardiac perfusion and then embedded in OCT solution (Cat#3801480; Leica, Wetzlar, Germany) to produce frozen tumor blocks. The frozen tumors were sectioned (4-µm; Leica CM3050S; Leica) and permeabilized with washing buffer (PBS containing 0.03% Triton X-100) for 10 min, then blocked with 5% normal goat serum (Cat#S-1000; Vector Laboratories, Burlingame, CA, USA) or horse serum (Cat#16050122; Gibco) in the washing buffer. Tumor vessels were stained with rat anti-mouse CD31 (1:100, Cat#553370; BD, Franklin Lakes, NJ, USA) and goat anti-mouse VEGFR-2 antibody (1:100, Cat#AF644; R&D Systems, Minneapolis, MN, USA), respectively. Apoptotic cells in the tumors were stained with rabbit anti-mouse/human activated caspase-3 antibody (1:200, Cat#AF835; R&D Systems). DLL4 levels were detected with goat anti-mouse DLL4 antibody (1:100, Cat#AF1389; R&D Systems), which is cross-reactive (about 50%) with human DLL4. After being washed three times, the sections were stained for each secondary antibody, Alexa-568-conjugated goat anti-rat IgG (1:250, Cat#A11077), donkey anti-goat IgG (1:250, Cat#A11057), Alexa-488-conjugated goat anti-rabbit IgG (1:500, Cat#A11008), or donkey anti-rat (1:500 or 1:250, Cat#A21208), all from Thermo Fisher Scientific (Waltham, MA, USA). Stained tumors were mounted with Vectashield (Vector Laboratories) containing DAPI (4′,6-diamidino-2-phenylindole), and digital images of the tumors were captured using a Zeiss fluorescence microscope (Axio observer.7, Carl Zeiss, Oberkochen, Germany) with a camera (Axiocam, Carl Zeiss). Digital fluorescence images were analyzed using a Zeiss analysis software program (ZEN 2.6, Carl Zeiss).

4.6. Statistics

Graph creation and statistical analysis were performed using GraphPad Prism (GraphPad software Inc., San Diego, CA, USA) version 8.4.3. Values were expressed as the means $\pm$ SEM. Normality of data was tested using the Shapiro–Wilk test or Anderson–Darling test. Comparison between two groups was performed using the Student's *t*-test. Multiple group comparisons were made parametric one-way ANOVA followed post hoc test (Tukey's test, $p < 0.0001$, $p < 0.001$, $p < 0.01$, $p < 0.05$ values were considered as significant). The nonparametric Kruskal–Wallis test was used for the other cases.

Author Contributions: Conceptualization, S.H.L. and W.-K.Y.; methodology, D.-H.Y. and Y.-S.L.; software, D.-H.Y. and Y.-S.L.; formal analysis, D.-H.Y., H.-B.L., S.L. and B.S.; investigation, E.H. and J.-H.A.; resources, I.R., D.K.; data curation, D.-H.Y. and J.-H.A.; writing—original draft preparation, D.-H.Y. and W.-K.Y.; writing—review and editing, Y.-S.C. and W.-K.Y.; visualization, Y.-S.L. and W.-K.Y.; supervision, W.-K.Y. and S.H.L. All authors have read and agreed to the published version of the manuscript.

Funding: This research received no external funding.

Institutional Review Board Statement: The study was conducted according to the guidelines of the Declaration of Helsinki, and all experimental protocols were approved by IACUC (approval number: IACUC180067; approved date: 17 April 2018).

Informed Consent Statement: Not applicable.

Data Availability Statement: Data is contained within the article.

Acknowledgments: This work was supported by the National OncoVenture Program (No. HI11C1191).

Conflicts of Interest: The authors declare no conflict of interest.

Abbreviations

DLL4	Delta-like-ligand 4
VEGF	Vascular Endothelial Growth Factor
VEGFR	Vascular Endothelial Growth Factor Receptor
FDA	Food and Drug Administration
PDX	Patient-Derived Xenograft
CSC	Cancer stem cell
scFv	Single-chain Fv
IV	Intravenous
MTD	Maximum Tolerated Dose
DLT	Dose-limiting Toxicity
AEs	Adverse Events
SD	Stable Disease
PR	Partial Response
%TGI	% Tumor Growth Inhibition
IACUC	Institutional Animal Care and Use Committee
HCC	Hepatocellular Carcinoma
NSCLC	Non-Small Cell Lung Cancer

References

1. Kerbel, R.S. Tumor angiogenesis. *N. Engl. J. Med.* **2008**, *358*, 2039–2049. [CrossRef] [PubMed]
2. Neufeld, G.; Cohen, T.; Gengrinovitch, S.; Poltorak, Z. Vascular endothelial growth factor (VEGF) and its receptors. *FASEB J.* **1999**, *13*, 9–22. [CrossRef] [PubMed]
3. Meadows, K.L.; Hurwitz, H.I. Anti-VEGF therapies in the clinic. *Cold Spring Harb. Perspect. Med.* **2012**, *2*, a006577. [CrossRef] [PubMed]
4. Shams, N.; Ianchulev, T. Role of vascular endothelial growth factor in ocular angiogenesis. *Ophthalmol. Clin. N. Am.* **2006**, *19*, 335–344.
5. Kaur, H.; Bruno, J.G.; Kumar, A.; Sharma, T.K. Aptamers in the therapeutics and diagnostics pipelines. *Theranostics* **2018**, *8*, 4016. [CrossRef]
6. Ruckman, J.; Green, L.S.; Beeson, J.; Waugh, S.; Gillette, W.L.; Henninger, D.D.; Claesson-Welsh, L.; Janjic, N. 2′-Fluoropyrimidine RNA-based aptamers to the 165-amino acid form of vascular endothelial growth factor (VEGF165) inhibition of receptor binding and VEGF-induced vascular permeability through interactions requiring the exon 7-encoded domain. *J. Biol. Chem.* **1998**, *273*, 20556–20567. [CrossRef]
7. Zhou, B.; Wang, B. Pegaptanib for the treatment of age-related macular degeneration. *Exp. Eye Res.* **2006**, *83*, 615–619. [CrossRef]
8. Ohr, M.; Kaiser, P.K. Intravitreal aflibercept injection for neovascular (wet) age-related macular degeneration. *Expert Opin. Pharmacother.* **2012**, *13*, 585–591. [CrossRef]
9. Bergers, G.; Hanahan, D. Modes of resistance to anti-angiogenic therapy. *Nat. Rev. Cancer* **2008**, *8*, 592–603. [CrossRef]
10. Ebos, J.M.; Lee, C.R.; Cruz-Munoz, W.; Bjarnason, G.A.; Christensen, J.G.; Kerbel, R.S. Accelerated metastasis after short-term treatment with a potent inhibitor of tumor angiogenesis. *Cancer Cell* **2009**, *15*, 232–239. [CrossRef]

11. Hashizume, H.; Falcón, B.L.; Kuroda, T.; Baluk, P.; Coxon, A.; Yu, D.; Bready, J.V.; Oliner, J.D.; McDonald, D.M. Complementary actions of inhibitors of angiopoietin-2 and VEGF on tumor angiogenesis and growth. *Cancer Res.* **2010**, *70*, 2213–2223. [CrossRef] [PubMed]
12. You, W.-K.; Sennino, B.; Williamson, C.W.; Falcón, B.; Hashizume, H.; Yao, L.-C.; Aftab, D.T.; McDonald, D.M. VEGF and c-Met blockade amplify angiogenesis inhibition in pancreatic islet cancer. *Cancer Res.* **2011**, *71*, 4758–4768. [CrossRef] [PubMed]
13. Gale, N.W.; Dominguez, M.G.; Noguera, I.; Pan, L.; Hughes, V.; Valenzuela, D.M.; Murphy, A.J.; Adams, N.C.; Lin, H.C.; Holash, J.; et al. Haploinsufficiency of delta-like 4 ligand results in embryonic lethality due to major defects in arterial and vascular development. *Proc. Natl. Acad. Sci. USA* **2004**, *101*, 15949–15954. [CrossRef] [PubMed]
14. Noguera-Troise, I.; Daly, C.; Papadopoulos, N.J.; Coetzee, S.; Boland, P.; Gale, N.W.; Lin, H.C.; Yancopoulos, G.D.; Thurston, G. Blockade of Dll4 inhibits tumour growth by promoting non-productive angiogenesis. *Nature* **2006**, *444*, 1032–1037. [CrossRef] [PubMed]
15. Sainson, R.C.; Harris, A.L. Anti-Dll4 therapy: Can we block tumour growth by increasing angiogenesis? *Trends Mol. Med.* **2007**, *13*, 389–395. [CrossRef] [PubMed]
16. Miles, K.M.; Seshadri, M.; Ciamporcero, E.; Adelaiye, R.; Gillard, B.; Sotomayor, P.; Attwood, K.; Shen, L.; Conroy, D.; Kuhnert, F.; et al. Dll4 blockade potentiates the anti-tumor effects of VEGF inhibition in renal cell carcinoma patient-derived xenografts. *PLoS ONE* **2014**, *9*, e112371. [CrossRef]
17. Kuramoto, T.; Goto, H.; Mitsuhashi, A.; Tabata, S.; Ogawa, H.; Uehara, H.; Saijo, A.; Kakiuchi, S.; Maekawa, Y.; Yasutomo, K.; et al. Dll4-Fc, an inhibitor of Dll4-notch signaling, suppresses liver metastasis of small cell lung cancer cells through the downregulation of the NF-κB activity. *Mol. Cancer Ther.* **2012**, *11*, 2578–2587. [CrossRef]
18. Jenkins, D.W.; Ross, S.; Veldman-Jones, M.; Foltz, I.N.; Clavette, B.C.; Manchulenko, K.; Eberlein, C.; Kendrew, J.; Petteruti, P.; Cho, S.; et al. MEDI0639: A novel therapeutic antibody targeting Dll4 modulates endothelial cell function and angiogenesis in vivo. *Mol. Cancer Ther.* **2012**, *11*, 1650–1660. [CrossRef]
19. Li, J.-L.; Sainson, R.C.; Oon, C.E.; Turley, H.; Leek, R.; Sheldon, H.; Bridges, E.; Shi, W.; Snell, C.; Bowden, E.T.; et al. DLL4-Notch signaling mediates tumor resistance to anti-VEGF therapy in vivo. *Cancer Res.* **2011**, *71*, 6073–6083. [CrossRef]
20. Kuhnert, F.; Chen, G.; Coetzee, S.; Thambi, N.; Hickey, C.; Shan, J.; Kovalenko, P.; Noguera-Troise, I.; Smith, E.; Fairhurst, J.; et al. Dll4 blockade in stromal cells mediates antitumor effects in preclinical models of ovarian cancer. *Cancer Res.* **2015**, *75*, 4086–4096. [CrossRef]
21. Hoey, T.; Yen, W.-C.; Axelrod, F.; Basi, J.; Donigian, L.; Dylla, S.; Fitch-Bruhns, M.; Lazetic, S.; Park, I.-K.; Sato, A.; et al. DLL4 blockade inhibits tumor growth and reduces tumor-initiating cell frequency. *Cell Stem Cell* **2009**, *5*, 168–177. [CrossRef]
22. Marvin, J.S.; Zhu, Z. Recombinant approaches to IgG-like bispecific antibodies. *Acta Pharmacol. Sin.* **2005**, *26*, 649–658. [CrossRef] [PubMed]
23. Lee, D.; Kim, D.; Choi, Y.B.; Kang, K.; Sung, E.-S.; Ahn, J.-H.; Goo, J.; Yeom, D.-H.; Jang, H.S.; Moon, K.D.; et al. Simultaneous blockade of VEGF and Dll4 by HD105, a bispecific antibody, inhibits tumor progression and angiogenesis. *MAbs* **2016**, *8*, 892–904. [CrossRef] [PubMed]
24. Kim, D.-H.; Lee, S.; Kang, H.G.; Park, H.-W.; Lee, H.-W.; Kim, D.; Yoem, D.-H.; Ahn, J.-H.; Ha, E.; You, W.-K.; et al. Synergistic antitumor activity of a DLL4/VEGF bispecific therapeutic antibody in combination with irinotecan in gastric cancer. *BMB Rep.* **2020**, *53*, 533. [CrossRef] [PubMed]
25. Lee, J.; Kim, S.; Lee, S.J.; Park, S.H.; Park, J.O.; Ha, E.; Park, D.-H.; Park, N.; Kim, H.-K.; Lee, S.H.; et al. Phase 1a study results investigating the safety and preliminary efficacy of ABL001 (NOV1501), a bispecific antibody targeting VEGF and DLL4 in metastatic gastrointestinal (GI) cancer. *J. Clin. Oncol.* **2019**, *37*, 3023. [CrossRef]
26. Teicher, B.A. A systems approach to cancer therapy. *Cancer Metastasis Rev.* **1996**, *15*, 247–272. [CrossRef] [PubMed]
27. Comunanza, V.; Bussolino, F. Therapy for cancer: Strategy of combining anti-angiogenic and target therapies. *Front. Cell Dev. Biol.* **2017**, *5*, 101. [CrossRef]
28. Wildiers, H.; Guetens, G.; De Boeck, G.; Verbeken, E.; Landuyt, B.; Landuyt, W.; De Bruijn, E.; Van Oosterom, A. Effect of antivascular endothelial growth factor treatment on the intratumoral uptake of CPT-11. *Br. J. Cancer* **2003**, *88*, 1979–1986. [CrossRef]
29. Zhang, Q.; Bindokas, V.; Shen, J.; Fan, H.; Hoffman, R.M.; Xing, H.R. Time-course imaging of therapeutic functional tumor vascular normalization by antiangiogenic agents. *Mol. Cancer Ther.* **2011**, *10*, 1173–1184. [CrossRef]
30. Zirlik, K.; Duyster, J. Anti-angiogenics: Current situation and future perspectives. *Oncol. Res. Treat.* **2018**, *41*, 166–171. [CrossRef]
31. Jászai, J.; Schmidt, M.H. Trends and challenges in tumor anti-angiogenic therapies. *Cells* **2019**, *8*, 1102. [CrossRef]
32. Han, J.; Gao, L.; Wang, J.; Wang, J. Application and development of aptamer in cancer: From clinical diagnosis to cancer therapy. *J. Cancer* **2020**, *11*, 6902. [CrossRef] [PubMed]
33. Kang, M.; Jiang, B.; Xu, B.; Lu, W.; Guo, Q.; Xie, Q.; Zhang, B.; Dong, X.; Chen, D.; Wu, Y. Delta like ligand 4 induces impaired chemo-drug delivery and enhanced chemoresistance in pancreatic cancer. *Cancer Lett.* **2013**, *330*, 11–21. [CrossRef] [PubMed]
34. Mancuso, M.R.; Davis, R.; Norberg, S.M.; O'Brien, S.; Sennino, B.; Nakahara, T.; Yao, V.J.; Inai, T.; Brooks, P.; Freimark, B.; et al. Rapid vascular regrowth in tumors after reversal of VEGF inhibition. *J. Clin. Investig.* **2006**, *116*, 2610–2621. [CrossRef] [PubMed]
35. Li, J.-L.; Harris, A.L. Crosstalk of VEGF and Notch pathways in tumour angiogenesis: Therapeutic implications. *Front. Biosci. (Landmark Ed.)* **2009**, *14*, 3094–3110. [CrossRef] [PubMed]

36. Mpekris, F.; Voutouri, C.; Baish, J.W.; Duda, D.G.; Munn, L.L.; Stylianopoulos, T.; Jain, R.K. Combining microenvironment normalization strategies to improve cancer immunotherapy. *Proc. Natl. Acad. Sci. USA* **2020**, *117*, 3728–3737. [CrossRef]
37. Campesato, L.F.; Merghoub, T. Antiangiogenic therapy and immune checkpoint blockade go hand in hand. *Ann. Transl. Med.* **2017**, *5*, 497. [CrossRef]
38. Tang, J.; Shalabi, A.; Hubbard-Lucey, V. Comprehensive analysis of the clinical immuno-oncology landscape. *Ann. Oncol.* **2018**, *29*, 84–91. [CrossRef]
39. Yu, J.X.; Hodge, J.P.; Oliva, C.; Neftelinov, S.T.; Hubbard-Lucey, V.M.; Tang, J. Trends in clinical development for PD-1/PD-L1 inhibitors. *Nat. Rev. Drug Discov.* **2020**, *19*, 163–164.
40. Socinski, M.A.; Jotte, R.M.; Cappuzzo, F.; Orlandi, F.; Stroyakovskiy, D.; Nogami, N.; Rodríguez-Abreu, D.; Moro-Sibilot, D.; Thomas, C.A.; Barlesi, F. Atezolizumab for first-line treatment of metastatic nonsquamous NSCLC. *N. Engl. J. Med.* **2018**, *378*, 2288–2301. [CrossRef]
41. Motzer, R.J.; Penkov, K.; Haanen, J.; Rini, B.; Albiges, L.; Campbell, M.T.; Venugopal, B.; Kollmannsberger, C.; Negrier, S.; Uemura, M. Avelumab plus axitinib versus sunitinib for advanced renal-cell carcinoma. *N. Engl. J. Med.* **2019**, *380*, 1103–1115. [CrossRef] [PubMed]
42. Rini, B.I.; Plimack, E.R.; Stus, V.; Gafanov, R.; Hawkins, R.; Nosov, D.; Pouliot, F.; Alekseev, B.; Soulières, D.; Melichar, B. Pembrolizumab plus axitinib versus sunitinib for advanced renal-cell carcinoma. *N. Engl. J. Med.* **2019**, *380*, 1116–1127. [CrossRef] [PubMed]
43. Finn, R.S.; Qin, S.; Ikeda, M.; Galle, P.R.; Ducreux, M.; Kim, T.-Y.; Kudo, M.; Breder, V.; Merle, P.; Kaseb, A.O. Atezolizumab plus bevacizumab in unresectable hepatocellular carcinoma. *N. Engl. J. Med.* **2020**, *382*, 1894–1905. [CrossRef] [PubMed]

International Journal of
Molecular Sciences

MDPI

Article

Blocking of the IL-33/ST2 Signaling Axis by a Single-Chain Antibody Variable Fragment (scFv) Specific to IL-33 with a Defined Epitope

Soo Bin Park, Sun-Jick Kim, Sang Woo Cho, Cheol Yong Choi and Sangho Lee *

Department of Biological Sciences, Sungkyunkwan University, Suwon 16419, Korea; stephanie7007@daum.net (S.B.P.); godmouse@skku.edu (S.-J.K.); aksgdlwkd@skku.edu (S.W.C.); choicy@skku.ac.kr (C.Y.C.)

* Correspondence: sangholee@skku.edu; Tel.: +82-31-290-5913

Received: 28 August 2020; Accepted: 16 September 2020; Published: 22 September 2020

Abstract: Interleukin 33 (IL-33) is an IL-1 family cytokine that plays a central role in immune system by regulating and initiating inflammatory responses. The binding of IL-33 to the suppressor of tumorigenicity 2 (ST2) receptor induces mitogen-activated protein kinases (MAPK) and nuclear factor κB (NF-κB) pathways, thereby leading to inflammatory cytokines production in type 2 helper T cells and type 2 innate lymphoid cells. To develop an antibody specific to IL-33 with a defined epitope, we characterized a single-chain antibody variable fragments (scFvs) clone specific to IL-33, C2_2E12, which was selected from a human synthetic library of scFvs using phage display. Affinity (K_d) of C2_2E12 was determined to be 38 nM using enzyme-linked immunosorbent assay. C2_2E12 did not show cross-reactivity toward other interleukin cytokines, including closely related IL-1 family cytokines and unrelated proteins. Mutational scanning analysis revealed that the epitope of IL-33 consisted of residues 149–158 with key residues being L150 and K151 of IL-33. Structural modeling suggested that L150 and K151 residues are important for the interaction of IL-33 with C2_2E12, implicating that C2_2E12 could block the binding of ST2 to IL-33. Pull-down and in-cell assays supported that C2_2E12 can inhibit the IL-33/ST2 signaling axis. These results suggest that the scFv clone characterized here can function as a neutralizing antibody.

Keywords: interleukin 33; ST2 receptor; scFv; C2_2E12

---

1. Introduction

Interleukin-1 (IL-1) family cytokines play important roles in regulating and initiating inflammatory and immunological responses [1]. The IL-1 family includes eleven cytokines comprising seven agonist ligands, three receptor antagonists, and an anti-inflammatory cytokine [2]. Interleukin 33 (hereafter called as "IL-33") cytokine is identified as one of the IL-1 family agonist ligands [3]. It was first regarded as an alarmin that is released to signal immune system when a cell or tissue is damaged or stressed [4]. Recently, IL-33 has been considered as an important factor of the immune system involved in allergic inflammation and chronic diseases such as asthma, atopic dermatitis, and allergic rhinitis [5–7].

IL-33, expressed in endothelial cells, fibroblasts, epithelial cells, and other cells, binds to its receptor suppressor of tumorigenicity 2 (ST2)/interleukin 1 receptor-like 1 (IL1RL1), which formed heterodimer with co-receptor, IL-1 receptor accessory protein (IL1RAcP) [4,8]. There are two types of ST2 isoforms: the transmembrane form, ST2, and soluble form, sST2, covering residues 19 through 321 of the ectodomain (hereafter, we call all isoforms as simply "ST2"). The ST2 is expressed on various immune cells including innate lymphoid group 2 cells (ILC2s), mast cells, dendritic cells, macrophages, basophils, and type 2 helper T cells (T_h2), and it is linked to T_h2 effector functions [9,10]. IL-33 exerts its biological functions followed by binding to ST2 expressed in immune cells, and it is mainly associated with T_h2 responses through the production of inflammatory cytokines IL-5 and IL-13 [3,11]. The heterodimer complex formation activates downstream signaling complex formation. Myeloid differentiation primary response 88 (MyD88) first binds to heterodimeric receptor and leads to the recruitment of interleukin-1 receptor-associated kinase 1 (IRAK1), IRAK4 and tumor necrosis factor (TNF) receptor-associated factor 6 (TRAF6), and these subsequently activate mitogen-activated protein kinases (MAPKs) and nuclear factor κB (NF-κB) signaling pathways to promote inflammatory cytokine production [9,12,13]. It seems that IL-33 has the potential to activate T_h2 cytokine-mediated allergic inflammation and related diseases, suggesting that blockade of the IL-33/ST2 signaling axis can be a new therapeutic strategy for allergic inflammation and chronic inflammatory diseases [14–16].

Several strategies have been developed to suppress the IL-33 mediated downstream signaling pathway to prevent chronic diseases and allergic inflammation: antagonists against IL-33, and antagonists against ST2 or sST2 binding to IL-33 [17]. Here, we describe the discovery and characterization of single-chain variable fragment (scFv) monoclonal antibodies (mAbs) directly targeting IL-33 to inhibit IL-33 binding to ST2. Although there are diverse antibodies against IL-33 for various purposes, they are mainly derived from immunizing living organisms with immunoglobulin G forms [16,18] or monoclonal antibodies for IL-33 detection [15,19]. Since immunoglobulin G (IgG) forms of antibodies are hard to handle and not suitable to further engineering, we used a human synthetic single-chain variable fragment (scFv) antibody library to screen IL-33 specific mAbs in vitro.

The discovery of mAbs using phage display library was performed with five rounds of biopanning, and enzyme-linked immunosorbent assay (ELISA) was used to determine the antibodies affinity. Using immunoblotting, we observed their cross-reactivity, and two types of mutant-based epitope mapping were implemented to identify the binding epitope domains. The inhibition effect of antibody was verified by glutathione *S*-transferase (GST) pull-down assay and human cell-expressing ST2 and IL1RAcP-based assay. The antibody seems to have therapeutic function by interfering with IL-33 binding to the ST2 receptor, heterodimeric receptor complex formation, and blocking the IL-33/ST2 signaling axis.

2. Results

2.1. Selection of scFvs Specific to IL-33

Human IL-33 is composed of three domains: N-terminal nuclear domain (residues 1–65), central domain (residues 66–111) and C-terminal IL-1-like cytokine domain (residues 112–270) [3,8,20]. The N-terminal and central domains of IL-33 are cleaved by caspase-1 to produce the mature form [3]. IL-33 is susceptible to oxidation by forming disulfide bonds among cysteine residues (C208, C227, C232, and C259). IL-33 oxidation reportedly drives a conformational change and inactivates its ST2-dependent cytokine activities [21,22]. To prevent from oxidation, we mutated C208 and C232 to serine and compared the activity of C208S/C232S mutant with that of IL-33 wild-type (WT). The purity of WT and C208S/C232S mutant was confirmed by SDS-PAGE (Figure S1A,B). The recognition of IL-33 WT and C208S/C232S mutant by a selected scFv (see next section) was comparable as corroborated by SDS-PAGE and immunoblot analyses (Figure S1C). We used GST-IL-33 WT for biopanning and characterizations and IL-33 C208S/C232S mutant for cell signaling analysis.

We performed five rounds of biopanning to select scFvs specific to IL-33 using a large synthetic human scFv library in two distinct conditions according to the number of negative selections (Table S1). GST-IL-33 and GST were used as antigens for positive and negative selections of biopanning, respectively. Ten scFv clones with high OD_{450} values in response to IL-33 compared to the negative selection were selected by ELISA screening (Figure S2A). Of the ten clones, clones with mutations in the backbone frame or duplicated sequences were excluded through multiple protein sequence alignment (Figure S2B). Finally, six clones (C1_1E1, C2_1D5, C2_2A10, C2_2E1, C2_2E12, and C2_2H5) were chosen based on their high binding signals at 450 nm without mutations in the amino acid sequences. Multiple sequence alignment revealed that these six clones have different amino acid residues mostly in the third complementarity determining region in heavy chain (CDR-H3) and the second complementarity determining region in light chain (CDR-L2).

The *E. coli* cell lysates containing overexpressed His_6-tagged scFvs were prepared to determine the binding affinity of selected scFvs with IL-33. The dissociation constants (K_d) values of C1_1E1, C2_1D5, C2_2A10, C2_2E1, C2_2E12, and C2_2H5 by ELISA were estimated to be 48, 36, 57, 35, 28, and 31 nM, respectively (Figure 1A). The K_d value of C2_2E12 that showed the highest affinity using cell lysate was further measured using the purified proteins by ELISA (Figure S2C and Figure S1B). The K_d value of the purified C2_2E12 was 38 nM (Figure 1B), which is consistent with the value estimated using the cell lysate. We selected C2_2E12 for further characterizations.

The cross-reactivity of C2_2E12 was checked for two interleukins belonging to the same subfamily (GST-IL-1β and IL-6) and three unrelated proteins (GST, bovine serum albumin (BSA) and IlvC). Immunoblot assay results showed that C2_2E12 only reacted with IL-33 (Figure 1C). It is interesting that C2_2E12 did not react with IL-1β and IL-6, since IL-33, IL-1β, and IL-6 belong to the same subfamily. Human IL-33 shows low sequence identities to IL-1β and IL-6 despite all three belonging to the same subfamily: 13.5% with IL-1β and 12.9% with IL-6, respectively (Figure 1D). The structure of IL-1β (PDB ID: 1L2H) is similar to that of IL-33 (PDB ID: 4KC3) with a root mean square deviation (r.m.s.d.) of 1.93 Å, while the structure of IL-6 (PDB ID: 1ALU) is completely different from that of IL-33. Given the low sequence similarities and structural differences, no cross-reactivity of C2_2E12 for IL-1β and IL-6 seems to be reasonable. The cross-reactivity results clearly demonstrate that C2_2E12 specifically binds to IL-33.

2.2. Epitope Mapping

To determine the epitope region in IL-33 for C2_2E12, a series of GST-IL-$33_{112\text{-}270}$ N-terminal deletion mutants were constructed by the insertion of a stop codon at the end of each α-helix or β-strand of IL-33 based on the crystal structure of human IL-33 (PDB ID: 4KC3) [23] (Figure 2A). Immunoblot analysis revealed that residues 149–158 of the IL-33 comprised the epitope region, which corresponded to its receptor ST2 binding site in the crystal structure of the IL-33:ST2 complex (PDB ID: 4KC3). We found that the other five scFv clones (C1_1E1, C2_1D5, C2_2A10, C2_2E1, C2_2E12, and C2_2H5) also recognized the same epitope region in the IL-33 (Figure 2B). Alanine scanning mutagenesis was performed to determine the critical residue(s) in the epitope region (Figure 2C). Each residue in GST-IL-$33_{149\text{-}158}$ was substituted to alanine by site-directed mutagenesis PCR. The effects of the IL-33 mutants were analyzed by immunoblots with C2_2E12 as the primary antibody. Alanine substitutions of L150 and K151 of IL-33 reduced the binding with C2_2E12, rendering these the key residues in the epitope region. To obtain further insights on alanine scanning results at the molecular level, we performed molecular docking between IL-33 and C2_2E12 using the HADDOCK server with restraints that only L150 and K151 residues of IL-33 and CDR residues of C2_2E12 should participate in interactions. Although alanine scanning data showed that L150 of IL-33 is a key residue of IL-33 and C2_2E12 binding, L150 seemed to not interact with any residue of C2_2E12. Alternatively, L150 seemed to possibly interact with the surrounding hydrophobic residues of the 149–158 epitope region of IL-33, and it also seemed to play an important role in maintaining the shape of the loop (Figure 2D). It seems that the L150A mutant inhibits the interaction between IL-33 and C2_2E12 by local conformational changes of the loop. The docked structural model of IL-33:C2_2E12 suggested that K151 of IL-33 seemed to interact electrostatically with the acidic pocket of C2_2E12 composed of D164, S166, Y168, A218, and Y230 (Figure 2E). This structural analysis with a docked model between IL-33 and C2_2E12 supports that L150 and K151 residues of IL-33 are important for their binding to C2_2E12.

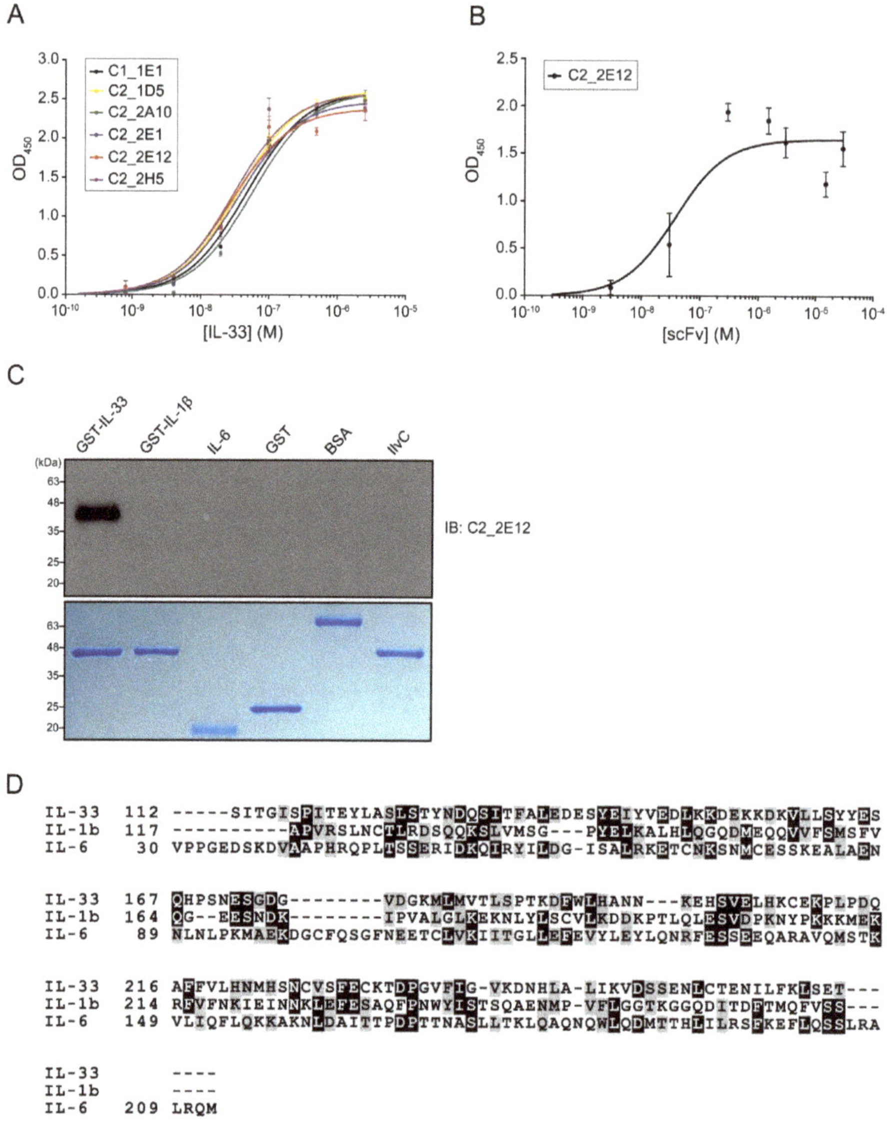

Figure 1. Molecular characterizations of anti-IL-33 single-chain antibody variable fragments (scFvs). Enzyme-linked immunosorbent assay (ELISA)-based affinity determination of anti-IL-33 scFvs. (**A**) Affinity determination of the top six clones that exhibited high binding signals against IL-33. (**B**) Affinity determination of the purified C2_2E12, which seems to have the highest binding signal and good protein condition among six clones. K_d values of C1_1E1, C2_1D5, C2_2A10, C2_2E1, C2_2E12, and C2_2H5 were estimated by kinetic analysis. ELISA was repeated three times. (**C**) Immunoblot analysis of the recombinant proteins using C2_2E12 for primary antibody (0.5 mg·mL^{-1}, 1:100 dilution) and anti-hemagglutinin-horse radish peroxidase (anti-HA-HRP) for secondary antibody (0.2 mg·mL^{-1}, 1:5000 dilution). Expression of recombinant interleukin cytokines (GST-IL-33, GST-IL1β, and GST-IL6) and unrelated proteins (GST, BSA, and IlvC) in *E. coli* BL21 (DE3) as revealed by SDS-PAGE analysis. IB, immunoblot. (**D**) Multiple protein sequence alignment of IL-33, IL1β, and IL6. BSA: bovine serum albumin, IL: interleukin.

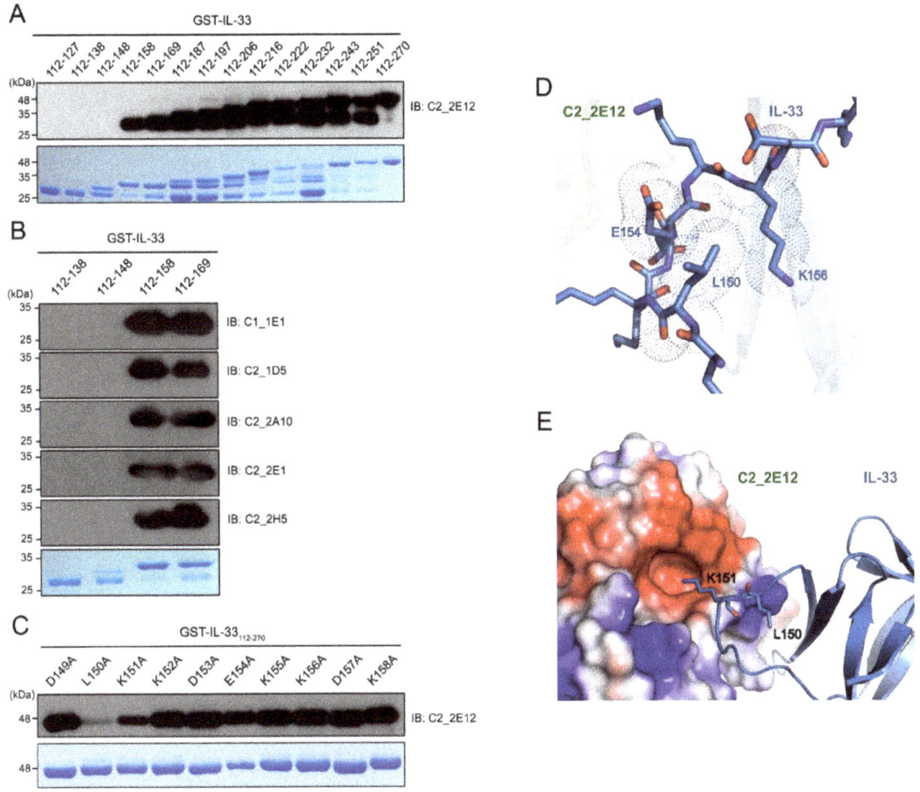

Figure 2. Epitope mapping of C2_2E12. (**A**) Immunoblot analysis of 14 GST-IL-33 deletion mutants to map the IL-33 epitope at secondary structural element level for scFv clone C2_2E12. Residue numbers of the mutants are shown. (**B**) Immunoblot analysis of four GST-IL-33 deletion mutants to map the IL-33 epitopes for scFv clones C1_1E1, C2_1D5, C2_2A10, C2_2E1, and C2_2H5. (**C**) Immunoblot analysis of alanine scanning for GST-IL-$33_{149-158}$ for recognition by the scFv clone C2_2E12. Residue numbers and identities are shown. In panels (**A**) through (**C**), Coomassie Blue stained gel is shown at the bottom. Amount of the loaded protein per lane was 1 μg. The scFv clones were used as the primary antibody (0.5 mg·mL^{-1}, 1:100 dilution), and anti-HA-HRP was used as the secondary antibody (0.2 mg·mL^{-1}, 1:5000 dilution). (**D**,**E**) The HADDOCK-derived molecular docking of C2_2E12 (green) to IL-33 (PDB: 4KC3, blue) complex. A homology structural model for C2_2E12 was generated using SwissModel [24]. Both proteins are depicted as cartoon diagrams. (**D**) Residues of IL-33 in the epitope region recognized by C2_2E12 are represented as stick models. Dash lines represent van der Waals atomic distances in Å. (**E**) Electrostatic interactions between C2_2E12 and IL-33. The acidic pocket in C2_2E12 consists of N163, D164, S166, Y168, A218, and Y230. L150 and basic K151, the two key residues in the epitope region of IL-33 are depicted as stick models. The figures in the panels (**D**) and (**E**) were generated using PyMOL (Schrödinger).

2.3. Competitive Binding of C2_2E12 to IL-33:ST2 Complex

Residues 149–152 and 156 in the epitope of IL-33 for C2_2E12 are reportedly involved in the interaction with the ectodomain (residues 19–321) of ST2, which is present in both the transmembrane and soluble isoforms [23]. Since the epitope of IL-33 for C2_2E12 overlaps with the ST2 binding site, we hypothesized that the C2_2E12 could function as a blocking antibody in the IL-33/ST2 signaling axis. To test the hypothesis, in vitro GST pull-down assay was performed. The antibody fragment crystallizable (Fc) fusion of ST2, ST2-Fc, interacted with immobilized GST-IL-33 as expected. By contrast, ST2-Fc did not bind to the immobilized GST-IL-33 in the presence of C2_2E11 (Figure 3A). To investigate whether C2_2E12 inhibits IL-33:ST2 interaction in a dose-dependent manner, a series of concentrations of C2_2E12 were used for competitive binding assay GST pull-down assay. The IL-33:ST2 interaction was reduced at 100-fold molar excess of C2_2E12 (Figure 3B). Quantification of the IL-33:ST2 interaction in the presence of increasing concentrations of C2_2E12 showed that the IL-33:ST2 interaction decreased in a concentration-dependent manner, leading to about 40% level at 100-fold molar excess of C2_2E12 (Figure 3C). These results suggest that C2_2E12 can act as a neutralizing antibody in the IL-33/ST2 signaling axis in vitro.

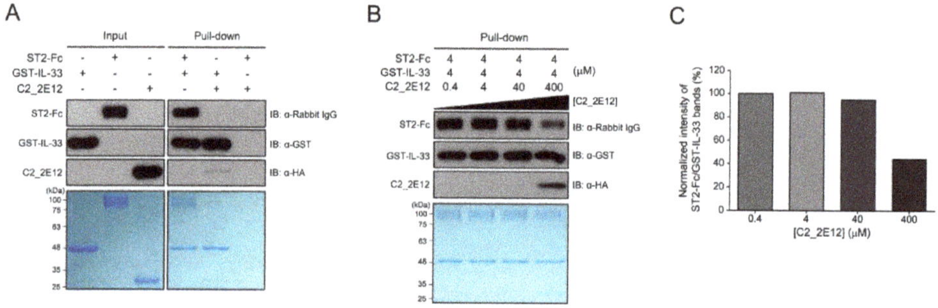

Figure 3. Interfering with IL-33 and suppressor of tumorigenicity 2 (ST2) complex formation by C2_2E12. GST pull-down assay was used to observe the interaction of C2_2E12 with IL-33 competitively with ST2 receptor in vitro. Pull-down assay was performed step by step. Immobilize GST-IL-33 in Glutathione Sepharose 4B and add ST2-Fc fusion proteins. Then, put C2_2E12 in a dose-dependent manner. Binding was performed for 30 min every step. Molar concentration of the proteins for binding were GST-IL-33: ST2-Fc: C2_2E12 = 1: 1: 0.1, 1:1:1, 1:1:10, and 1:1:100 (M). (**A**) Input loading (GST-IL-33 in lane 1, ST2-Fc in lane 2, and C2_2E12 in lane 3) and proteins binding test (lane 4, 5, and 6) with pull-down assay were visualized by immunoblot and SDS-PAGE. (**B**) Inhibition of IL-33 and ST2 binding by anti-IL-33 antibody in a dose-dependent manner. After 4 μM of GST-IL-33 was immobilized in resin and 4 μM of ST2-Fc was added to the resin, C2_2E12 (0.4, 4, 40, and 400 μM in lane 1, 2, 3, and 4) was added in a dose-dependent manner and visualized by immunoblot analysis and SDS-PAGE. (**C**) Quantification of the inhibitory effects of C2_2E12 for the IL-33:ST2 interaction. Band intensities of ST2-Fc in panel (**B**) were quantified using ImageJ and normalized by dividing them by those of GST-IL-33. Relative intensities in reference to that of ST2-Fc with 0.4 μM C2_2E12 are shown as a bar graph.

2.4. C2_2E12 Can Neutralize IL-33/ST2 Axis Driving Downstream Signaling Pathway in Human Cell Line

To corroborate the neutralizing effects of C2_2E12 in the IL-33/ST2 signaling axis in cells, we tested IL-33 induced MAPK and NF-κB pathways activation in human mast cells (HMC-1). HMC-1 cells expressed endogenous ST2 receptor and IL-1RAcP co-receptor, unlike HeLa cells (Figure 4A). The levels of phosphorylated extracellular signal-regulated kinase (ERK) and c-Jun N-terminal kinase (JNK) in the MAPK pathway were increased by the IL-33 C208S/C232S:ST2 complex while the level of inhibitor of NF-κB α subunit (IκBα) in the NF-κB pathway was reduced, supporting that IL-33 activates both MAPK and NF-κB pathways (Figure 4A). Subsequently, we treated the HMC-1 cells with IL-33 C208S/C232S alone or pre-incubated with C2_2E12 and analyzed phosphorylation levels of ERK, JNK, and IκBα (Figure 4B,C). The relative phosphorylation level of IκBα is decreased by C2_2E12 in a dose-dependent manner, indicating the suppression of the NF-κB signaling pathway. Relative phosphorylation levels of ERK and JNK were reduced by C2_2E12 in a dose-dependent manner, implicating the suppression of the MAPK pathway. Analysis of the results indicated that C2_2E12 can neutralize IL-33 and ST2 interaction by binding with IL-33 in a dose-dependent manner (Figure 4B,C). Taken together, our results demonstrate that C2_2E12 treatment can reduce IL33/ST2 complex formation by interfering with IL-33 and ST2 binding and thus act as a neutralizing antibody for the suppression of the IL-33/ST2 signaling axis in cells.

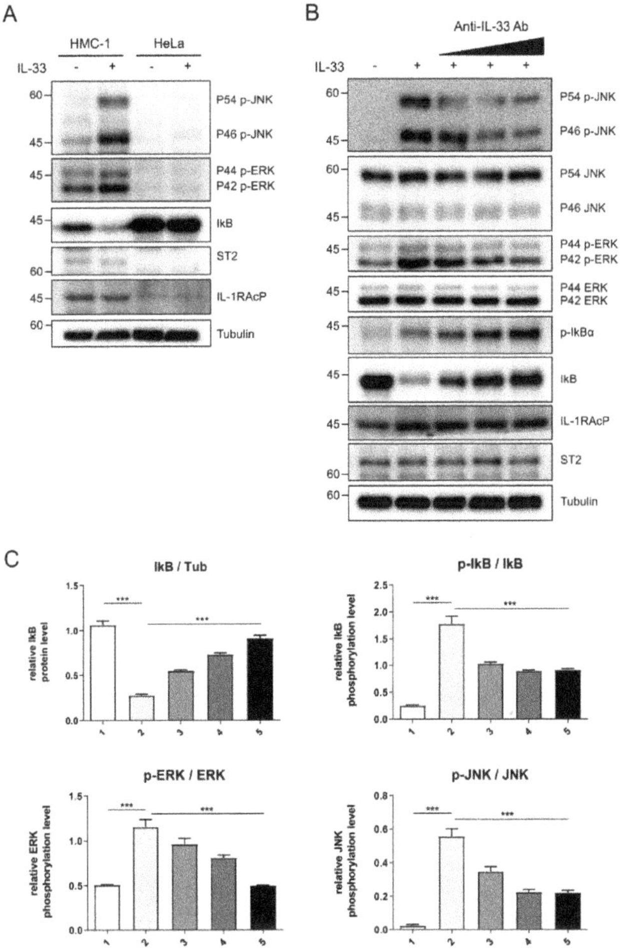

Figure 4. Intervention of IL-33/ST2 signaling axis by C2_2E12 antibody. (**A**) IL-33-mediated activation of nuclear factor κB (NF-κB) signaling in human mast cells (HMC-1) cells, but not in HeLa cells where ST2 and IL-1RAcP were not expressed. HMC-1 and HeLa cells were stimulated with mock or human IL-33 (1 ng·mL^{-1}, 8 min), and cell lysates were analyzed by immunoblotting with the indicated antibodies. (**B**) The inhibition of IL-33-induced NF-κB signaling by C2_2E12 antibody in a dose-dependent manner. HMC-1 cells were treated with IL-33 alone or IL-33 pre-incubated with the increasing amounts of C2_2E12 antibody. Cell lysates were analyzed by immunoblotting with the indicated antibodies. IL-33 (1 ng·mL^{-1}) was pre-incubated with increasing amounts of the C2_2E12 antibody (0.1, 0.5, and 2.0 ng·mL^{-1} in lanes 3, 4, and 5, respectively) for 15 min and treated to HMC-1 cells for 8 min. (**C**) Quantification of protein levels shown in (**B**). Band intensities in immunoblots were quantified using ImageJ. Data are expressed as the mean ± SEM. The statistical significance of differences was analyzed by one-way analysis of variance (ANOVA) followed by Bonferroni's multiple comparison test (*** $p < 0.001$ compared to the indicated points; $n = 3$).

3. Discussion

IL-33 has been associated with several chronic diseases such as asthma, atopic dermatitis, and inflammatory allergy, and recently, it was discovered that it plays important roles in regulatory immune responses. Neutralizing antibodies against IL-33 or ST2 have been developed to hinder IL-33 and ST2 binding. In this study, we discovered an scFv that specifically binds to IL-33 and subsequently interferes with IL-33 and ST2 complex formation. The IL-33 epitope region with C2_2E12 overlaps the ST2 binding domain in IL-33, implicating that C2_2E12 can act as a neutralizing antibody by competitive binding to IL-33. Pull-down assay and human cell line analysis verified that C2_2E12 has neutralizing efficacy. IL-33 and ST2 interaction stimulates the activation of immune cells such as mast cells, T-helper type 2 cells, and dendritic cells, thereby causing allergic inflammatory responses. Therefore, future evaluation of C2_2E12 and its refined clone(s) would desirably include the determination of efficacies in the keratinocyte/dendritic cells or epithelium/dendritic cell co-cultures. IL-33 is also known to stimulate type 2 innate lymphoid cells to release cytokines such as IL-5 and IL-13 [25]. Determination of the secreted IL-5 and IL-13 in response to the intervention of IL-33/ST-2 signaling axis by C2_2E12 would require future studies. C2_2E12 is not only a neutralizing antibody binding to IL-33, but also a monoclonal antibody discovered from human synthetic library of scFvs in vitro. The identification of epitope at the residue level, neutralizing the efficacy and human origin of C2_2E12 renders it a suitable candidate for further engineering. Our preliminary comparative data reveal that C2_2E12 shows an affinity only marginally inferior to that of a commercial antibody (data not shown). After further improving the affinity of C2_2E12 by affinity maturation and going through an in vivo test, C2_2E12 and its refined clone(s) could be used as a therapeutic antibody against IL-33 for treating allergic inflammatory diseases.

4. Materials and Methods

4.1. Plasmid Constructs Cloning

Genes encoding the mature form of IL-33 (residues 112–270), hereafter called simply "IL-33", and the ectodomain of ST2 (residues 19–321) were synthesized (Cosmo Genetech, Seoul, Korea) and cloned into BamHI/StuI sites of parallel GST-2 vector [26] and *Not*I/*Nco*I sites of the pSF vector, respectively. CH2 and CH3 domains of human the IgG Fc region were cloned into XhoI/BsgI sites of pSF-ST2 plasmid for ST2-Fc fusion protein expression. Plasmids encoding IL-33 mutants (deletion mutants, alanine-scanning mutants, and an oxidation-resistant mutant C208S/C232S) were prepared by following the protocol for QuikChange kit (Agilent, Santa Clara, CA, USA). Identities of all the constructs were verified by DNA sequencing.

4.2. Expression and Purification of Recombinant Proteins

The plasmid encoding GST-IL-33 was transformed into *E. coli* BL21 (DE3) cells. A single colony was inoculated into 10 mL Luria broth (LB) media containing 100 $\mu g \cdot mL^{-1}$ ampicillin and grown at 37 °C overnight. After 16–18 h, the pre-cultured cells were transferred to 500 mL LB media containing 100 $\mu g \cdot mL^{-1}$ of ampicillin, grown at 37 °C until OD_{600} 0.6–1.0, induced with 0.6 mM isopropyl-β-D-1-thiogalactopyranoside (IPTG), and further grown at 25 °C overnight with gentle shaking. Cells were harvested by centrifugation and re-suspended in lysis buffer (50 mM Tris-HCl pH = 7.5 and 150 mM NaCl). Cells were disrupted by ultrasonication, cleared by centrifugation, and the supernatant containing GST-IL-33 was transferred to Glutathione Sepharose 4B resin (GE Healthcare, Chicago, IL, USA) pre-equilibrated with the lysis buffer. After washing the resin with the lysis buffer, GST-IL-33 was eluted in GST elution buffer (50 mM Tris-HCl pH 8.0, 150 mM NaCl, and 10 mM reduced glutathione). IL-33 was relieved from the GST fusion protein using a recombinant His_6-tagged tobacco etch virus (TEV) protease during dialysis at 4 °C overnight. The resulting IL-33 was further purified on a Superdex 75 10/300 GL size-exclusion chromatography column (GE HealthCare, Chicago, IL, USA) pre-equilibrated with the lysis buffer. A ST2-Fc fusion protein, containing the ectodomain (residues

19–321) of ST2 and Fc from human IgG, was expressed in Expi293F cells (Thermo Fisher Scientific, Waltham, MA, USA) maintained in Expi293 expression medium (Thermo Fisher Scientific, Waltham, MA, USA). The day before transfection, cells were seeded to a final density of 2×10^6 viable cells ml^{-1} in a 125 mL Erlenmeyer flask and grown at 37 °C for 24 h. After 24 h, cells were transfected with 30 µg of pSF-ST2-Fc plasmid DNA diluted in Opti-MEM™ I Medium (Thermo Fisher Scientific, Waltham, MA, USA) supplemented with 80 µL of ExpiFectamine™ 293 Reagent (Thermo Fisher Scientific, Waltham, MA, USA). Four days post-transfection, the cells were harvested by centrifugation, and its supernatant containing ST2-Fc was transferred to protein A agarose (Thermo Fisher Scientific, Waltham, MA, USA) pre-equilibrated by phosphate-buffered saline (PBS). The resin was washed using PBS, and ST2-Fc was eluted in Fc elution buffer (100 mM glycine pH = 3 with 1/10 volume of 1 M Tris-HCl pH = 8.0). The eluted ST2-Fc was dialyzed in the lysis buffer at 4 °C overnight.

4.3. Biopanning Using Phage Display

A synthetic human scFv library encoding His_6- and HA-tagged scFv clones was used for biopanning [27]. Biopanning was performed as described previously with some modifications [28]. Library biopanning was performed in immuno tubes coated with the recombinant GST–IL-33 as an antigen in two conditions: inclusion of a negative selection with GST in every round (condition 1), and in the first round only (condition 2). In condition 1, five rounds of biopanning were performed in immuno tubes coated with GST protein for a negative selection and the recombinant GST-IL-33 at a gentle decrease in antigen concentrations (50, 10, 7.5, 5, and 2.5 $\mu g \cdot mL^{-1}$). In condition 2, the negative selection using GST protein is performed only in the first round of biopanning and coated with GST-IL-33 in the other four rounds of biopanning using the same concentration with condition 1. To select scFv clones that specifically bind to IL-33, single colonies from the final round of a biopanning output plate were grown in a 96-well cell culture plate until OD_{600} reached 0.6–1.0 and induced with 1 mM IPTG grown overnight at 30 °C with shaking. The harvested cells in each 96-well were re-suspended in cold 1× TES buffer (50 mM Tris-HCl pH = 8.0, 1 mM ethylenediaminetetraacetic acid (EDTA) and 20% (*w*/*v*) sucrose) for 30 min on ice, and cold 0.2×TES buffer was added to the re-suspended cells for 1 h on ice. The recombinant GST-IL-33 protein at 10 $\mu g \cdot mL^{-1}$ in PBS was coated on a 96-well ELISA plate. ELISA assay for scFv screening with horseradish peroxidase (HRP) conjugated anti-HA secondary antibody (1:3000 dilution, Santa Cruz Biotechnology, Dallas, TX, USA) was performed with a final reading of signals recorded at OD_{450}. The OD_{450} values with GST-IL-33 were divided by the OD_{450} value with GST, and the ratio of OD_{450} values was compared.

4.4. Expression and Purification of scFvs in E. coli

Cells were pre-cultured from the single colonies of scFv-expressing *E. coli* BL21 (DE3) at 37 °C overnight, transferred to 500 mL super broth (SB) media containing 100 $\mu g \cdot mL^{-1}$ ampicillin. Cells were grown at 37 °C until OD_{600} 0.5–0.8 and induced with 1 mM IPTG at 30 °C with vigorous shaking. After 16–18 h, cells were harvested by centrifugation and re-suspended in cold 1× TES buffer for 30 min on ice, and cold 0.2× TES buffer was added to the re-suspended cells for 1 h on ice. The re-suspended cells supplemented with 5 mM $MgCl_2$ to block EDTA were centrifuged, and their supernatants containing each scFvs were transferred to Ni-NTA agarose resin (Qiagen, Hilden, Germany). Each resin was washed by wash buffer A (PBS supplanted with 20 mM imidazole and 0.5 mM DTT) and scFvs were eluted by His-tag elution buffer A (PBS supplemented with 300 mM imidazole and 0.5 mM DTT). Size exclusion chromatography was performed on a Superdex 75 increase 10/300 GL column (GE HealthCare, Chicago, IL, USA) pre-equilibrated with PBS.

4.5. Reformatting, Expression, and Purification of C2_2E12 in Mammalian Cells

The gene encoding C2_2E12 in the pComb3X vector [27] was cloned into the pSF vector to express three different formats of C2_2E12 in mammalian cells: scFv, antigen-binding fragment (Fab), and immunoglobulin G (IgG). The C2_2E12 scFv was cloned into NotI/XhoI sites of the pSF vector for expression in Expi293F cells (Thermo Fisher Scientific, Waltham, MA, USA) maintained in Expi293 expression medium (Thermo Fisher Scientific, Waltham, MA, USA). A variable heavy chain and variable light chain of C2_2E12 were cloned into NotI/NcoI sites and HindIII/XhoI sites of the pSF vector, respectively, for the expression of Fab and IgG formats in Expi293F cells (Thermo Fisher Scientific, Waltham, MA, USA). Transfection and preparation steps for Fab and IgG were the same with those for scFv except for the amount and ratio of DNA plasmid used for transfection. The expression of scFv, Fab, and IgG formats of C2_2E12 in mammalian cells was performed in the same way as for ST2-Fc. Supernatants containing C2_2E12 scFv and Fab were transferred to Ni-NTA agarose resin (Qiagen, Hilden, Germany) pre-equilibrated with PBS. Each resin was washed by wash buffer B (PBS supplemented with 20 mM imidazole) and eluted by His-tag elution buffer B (PBS supplemented with 300 mM imidazole). Supernatant containing C2_2E12 IgG was transferred to a protein A agarose (Thermo Fisher Scientific, Waltham, MA, USA) pre-equilibrated by PBS. The resin was washed using PBS, and the C2_2E12 IgG was eluted in the Fc elution buffer. The antibodies were dialyzed at 4 °C overnight, concentrated, and loaded to a Superdex 75 10/300 GL size-exclusion chromatography column (GE HealthCare, Chicago, IL, USA) pre-equilibrated with PBS.

4.6. Immunoblot

Purified proteins were subjected to 12% SDS-PAGE and transferred onto polyvinylidene difluoride (PVDF) membranes (Merck Millipore, Burlington, MA, USA). Membranes were blocked with 5% (*w*/*v*) skim milk in Tris-buffered saline (pH = 7.5) containing 0.1% (*v*/*v*) tween-20 for 1 h at room temperature. Different primary antibodies were incubated at 4 °C overnight, and secondary antibodies were incubated at room temperature for 1 h. The bound antibody was detected by enhanced chemiluminescence (ECL) reaction with EZ-Western Lumi Pico kit (DoGen, Seoul, Korea).

4.7. Enzyme-Linked Immunosorbent Assay (ELISA)

GST-IL-33 was coated on half the total area of a Costar® 96-well plate in the clear flat bottom polystyrene high bind microplate (Corning, Corning, NY, USA) and incubated at 4 °C for overnight. In the next day, the resulting culture was washed using PBST (PBS supplemented with 0.1% (*v*/*v*) tween-20) and blocked using blocking buffer (5% (*w*/*v*) skim milk in PBST). Serial dilutions of purified scFvs as the primary antibody with approximately 8 ng·mL^{-1} to 0.8 mg·mL^{-1} were added to the wells. The plate was incubated at ambient temperature for 1 h and washed using PBST. Subsequently, HRP-conjugated anti-HA antibody as the secondary antibody (1:3000 dilution, Santa Cruz Biotechnology) was added to the wells and incubated at ambient temperature for 1 h. The incubated plate was washed using PBST, and tetramethylbenzidine (TMB) substrate solution (GenDEPOT, Katy, TX, USA) was added for color development. After incubation for 10 min, 1 M H_2SO_4 was added to the plate to stop the color development reaction. The final signal readings were recorded at 450 nm and plotted using Prism 5 (GraphPad, San Diego, CA, USA).

4.8. Biolayer Interferometry (BLI)

Binding kinetics was measured by BLI experiments using a BLItz system (ForteBio, Fremont, CA, USA). *E. coli* cell lysate containing His$_6$-tagged antibodies was prepared in 0.5× TES buffer. GST-IL-33 was prepared in BLI buffer (PBS supplemented with 20 mM imidazole, 0.05% (*v*/*v*) Triton X-100 and 0.1 mg·mL^{-1} BSA) to reduce the nonspecific binding signal. The BLI buffer was also used as the kinetics buffer. The cell lysate was immobilized to Ni-NTA biosensors (ForteBio, Fremont, CA, USA) and washed using the kinetics buffer. The sensors were subsequently reacted with various concentrations (2, 1, 0.5, and 0.25 μM) of GST-IL33 (association step) and washed using the kinetics buffer (dissociation step). These assays were performed twice each. All real-time recorded sensograms were analyzed by the 'global fitting' method in BLItz Pro 1.2 (ForteBio, Fremont, CA, USA) to calculate k_{on} (association rate constant) and k_{off} (dissociation rate constant) values. The K_d (dissociation constant) value of each antibody was calculated using the following equation:

$$K_d = k_{off}/k_{on}. \quad (1)$$

r^2 analysis, an indication of goodness of graph curve fitting, was performed using BLItz Pro 1.2, and the r^2 values of all experiments were above 0.98. The graphs of raw sensograms were prepared by Prism 5 (GraphPad, San Diego, CA, USA).

4.9. Structural Modeling

A homology structural model for C2_2E12 that was generated using the SWISS-MODEL server [24] and the crystal structure of IL-33:ST2 complex (PDB ID: 4KC3) were used as templates for the docking of C2_2E12 to IL-33. Protein–protein docking modeling was performed using the HADDOCK server [29]. To perform the HADDOCK modeling, a restraint was applied such that the two key epitope residues of IL-33, L150 and K151, must interact with the complementary determination region of C2_2E12. The Z-score of clustering and other modeling parameters are listed in Table S2. Structural analysis of the interface between C2_2E12 and IL-33 was performed using PyMOL 1.8 (Schrödinger, New York, NY, USA).

4.10. Pull-Down Assay

Pull-down assay was performed using Glutathione Sepharose 4B resin (GE Healthcare, Chicago, IL, USA). First, 4 µM of GST-IL-33 was added to the resin and incubated for 30 min at 4 °C with gentle shaking. The resin was washed 4 times with wash buffer C (50 mM Tris-HCl pH = 7.5 and 150 mM NaCl) and incubated for 30 min at 4 °C with gentle shaking upon the addition of 4 µM of ST2-Fc. Subsequently, C2_2E12 at a series of concentrations (0.4, 4, 40, and 400 µM) was added to the resulting resin with further incubation for 30 min at 4 °C. After 4 times of washing, proteins were separated by SDS-PAGE on a 12% gel, stained with Coomassie Brilliant Blue, or transferred onto a PVDF membrane (45 mA for 60 min). Protein bands on the PVDF membrane were visualized by immunoblotting by ECL reaction using anti-ST2 (1:5000 dilution, Abcam, Cambridge, United Kingdom) and mouse anti-rabbit IgG–HRP (1:10000 dilution, Santa Cruz Biotechnology, Dallas, TX, USA), anti-GST-HRP (1:10000 dilution, Santa Cruz Biotechnology, Dallas, TX, USA), and anti-His_6–HRP (1:10000 dilution, Santa Cruz Biotechnology, Dallas, TX, USA). Gels were quantified using ImageJ (National Institutes of Health, Bethesda, MD, USA).

4.11. Cell Signaling Analysis

HMC-1 cells were a kind gift from Prof. Soohyun Kim, Konkuk University, South Korea. HMC-1 cells were cultured in Iscove's modified Dulbecco's medium (IMDM) containing 10% FBS. HeLa cells were cultured in Dulbecco's modified Eagle's media (DMEM) containing 10% FBS. Cells were centrifuged at 800× *g* for 5 min at 4°C, and they were lysed with NETN lysis buffer (100 mM NaCl, 20 mM Tris-HCl pH = 8.0, 0.5 mM EDTA, 0.1% NP-40, 5 mM NEM, 10 mM NaF, 1 mM Na_3VO_4, a protein inhibitor cocktail) for 15 min on ice. Cell lysates were centrifuged at 15,000× *g* at 4°C for 10 min. Protein extracts were separated by SDS-PAGE and transferred onto PVDF membranes. Membranes were immunoblotted with the indicated antibodies, and the signals were visualized with ImageQuant™ LAS 4000 mini (GE Healthcare, Chicago, IL, USA). Anti-p-IkB (#2859), anti-IkB (#4814), anti-p-S6K (#9251), and anti-S6K (#9252) antibodies were purchased from Cell signaling. Anti-p-ERK (sc-7383), anti-ERK (sc-27129), and anti-IL-1RAcP (sc-376872) were purchased from Santa Cruz Biotechnology (Dallas, TX, USA). Anti-ST2 (#D065-3) were purchased from MBL (Woburn, MA, USA).

5. Patent

A patent application has been filed in South Korea (application number: 10-2020-0103135).

Supplementary Materials: Supplementary materials can be found at http://www.mdpi.com/1422-0067/21/18/6953/s1.

Author Contributions: Conceptualization, S.B.P. and S.L.; investigation, S.B.P., S.-J.K., S.W.C.; resources, C.Y.C.; writing—original draft preparation, S.B.P.; writing—review and editing, S.L.; visualization, S.B.P.; supervision, S.L.; project administration, S.L.; funding acquisition, S.L. All authors have read and agreed to the published version of the manuscript.

Funding: This research was funded by the Basic Science Research Program (NRF-2018R1A2B6004367), the Science Research Center Program (NRF-2017R1A5A1014560), and the Bio & Medical Technology Development Program (NRF-2020M3A9E4039217) through the National Research Foundation of Korea (NRF) grants and the Next-Generation BioGreen 21 program (PJ01367602) through the Rural Development Administration.

Acknowledgments: We thank Yong-Soo Bae, Yoe-Sik Bae, and Seok Hee Park at Sungkyunkwan University for discussion.

Conflicts of Interest: The authors declare no conflict of interest. The funders had no role in the design of the study; in the collection, analyses, or interpretation of data; in the writing of the manuscript, or in the decision to publish the results.

Abbreviations

IL-33	Interleukin-33
ST2	ST2, suppressor of tumorigenicity 2
scFv	Single-chain antibody variable fragment
GST	glutathione *S*-transferase
Fc	Antibody fragment crystallizable

References

1. Dinarello, C.A. Interleukin-1 in the pathogenesis and treatment of inflammatory diseases. *Blood* **2011**, *117*, 3720–3732. [CrossRef]
2. Garlanda, C.; Dinarello, C.A.; Mantovani, A. The interleukin-1 family: Back to the future. *Immunity* **2013**, *39*, 1003–1018. [CrossRef]
3. Schmitz, J.; Owyang, A.; Oldham, E.; Song, Y.; Murphy, E.; McClanahan, T.K.; Zurawski, G.; Moshrefi, M.; Qin, J.; Li, X.; et al. IL-33, an interleukin-1-like cytokine that signals via the IL-1 receptor-related protein ST2 and induces T helper type 2-associated cytokines. *Immunity* **2005**, *23*, 479–490. [CrossRef] [PubMed]
4. Gupta, R.K.; Gupta, K.; Dwivedi, P.D. Pathophysiology of IL-33 and IL-17 in allergic disorders. *Cytokine Growth Factor Rev.* **2017**, *38*, 22–36. [CrossRef]
5. Stolarski, B.; Kurowska-Stolarska, M.; Kewin, P.; Xu, D.; Liew, F.Y. IL-33 exacerbates eosinophil-mediated airway inflammation. *J. Immunol.* **2010**, *185*, 3472–3480. [CrossRef]
6. Savinko, T.; Matikainen, S.; Saarialho-Kere, U.; Lehto, M.; Wang, G.; Lehtimaki, S.; Karisola, P.; Reunala, T.; Wolff, H.; Lauerma, A.; et al. IL-33 and ST2 in atopic dermatitis: Expression profiles and modulation by triggering factors. *J. Investig. Dermatol.* **2012**, *132*, 1392–1400. [CrossRef]
7. Chan, B.C.L.; Lam, C.W.K.; Tam, L.S.; Wong, C.K. IL33: Roles in allergic inflammation and therapeutic perspectives. *Front. Immunol.* **2019**, *10*, 364. [CrossRef] [PubMed]
8. Liew, F.Y.; Girard, J.P.; Turnquist, H.R. Interleukin-33 in health and disease. *Nat. Rev. Immunol.* **2016**, *16*, 676–689. [CrossRef]
9. Griesenauer, B.; Paczesny, S. The ST2/IL-33 Axis in immune cells during inflammatory diseases. *Front. Immunol.* **2017**, *8*, 475. [CrossRef]
10. Townsend, M.J.; Fallon, P.G.; Matthews, D.J.; Jolin, H.E.; McKenzie, A.N. T1/ST2-deficient mice demonstrate the importance of T1/ST2 in developing primary T helper cell type 2 responses. *J. Exp. Med.* **2000**, *191*, 1069–1076. [CrossRef]
11. Milovanovic, M.; Volarevic, V.; Radosavljevic, G.; Jovanovic, I.; Pejnovic, N.; Arsenijevic, N.; Lukic, M.L. IL-33/ST2 axis in inflammation and immunopathology. *Immunol. Res.* **2012**, *52*, 89–99. [CrossRef]
12. Das, J.; Chen, C.H.; Yang, L.; Cohn, L.; Ray, P.; Ray, A. A critical role for NF-kappa B in GATA3 expression and TH2 differentiation in allergic airway inflammation. *Nat. Immunol.* **2001**, *2*, 45–50. [CrossRef]

13. Pinto, S.M.; Subbannayya, Y.; Rex, D.A.B.; Raju, R.; Chatterjee, O.; Advani, J.; Radhakrishnan, A.; Prasad, K.T.S.; Wani, M.R.; Pandey, A. A network map of IL-33 signaling pathway. *J. Cell Commun. Signal* **2018**, *12*, 615–624. [CrossRef]
14. Haenuki, Y.; Matsushita, K.; Futatsugi-Yumikura, S.; Ishii, K.J.; Kawagoe, T.; Imoto, Y.; Fujieda, S.; Yasuda, M.; Hisa, Y.; Akira, S.; et al. A critical role of IL-33 in experimental allergic rhinitis. *J. Allergy Clin. Immunol.* **2012**, *130*, 184–194. [CrossRef]
15. Yuan, Q.; Huang, L.; Wang, X.; Wu, Y.; Gao, Y.; Li, C.; Nian, S. Construction of human nonimmune library and selection of scFvs against IL-33. *Appl. Biochem. Biotechnol.* **2012**, *167*, 498–509. [CrossRef]
16. Kim, Y.H.; Yang, T.Y.; Park, C.S.; Ahn, S.H.; Son, B.K.; Kim, J.H.; Lim, D.H.; Jang, T.Y. Anti-IL-33 antibody has a therapeutic effect in a murine model of allergic rhinitis. *Allergy* **2012**, *67*, 183–190. [CrossRef]
17. Chen, W.Y.; Tsai, T.H.; Yang, J.L.; Li, L.C. Therapeutic strategies for targeting IL-33/ST2 signalling for the treatment of inflammatory diseases. *Cell Physiol. Biochem.* **2018**, *49*, 349–358. [CrossRef]
18. Liu, X.; Li, M.; Wu, Y.; Zhou, Y.; Zeng, L.; Huang, T. Anti-IL-33 antibody treatment inhibits airway inflammation in a murine model of allergic asthma. *Biochem. Biophys. Res. Commun.* **2009**, *386*, 181–185. [CrossRef]
19. Ye, Y.; Nian, S.; Xu, W.; Wu, T.; Wang, X.; Gao, Y.; Yuan, Q. Construction and expression of human scFv-Fc against interleukin-33. *Protein Expr. Purif.* **2015**, *114*, 58–63. [CrossRef]
20. Haraldsen, G.; Balogh, J.; Pollheimer, J.; Sponheim, J.; Kuchler, A.M. Interleukin-33—Cytokine of dual function or novel alarmin? *Trends Immunol.* **2009**, *30*, 227–233. [CrossRef]
21. Cohen, E.S.; Scott, I.C.; Majithiya, J.B.; Rapley, L.; Kemp, B.P.; England, E.; Rees, D.G.; Overed-Sayer, C.L.; Woods, J.; Bond, N.J.; et al. Oxidation of the alarmin IL-33 regulates ST2-dependent inflammation. *Nat. Commun.* **2015**, *6*, 8327. [CrossRef] [PubMed]
22. Cayrol, C.; Girard, J.P. Interleukin-33 (IL-33): A nuclear cytokine from the IL-1 family. *Immunol. Rev.* **2018**, *281*, 154–168. [CrossRef]
23. Liu, X.; Hammel, M.; He, Y.; Tainer, J.A.; Jeng, U.S.; Zhang, L.; Wang, S.; Wang, X. Structural insights into the interaction of IL-33 with its receptors. *Proc. Natl. Acad. Sci. USA* **2013**, *110*, 14918–14923. [CrossRef]
24. Waterhouse, A.; Bertoni, M.; Bienert, S.; Studer, G.; Tauriello, G.; Gumienny, R.; Heer, F.T.; de Beer, T.A.P.; Rempfer, C.; Bordoli, L.; et al. SWISS-MODEL: Homology modelling of protein structures and complexes. *Nucleic Acids Res.* **2018**, *46*, W296–W303. [CrossRef]
25. Mjosberg, J.M.; Trifari, S.; Crellin, N.K.; Peters, C.P.; van Drunen, C.M.; Piet, B.P.; Fokkens, W.J.; Cupedo, T.; Spits, H. Human IL-25- and IL-33-responsive type 2 innate lymphoid cells are defined by expression of CRTH2 and CD161. *Nat. Immunol.* **2011**, *12*, 1055–1062. [CrossRef]
26. Sheffield, P.; Garrard, S.; Derewenda, Z. Overcoming expression and purification problems of RhoGDI using a family of "parallel" expression vectors. *Protein Expr. Purif.* **1999**, *15*, 34–39. [CrossRef]
27. Yang, H.Y.; Kang, K.J.; Chung, J.E.; Shim, H. Construction of a large synthetic human scFv library with six diversified CDRs and high functional diversity. *Mol. Cells* **2009**, *27*, 225–235. [CrossRef]
28. Kim, D.; Jang, S.; Oh, J.; Han, S.; Park, S.; Ghosh, P.; Rhee, D.K.; Lee, S. Molecular characterization of single-chain antibody variable fragments (scFv) specific to Pep27 from Streptococcus pneumoniae. *Biochem. Biophys. Res. Commun.* **2018**, *501*, 718–723. [CrossRef]
29. Van Zundert, G.C.P.; Rodrigues, J.; Trellet, M.; Schmitz, C.; Kastritis, P.L.; Karaca, E.; Melquiond, A.S.J.; van Dijk, M.; de Vries, S.J.; Bonvin, A. The HADDOCK2.2 web server: User-friendly integrative modeling of biomolecular complexes. *J. Mol. Biol.* **2016**, *428*, 720–725. [CrossRef]

International Journal of
Molecular Sciences

MDPI

Review

Advances and Challenges of Antibody Therapeutics for Severe Bronchial Asthma

Yuko Abe [1,2], Yasuhiko Suga [1], Kiyoharu Fukushima [1,2,3,*], Hayase Ohata [1], Takayuki Niitsu [1,2], Hiroshi Nabeshima [2,3], Yasuharu Nagahama [2,3], Hiroshi Kida [4] and Atsushi Kumanogoh [1,5,6]

1 Department of Respiratory Medicine and Clinical Immunology, Osaka University Graduate School of Medicine, 2-2 Yamadaoka, Suita, Osaka 565-0871, Japan; y.abe@imed3.med.osaka-u.ac.jp (Y.A.); Yasu031055@imed3.med.osaka-u.ac.jp (Y.S.); haya.oohata@gmail.com (H.O.); mosatsu1987@gmail.com (T.N.); kumanogo@imed3.med.osaka-u.ac.jp (A.K.)

2 Laboratory of Host Defense, World Premier Institute Immunology Frontier Research Center (WPI-IFReC), Osaka University, Osaka 565-0871, Japan; h-nabeshima@ifrec.osaka-u.ac.jp (H.N.); y-nagahama@ifrec.osaka-u.ac.jp (Y.N.)

3 Department of Host Defense, Research Institute for Microbial Diseases (RIMD), Osaka University, Osaka 565-0871, Japan

4 Department of Respiratory Medicine, National Hospital Organization, Osaka Toneyama Medical Centre, 5-1-1 Toneyama, Toyonaka, Osaka 560-0852, Japan; kida.hiroshi.sv@mail.hosp.go.jp

5 Department of Immunopathology, World Premier Institute Immunology Frontier Research Center (WPI-IFReC), Osaka University, Osaka 565-0871, Japan

6 Integrated Frontier Research for Medical Science Division, Institute for Open and Transdisciplinary Research Initiatives, Osaka University, Osaka 565-0871, Japan

* Correspondence: fukushima@imed3.med.osaka-u.ac.jp; Tel./Fax: +81-6-6879-3831

Abstract: Asthma is a disease that consists of three main components: airway inflammation, airway hyperresponsiveness, and airway remodeling. Persistent airway inflammation leads to the destruction and degeneration of normal airway tissues, resulting in thickening of the airway wall, decreased reversibility, and increased airway hyperresponsiveness. The progression of irreversible airway narrowing and the associated increase in airway hyperresponsiveness are major factors in severe asthma. This has led to the identification of effective pharmacological targets and the recognition of several biomarkers that enable a more personalized approach to asthma. However, the efficacies of current antibody therapeutics and biomarkers are still unsatisfactory in clinical practice. The establishment of an ideal phenotype classification that will predict the response of antibody treatment is urgently needed. Here, we review recent advancements in antibody therapeutics and novel findings related to the disease process for severe asthma.

Keywords: asthma; refractory asthma; antibody therapeutics; biomarker

Citation: Abe, Y.; Suga, Y.; Fukushima, K.; Ohata, H.; Niitsu, T.; Nabeshima, H.; Nagahama, Y.; Kida, H.; Kumanogoh, A. Advances and Challenges of Antibody Therapeutics for Severe Bronchial Asthma. *Int. J. Mol. Sci.* **2022**, *23*, 83. https://doi.org/10.3390/ijms23010083

Academic Editor: Yong-Seok Heo

Received: 7 September 2021
Accepted: 20 December 2021
Published: 22 December 2021

1. Introduction

Asthma is a disorder ordinarily characterized by allergic chronic airway inflammation. Usually, this condition is sensitive to corticosteroids and the widespread use of inhaled corticosteroids (ICS) has markedly reduced asthma emergencies. However, 5–10% of asthma patients are refractory to the maximum combination treatment of high-dose ICS, long-acting β_2-agonists, and long-acting muscarinic antagonists. In 2014, the American Thoracic Society and European Respiratory Society published guidelines defining severe asthma as a condition that requires treatment with high-dose ICS, plus other long-term control medications (and/or oral corticosteroids (OCS)), or is poorly controlled regardless of these treatments [1]. These guidelines indicate that a diagnosis of severe asthma requires a correct diagnosis of asthma, confirmation of the presence of comorbidities (sinus disease, obesity, aspirin asthma, chronic obstructive pulmonary disease), and appropriate assessment of asthma control.

Newly developed antibody therapies targeting cytokines involved in the pathophysiological process of asthma have led to reduced exacerbations and improved symptom control and lung function in a subgroup of severe asthmatics. However, the efficacies of current antibody therapeutics are still unsatisfactory in clinical practice. This is, in part, because of the heterogeneity of severe asthma. Here, we review recent advancements in antibody therapeutics and novel findings related to the disease process of severe asthma.

2. Current Understanding of Severe Bronchial Asthma

Asthma is a disease characterized by chronic airway inflammation and usually reversible airflow limitation. However, uncontrolled disease activity leads to sustained airway inflammation, and increased airway hyperresponsiveness (AHR) and airway remodeling, resulting in persistent respiratory symptoms. Airway inflammation, airway remodeling, and airway hyperresponsiveness differentially contribute to the clinical features of each patient with severe asthma [2] (Figure 1). Typically, airway inflammation is a triggering/exacerbation factor for airway hypersensitivity and airway remodeling, but the interaction of each of the three factors becomes a further exacerbation factor as asthma progresses. Therefore, treatment strategies targeting airway inflammation as well as airway hyperresponsiveness and airway remodeling would be more effective than targeting only airway inflammation.

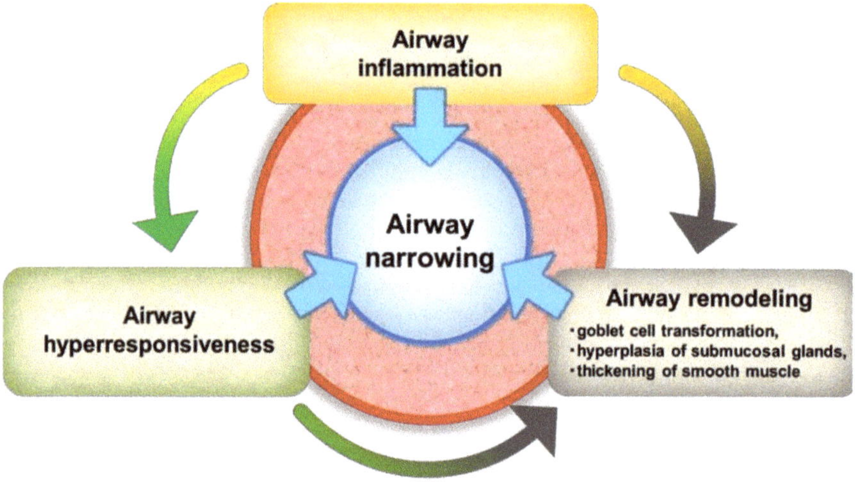

Figure 1. Mechanisms of the onset and exacerbation of severe asthma.

Chronic airway inflammation in asthma is typically characterized by eosinophil infiltration, overproduction of IgE, and Th2 cytokines, including IL-4, IL-5, and IL-13. IL-5, which is essential for eosinophil activation and proliferation and is derived from Th2 cells and Group 2 innate lymphoid cells (ILC2s). IL-4 and IL-13, derived from Th2 cells, promote the production of specific IgE antibodies from B cells. IgE antibodies bind to the IgE receptor (FcεRI) on the surface of mast cells and prepare them for activation during allergen exposure. IL-13, secreted from Th2 cells and ILC2s, shares the IL-4 receptor and induces smooth muscle hyperplasia, goblet cell hyperplasia, and mucous secretion, leading to airway remodeling and decreased respiratory function. Lung ILC2s respond to the alarmin IL-33, or IL-25 and TSLP released by epithelial cells, which induce their activation and the production of large amounts of IL-5 and IL-13. Thus, IgE, IL-5, and IL-4/IL-13 are particularly important in the pathogenesis of type 2 asthma. Blood eosinophils have been proposed as a surrogate marker of airway eosinophilia [3]. Elevated numbers of blood eosinophils have been associated with more severe asthma and have shown to predict a higher risk of asthma exacerbation [4]. Measurement of FeNO is another non-invasive way to quantify Th2 high airway inflammation. Nitric oxide (NO) is produced by epithelial cells lining the airways. Inducible nitric oxide synthase (iNOS) is induced by Th2 type inflammation, where it is largely driven by IL-4 and IL-13, leading to the increased production of NO. Similar to elevated blood eosinophils, elevated FeNO is predictive of asthma exacerbations and asthma severity [5,6]. In addition, simultaneously increased FeNO and blood eosinophils were associated with a higher likelihood of AHR [6]. Because Th2 cytokines, including IL-13 and IL-4, act on goblet cell hyperplasia, fibroblast-to-myofibroblast transformation, collagen deposition, and airway smooth muscle contraction [7], high FeNO levels in patients with severe asthma may be affected by airway remodeling. In another study involving 310 young adult subjects with suspected cough variant asthma, FeNO levels and the eosinophil count percentage in induced sputum, in addition to the Forced expiratory flow at 25–75% of FVC (FEF25-75), were associated with AHR [8]. Of note, FeNO can be affected by many external variables including ambient air quality, smoking, sinus disease, allergic rhinitis, and virus infection. These factors need to be considered when interpreting results. As already described, IgE is a key factor in high Th2 inflammation. Total serum IgE and specific IgE are the most common risk factors for allergic asthma. In a cluster analysis by the National Institute of Health/National Heart, Lung, and Blood Institute Severe Asthma Research Program pediatric cohort, children with severe asthma had higher serum IgE levels and increased sensitization to aeroallergens [9].

Airway remodeling describes structural changes of the airway wall, including fibrosis, airway smooth muscle hypertrophy, and goblet cell hyperplasia. Among these, the molecular mechanism of goblet cell hyperplasia has been intensively studied. SAM (sterile α-motif) pointed domain containing ETS transcription factor (SPDEF) and forkhead box protein (Foxa3) are the main transcription factors that regulate differentiation into goblet cell hyperplasia [10]. These transcription factors are induced by Th2 cytokines in the airway epithelium and promote thymic stromal lymphopoietin (TSLP) production in airway epithelial cells, which exacerbates Th2 inflammation [11]. Epithelial-mesenchymal transition (EMT), and the migration and proliferation of cultured airway smooth muscle cells have been used as surrogate experimental models to investigate the molecular mechanisms involved in fibrosis and airway smooth muscle hypertrophy. By using these models, transforming growth factor (TGF)-β was shown to be an important factor in the airway remodeling in asthma [12–15]. Clinically, the standard assessment of remodeling is obtained by a biopsy of the lungs and airways by surgery or bronchoscopy. However, bronchial biopsy is invasive and not applicable to routine clinical settings. It also requires expert knowledge, therefore, indirect analytical methods using remodeling markers in the blood, urine, and sputum have also been developed [16]. Periostin is a matricellular protein secreted by bronchial epithelial cells and lung fibroblasts in response to the Th2 cytokines, IL-13, and IL-4 [17]. Periostin-high asthma patients had clinical characteristics including eosinophilia, high FeNO, aspirin intolerance, nasal disorders, and late-onset disease [18]. In addition, periostin was reported to be associated with hyporesponsiveness to ICS. Other alternatives, such as high-resolution computed tomography, endobronchial ultrasonography, and lung function measurements, can also be used as screening tools in clinical practice [19]. Computed tomography, a non-invasive process, allows the study of the airway lumen and wall dimensions, which might help evaluate airway remodeling in children and clinical studies [20]. This approach can be used to identify the airway tree and evaluate changes in remodeling after treatment, as well as determine air trapping. Endobronchial ultrasound (EBUS) is performed with an ultrasonographic probe through the working channel of a fiberoptic bronchoscope. It can access airways 4 mm in internal diameter and visualize multiple layers of the airway wall without the use of radiation [21]. Decreased values of V50 and V25 and increased values of the V50/V25 ratio are useful for the early detection of peripheral airway diseases [22]. Because persistent airflow obstruction is caused by airway remodeling, V50/V25, which indicates a peripheral airflow obstruction, can also be an indicator of airway remodeling. In our case of severe asthma, airway remodeling was diagnosed by low FEV1% (62.79%), highV50/V25 (5.48), and thickening of the airway wall assessed by CT. In this case, after one-year treatment by dupilumab, FEV1 (2.43 L → 3.48 L) was increased, and V50/25 (5.48 → 4.23) was decreased. Furthermore, the airway wall thickness was attenuated (Figure 2), which strongly suggests the improvement of airway remodeling by dupilumab.

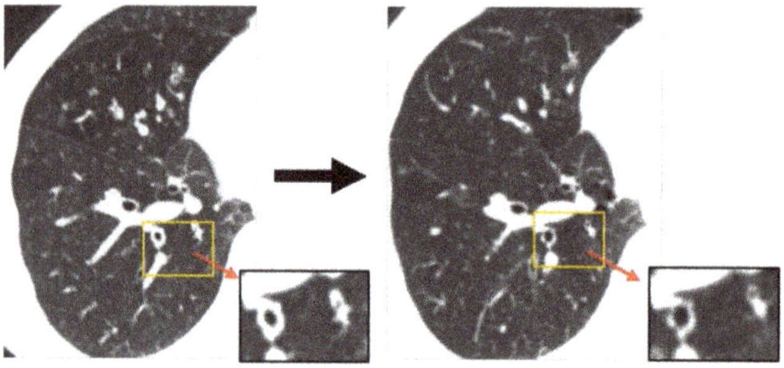

Figure 2. Chest CT before and one year after the start of dupilumab.

AHR is defined as the increased sensitivity and enhanced narrowing of the airways in response to physical or chemical stimuli. AHR is caused by abnormalities in the airway smooth muscle, which is primed by Th2 inflammation. Recent studies suggested that IL-13 and IL-4 signaling through the IL-4 receptor is responsible for these abnormalities, by upregulating the expressions of histamine receptor H1 (HRH1) and cysteinyl leukotriene receptor 1 (CYSLTR1) in airway smooth muscle cells [23]. Clinically, bronchial provocation tests (BPTs) are used to measure AHR, in which airway constrictors such as methacholine or cAMP are inhaled and their propensities to develop airflow obstruction are examined. BPTs are the gold standard test, but their methodology is complicated for general clinical practice, time consuming, and can induce severe bronchospasms. Therefore, alternative markers that reflect AHR have been explored. Kono et al. investigated a correlation between airway hyperresponsiveness measured by BPTs and the variables obtained by spirometry tests and reported that the FEF25-75% predicted showed the highest correlation with airway hyperresponsiveness [24]. Respiratory system resistance (Rrs) measured by the forced oscillation technique at 5 Hz (R5) and 20 Hz (R20) is a marker of airway caliber. A larger R5 reflects small airway dysfunction and was reported to be associated in part with airway hypersensitivity [25].

As described above, airway inflammation is often a triggering/exacerbation factor for airway hypersensitivity and airway remodeling, but the interaction of each of the three factors becomes a further exacerbation factor as asthma progresses. Therefore, monoclonal antibodies targeting airway inflammation as well as airway hyperresponsiveness and airway remodeling would be more effective than monoclonal antibodies targeting only airway inflammation.

3. Therapeutic Antibodies for Bronchial Asthma

There are four types of monoclonal antibodies available to treat bronchial asthma, including anti-IgE antibody, anti-IL-5 antibody, anti-IL-5 receptor α antibody, and anti-IL-4 receptor α antibody (Table 1).

Omalizumab, a humanized monoclonal IgG1κ antibody to IgE, inhibits the binding of IgE to high-affinity receptor, FcεRI, on mast cells or basophils and low-affinity receptor, FcεRII, on B cells, T cells, Langerhans cells, macrophages, monocytes, eosinophils, and platelets. Upon the cross-linking of membrane bound IgE by a specific allergen, mast cells or basophils degranulate and secrete mediators such as histamine, which induce bronchoconstriction in asthmatic patients. Omalizumab does not bind to IgE, which binds to its high-affinity receptor IgεRI, suggesting that there is no risk of the cross-linking of membrane-bound IgE [26]. Because FcεRI and FcεRII are stabilized by the binding of IgE, the administration of omalizumab reduces the expression of these receptors on inflammatory cells. Recently, it was reported that bronchial epithelial cells and airway smooth muscle cells from patients with bronchial asthma also expressed FcεRI and FcεRII [27]. An ex vivo study investigating the impact of omalizumab on specific and nonspecific AHR in proximal and distal human airways passively sensitized with serum from asthmatic donors showed it significantly suppressed the contractile response [28]. Therefore, omalizumab might directly affect the three components of asthma: airway inflammation, airway remodeling, and AHR.

Mepolizumab and reslizumab are humanized monoclonal IgG1κ and IgG4 antibodies, respectively, that bind with high affinity to human IL-5, thus preventing its interaction with the α subunit of the IL-5 receptor [29]. In patients with asthma, IL-5 is locally produced by Th2 lymphocytes, group 2 innate lymphoid cells (ILC2s), and epithelial cells in the airway mucosa. IL-5 stimulates the differentiation of eosinophils in the bone marrow and mobilization of eosinophils from the bone marrow. IL-5 also acts on basophils and stimulates the release of mediators, including histamine and leukotrienes. Therefore, mepolizumab and reslizumab inhibit airway inflammation in asthmatic patients. Although IL-5-deficient mice showed a reduction of airway remodeling in an ovalbumin-induced allergic airway inflammation model, the authors discussed that airway remodeling was caused by TGF-β produced by eosinophils and that the effect of IL-5 on airway remodeling was indirect [30].

A different mechanism of function characterizes the biological targeting of the IL-5 cascade. Benralizumab is a humanized IgG1κ monoclonal antibody, which binds to IL-5Rα. The IL-5 receptor is a heterodimer composed of IL-5-specific IL-5Rα and β subunits, which is commonly used by IL-5, IL-3, and GM-CSF. Benralizumab triggered apoptosis in eosinophils and basophils by antibody-dependent cell-mediated cytotoxicity (ADCC) associated with natural killer cells, a mechanism potentiated by afucosylation [31,32]. This effect is expected to reduce eosinophil counts, even in the presence of eosinophil activators such as IL-5, resulting in the rapid loss of peripheral blood eosinophils. Therefore, it can reduce eosinophilic airway inflammation. Ex vivo experiments demonstrated benralizumab suppressed AHR induced by histamine administered when significantly high cAMP levels were present, and that its effect was greater compared with mepolizumab [33]. This suggested that the improvement in the concentration of cAMP by inhibiting the IL-5/IL-5Rα pathway may converge to prevent AHR. An in vitro study using human ASM cells confirmed the beneficial role of benralizumab in reversing airway remodeling [34].

Dupilumab is a humanized IgG1k monoclonal antibody to the IL-4 receptor α subunit (IL-4Rα), common to both IL-4R complexes: type I (IL-4Rα/γc; IL-4 specific) and type II (IL-4Rα/IL-13Rα1; IL-4 and IL-13 specific). The type I IL-4R complex is expressed on hematopoietic cells and the type II IL-4R complex is expressed on hematopoietic and non-hematopoietic cells including epithelial cells and fibroblasts. In experimental mouse models of bronchial asthma using IL-4Rα-knockout mice and IL-13Rα1-knockout mice, the type I IL-4R complex is thought to activate Th2 inflammation, whereas the type II IL-4R complex inhibits Th2 inflammation but augments AHR and airway remodeling [35]. Although the precise mechanisms have not been reported, dupilumab is thought to function as a dual receptor antagonist of the type I and type II IL-4R complexes, by inhibiting their biological actions [36,37].

Table 1. Current strategies of biological therapies for severe asthma.

Target	Drug Name	Molecular Mechanisms	Pathophysiological Effect	Predictors of Efficacy	Changes in Clinical Parameters
FcεRI-binding domain of IgE	Omalizumab (Genentech/ Novartis)	Inhibit of IgE–mediated cascade	•Airway allergic inflammation •Airway hyperresponsiveness [38] •Airway remodeling [38]	•Specific IgE antibody positivity or skin prick test [39] •Increase of serum IgE at 4 week [40] •High eosinophils (blood) [41] •High FeNO [41]	•Decrease exacerbationrate [42] and FeNO [41] •Increase FEV1 and ACQ [43] •Reduce OCS [43]
IL-5	Mepolizumab (Glaxo Smithline)	Inhibit the activity of IL-5 by preventing IL-5 to bind IL-5R	•Airway eosinophilic inflammation •Airway hyperresponsiveness * [33] •Airway remodeling * [30]	•High eosinophils (sputum, blood) [44,45] • Nasal polyposis [46] • Lower BMI [46] • Lower OCS [46] • Lower CCL4/MIP-1β [47]	•Decrease exacerbation rate and eosinophils [44,45] •Increase FEV1 [45,48] and ACQ [44,45] •Reduce OCS [44]
	Reslizumab (Teva Pharmaceuticals)	Inhibit of IL-5 signaling			
IL-5Rα	Benralizumab (AstraZeneca)	Blockade of IL-5Rα, and ADCC-induced eosinophil apoptosis	•Airway eosinophilic inflammation •Airway hyperresponsiveness * [33] •Airway remodeling * [34]	•High eosinophils (sputum, blood) [49] • Nasal polyposis [49,50] • Low lung function [50] • age at diagnosis ≥18 years [50]	•Decrease exacerbation rate and eosinophils [51] •Increase FEV1 and ACQ [52] •Reduce OCS [52]
IL-4Rα	Dupilumab (Sanofi/ Regeneron)	Dual blockade of IL4/IL-4Rα and IL-13/IL-13Rα binding	Airway inflammation •Airway hyperresponsiveness [53] •Airway remodeling [54]	•High IgE [55] •High eosinophils [55,56] (sputum, blood) •High FeNO [55,56] • Chronic Sinusitis and nasal polyposis [57]	•Decrease circulating IgE, exacerbation rate, and FeNO [55] •Decrease blood eosinophils after transient increase [55] •Increase FEV1 and ACQ [55] •Reduce OCS [55]

FeNO: Fractional exhaled nitric oxide, FEV1: Forced expiratory volume in 1, ACQ: asthma control score, OCS: oral corticosteroids, CCL4: chemokine (C-C motif) ligand 4, MIP-1β: macrophage inflammatory protein-1β. * This was suggested to be effective ex vivo or in animal models.

4. Clinical Effects of Antibodies for Bronchial Asthma Patients

4.1. Omalizumab

Randomized controlled trials (RCTs) and a systematic review indicated that omalizumab reduced asthma exacerbation and OCS intake, improved quality of life, and contributed to symptom control [42,43,51]. Omalizumab also has a good safety profile. An RCT reported that omalizumab improved AHR measured by cAMP after 4 weeks of treatment [38]. In real-world studies and a systematic review, omalizumab reduced asthma exacerbation, contributed to the step-down of asthma treatment, and improved the quality of life in long-term users without compromising safety [58,59]. Since omalizumab was first licensed as a therapeutic antibody for bronchial asthma two decades ago, some studies have addressed omalizumab discontinuation after long-term treatment. Two RCTs and one real-world study showed that a proportion of patients could withdraw from long-term omalizumab treatment without relapse [60–62].

4.2. Mepolizumab

RCTs confirmed that mepolizumab reduced asthma exacerbation, emergency department visits, and hospitalization [44]. These studies also demonstrated that mepolizumab improved health-related quality of life (HRQOL) among patients with severe asthma [63]. In real-world settings, treatment with mepolizumab reduced asthma exacerbation, OCS requirement, and the rescue use of short-acting β-agonists, resulting in the step-down of maintenance therapy of asthma [53]. It also improved the HRQOL. Regarding its effectiveness for AHR, an RCT showed that mepolizumab had no significant effect on AHR measured by BPT using methacholine [64].

4.3. Reslizumab

RCTs reported that reslizumab reduced asthma exacerbation and improved lung function, symptoms, and HRQOL [45,65,66]. A real-world study supported the results of the RCTs showing reslizumab reduced asthma exacerbations, maintenance OCS use, and health-care resource use. Reslizumab was also shown to improve asthma symptoms and lung function [67]. Although mepolizumab is an IgG1κ antibody and reslizumab is an IgG4 antibody, both reduced asthma exacerbation and improved the FEV1 [45].

4.4. Benralizumab

RCTs and a systematic review reported that benralizumab was effective at reducing asthma exacerbations, improving prebronchodilator FEV_1, asthma symptoms, HRQOL, and reducing OCS intake in patients with severe asthma [49,52,68,69]. Real-world studies re-confirmed these clinical benefits. Benralizumab reduced asthma exacerbations and OCS dose, and improved HRQOL [70]. Despite the improvement in AHR in an ex vivo model [33], a clinical trial reported benralizumab did not significantly improve AHR measured by BPT using histamines [71]. Regarding its effectiveness on airway remodeling, benralizumab reduced airway smooth muscle mass using a computational modeling approach [34].

4.5. Dupilumab

RCTs reported that dupilumab decreased asthma exacerbations and improved prebronchodilator FEV_1 and asthma symptoms [55,72]. Unlike other therapeutic antibodies, the RCTs included patients with moderate disease, making dupilumab available for patients with moderate asthma. Real-world data supported the results of the RCTs, showing that dupilumab reduced asthma exacerbations, the daily dose of OCS, and FeNO levels, and improved asthma symptoms [73,74].

5. Clinical Predictors of Good Responders to Each Antibody Therapy

As described above, currently approved monoclonal antibodies have been shown to have many clinical effects. However, these treatments are not successful in all patients, and super-responders to specific therapeutic antibodies have been reported. Therefore, studies investigating clinical predictors of good responders to each antibody therapy have been initiated.

In patients treated with omalizumab, the baseline total IgE does not predict likelihood of response, allergen-specific IgE, or the reduction of total IgE 4-weeks after the initiation of omalizumab might predict response [75]. In a real-world study, each of the three Th2-inflammation markers, including FeNO, peripheral blood eosinophil, and serum periostin, or their combinations, predicted response to omalizumab [37]. The biomarkers for withdrawal of mepolizumab also have been proposed. The downregulation of basophil allergen sensitivity (CD-sens) and regulatory T cells were reported to be the candidates for the cessation criteria [76,77]

In an RCT of mepolizumab, high blood eosinophil counts predicted a good response [44]. Although a post hoc analysis of two RCTs could not identify the additional baseline characteristics associated with a response to mepolizumab [78], a retrospective review of patients who received at least 16 weeks of treatment with mepolizumab showed that the presence of nasal polyposis, a lower BMI, and a significantly lower prednisolone dose at baseline might predict a good response to mepolizumab [46]. Another study following patients receiving anti-IL-5 treatment for two years, showed that adult onset, absence of nasal polyposis, FEV1 $\geq$ 80% predicted, asthma duration < 10 years, and BMI < 25 were baseline characteristics that predicted a super-response to anti-IL-5 treatment [79]. It was also reported that the responders to mepolizumab had a significantly lower level of CCL4/MIP-1β at baseline compared with non-responders [47].

RCTs of benralizumab showed that high blood eosinophil counts predicted a good response [49,52]. A post hoc analysis of two RCTs showed that nasal polyposis, prebronchodilator FVC < 65% of predicted, and age at diagnosis ≥ 18 years were the most important factors that influenced benralizumab responsiveness for improving lung function [50]. A real-world study reported a strongly eosinophilic phenotype, high blood eosinophil count, and elevated FeNO levels, as well as less severe disease were associated with super-responders [70]. Exploratory studies reported that low baseline levels of serum inflammatory cytokines and a serum miRNA response 8 weeks after the initiation of benralizumab were potential predictors of a good response [80,81].

The treatment effects of dupilumab were greater in patients with elevated Th2 biomarkers at baseline (blood eosinophils (≥150/uL) or FeNO (≥25 ppb)) [55].

6. Prospects for Severe Asthma Treatment

New potential targets for asthma treatments are being investigated globally. Alarmins including thymic stromal lymphopoietin (TSLP), IL-25, and IL-33, have an important role in T2-high asthma [82].

TSLP induces the strong activation of dendritic cells (DCs) [83], and DCs stimulated by TSLP drive naïve Th lymphocytes towards differentiation into active T2 cells producing IL-4, IL-5, and IL-13 [84]. TSLP also stimulates basophils, mast cells, and ILC2 [82,85,86]. Recent clinical trials have shown the effectiveness of anti-TSLP antibody for asthma [87]. TSLP is also a key airway remodeling mediator that promotes airway smooth muscle cells to increase airway smooth muscle mass migration [88]. TSLP might promote asthmatic airway remodeling by activating the p38 MAPK-STAT3 axis [89]. Tezepelumab is an anti-TSLP human monoclonal antibody that binds to TSLP and prevents TSLP binding to its receptor complex [90]. The first study of tezepelumab was conducted in patients with mild allergic asthma [91]. In that study, tezepelumab minimized the allergen-induced decline in the FEV1. It also reduced the level of post-allergen blood/sputum eosinophils and FeNO levels. In a phase IIb study of 584 adult patients, tezepelumab decreased the asthma exacerbation rate by 60–70% per year and improved the FEV1 without the use of bronchodilators, regardless of blood eosinophil numbers [92]. That study confirmed the ability of tezepelumab to suppress serum IgE concentrations, blood eosinophil counts, and FeNO levels. The safety and efficacy of tezepelumab to decrease airway inflammation and OCS intake are now being evaluated in phase II and III trials [82]. Tezepelumab is also expected to be effective in airway remodeling, but at present, there are no available studies of its in vitro or in vivo effects on airway remodeling. An RCT showed that tezepelumab induced a numerical improvement in the provoking dose of mannitol causing a 15% reduction in FEV1 (PD15) compared with placebo, and at the end of the treatment period, the proportion of patients without AHR to mannitol was significantly ($p < 0.05$) higher in the tezepelumab group than in the placebo group [93].

Although IL-25 has a pathogenic role in allergic inflammation, there has been no clinical study of anti-IL-25 monoclonal antibodies for the treatment of severe asthma.

IL-33 activates Th2 and group 2 innate lymphoid cells and induces allergic diseases including allergic rhinitis, spontaneous dermatitis, and asthma [94,95]. IL-33 stimulates ILC2 and mast cells to release IL-13 and induces airway hyperresponsiveness [96,97]. A phase II trial reported that an anti-IL-33 monoclonal antibody, REGN3500, improved the QOL of patients and controlled the symptoms of severe asthma [82].

Another potential target molecule is IL-13 and IL-13 blockade therapies, which are being investigated in clinical trials. Tralokinumab and lebrikizumab are mAbs that target IL-13 [98,99]. Phase 2 studies reported that anti-IL-13 antibodies improved the annual asthma exacerbation rate at week 52 [100]. However, the results of phase 3 studies were not satisfactory [101–103]. In those trials, anti-IL-13 antibodies had no benefit for reducing asthma exacerbation and sparing steroid intake.

Another key mediator of type-2 asthma is prostaglandin D2 (PGD2), an upstream mediator of T2 inflammation. PGD2 is mainly produced by mast cells [104]. Fevipiprant, which targets PGD2, is being investigated in phase 3 trials; however, it showed a poor improvement in the FEV1 and no significant reduction in the AER [105,106].

IL-13-dependent chemokines may be involved in severe asthma. CCL-26/eotaxin-3 is important for the migration of eosinophils from the blood to tissues and an approach that blocks CCL-26/eotaxin-3 might reduce eosinophil numbers in the lungs [57,107]. CCL17 and CCL22 chemokines, secreted by DCs, interact with CCR4 receptors expressed by mature Th2 lymphocytes, thus promoting their migration from thoracic lymph nodes to the airways [108]. Because these chemokines and chemokine receptors are involved in the signal cascade of asthma, they may be candidate therapeutic targets for severe asthma in the future.

Regarding therapeutic antibodies, attempts to generate bispecific antibodies targeting more than one cell or receptor are also being tested. Bispecific antibodies have become of increasing interest as therapeutic agents for asthma. Bispecific antibodies can be directed against different signaling pathways simultaneously by binding to two different targets, thus enhancing drug delivery. Compared with combination therapy using two monospecific agents, the use of bispecific antibodies can reduce the cost of development and clinical trials. A bispecific antibody targeting IL-4Ra/IL-5 is under preclinical investigation [109]. The monovalent bispecific antibody Zweimabs and the bivalent bispecific Doppelmab against TSLP/IL-13 have been developed to target Th2 responses [110]. These bispecific antibodies have a strong affinity for human target molecules compared with the parental antibody formats, but with comparable effects. An anti-IL-13/IL-17 antibody (BITS7201A), which can be used for mix-typed eosinophilic and neutrophilic inflammation, is being investigated in a phase I trial [111].

As described previously, mediators of Th2-dependent reactions have a key role in the pathogenesis of asthma. However, non-Th2 dominant type patients also exist, and the regulators of non-type 2 inflammation in asthma include Th17 cells and neutrophils (Figure 3). Th17 cells secrete proinflammatory cytokines such as IL-17A and IL-17F. IL-17A was elevated in the sputum of asthmatic patients and correlated with IL-8, neutrophils in the sputum, and asthma severity [11]. Therefore, asthma is a heterogeneous chronic inflammation with different pathophysiologies, and crosstalk between each cascade augments its severity and increases its intractability. Therefore, treatment strategies targeting non-Th2 type asthmatic components are urgently needed.

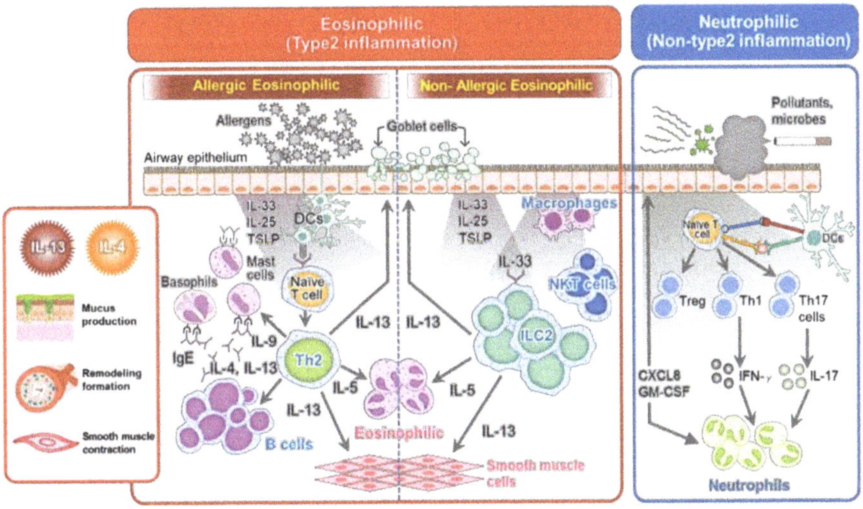

Figure 3. Schematic of the diverse signaling pathways determining bronchial asthma onset and development.

Bronchial thermoplasty (BT), a non-pharmacological treatment developed and performed worldwide for severe asthma, alleviates the symptoms of asthma patients. Bronchial smooth muscle is thickened by applying high-frequency energy from a probe inserted transbronchoscopically to the airway wall. It aims to reduce asthma attacks by reducing smooth muscle contractility. In the AIR2 Trial, a large randomized, double-blind study, BT improved the Asthma Quality of Life Questionnaire (AQLQ) and reduced the frequency of exacerbations in severe asthma patients [112]. These effects persisted for 5 years after treatment [113], indicating there is a population of severe asthmatics who are highly responsive to BT. However, no improvement in the FEV1 or airway hyperresponsiveness was observed, and no predictive markers for treatment responses have been identified. Although some experts propose that BT should be considered for severe asthma associated with non-type 2 inflammation or patients who fail to respond to biological therapies targeting type 2 inflammation, the position of BT for the management of severe asthma is still unclear [114]. Therefore, BT can only be positioned as a treatment option for asthma.

Regarding the future developments of asthma treatment, it will be important to fully understand the pathogenesis of asthma. Most importantly, biomarkers must be used to identify disease endotypes and to develop more effective therapeutic approaches.

7. Conclusions

Considerable advances have been made in antibody therapeutics for severe asthma over the last decade. Increasing numbers of biological therapies will be introduced to clinical settings. Therefore, it will be of great importance for clinicians to consider the target and mechanism of action of each therapeutic antibody when selecting an appropriate treatment option for individual patients with severe asthma. The current selection and treatment strategies of antibody therapeutics are primarily based on Th2 type disease and eosinophilic inflammation. Further studies are necessary to compare the effects of each antibody type and clarify their effects against airway remodeling and hypersensitivity, and to guide decision making regarding appropriate antibody therapeutics by establishing a real phenotype classification that will predict the response of patients to antibody treatments. Importantly, a better understanding of non-Th2 type immunological mechanisms is urgently required to help develop treatment strategies using antibodies against non-Th2 type signaling cascades.

Funding: This work was supported in part by Japan Agency for Medical Research and Development: JP20fk0108129; Japan Agency for Medical Research and Development: JP21lm0203007; GlaxoSmithKline (United States): A-32; Japan Society for the Promotion of Science: JP21K16118; Japan Society for the Promotion of Science: JP21K08194, the Japan Intractable Diseases (Nanbyo) Research Foundation: 2020B02, and Smoking Research Foundation: 2021Y007 Takeda Science Foundation.

Institutional Review Board Statement: The experimental protocol for data involving human participants followed the Ethical Guidelines of the Japan Ministries of Health and Labour for Medical and Health Research Involving Human Subjects. All experiments were conducted in accordance with the principles laid out in the Declaration of Helsinki.

Informed Consent Statement: The study was approved by the Institutional Review Board of the National Hospital Organization, Osaka Toneyama Medical Centre (TNH-P-2021007). The IRB committee waived the requirement for informed consent for a retrospective review of participant data. The opt-out recruitment method was applied to provide an opportunity to decline participation for all patients. Members of the IRB committee were as follows; Tsuyoshi Matsumura, Toshihiko Yamaguchi, Noriyuki Takeuchi, Yukiyasu Takeuchi, Taku Shiomi, Makiko Sawamoto, Hiroyuki Ueno, Akihiro Takechi, Teruaki Masumoto, Motomu Shimoda, Hironori Tsukada, and Minako Nakano.

Data Availability Statement: The datasets supporting the conclusions of this article are included within the article. The data sets generated and analyzed in this study are available from the corresponding author on reasonable request.

Acknowledgments: We thank E. Akiba for assistance with data collection and helpful discussions. We also thank J. Ludovic Croxford, from Edanz (https://jp.edanz.com/ac) (accessed on 7 September 2021) for editing a draft of this manuscript.

Conflicts of Interest: The authors declare no conflict of interest.

Abbreviations

ICS	Inhaled corticosteroids
OCS	Oral corticosteroids
SPDEF	SAM pointed domain containing ETS transcription factor
Foxa	Forkhead box protein
TSLP	Thymic stromal lymphopoietin
EMT	Epithelial-mesenchymal transition
TGF	Transforming growth factor
SARP	Severe Asthma Research Program
ILC2	Group 2 innate lymphoid cells
ILC3	Group 2 innate lymphoid cells
BAL	Bronchoalveolar lavage
FeNO	Fractional exhaled nitric oxide
FEV1	Forced expiratory volume in 1 s
ADCC	Antibody-dependent cell-mediated cytotoxicity
BPT	Bronchial provocation test
FEF	Forced expiratory flow
FOT	Forced oscillation technique
BMI	Body mass index
R5	Respiratory reactance at 5 Hz
R20	Respiratory reactance at 20 Hz
DC	Dendritic cell
PGD2	Prostaglandin D2
BT	Bronchial thermoplasty
AQLQ	Asthma Quality of Life Questionnaire

References

1. Chung, K.F.; Wenzel, S.E.; Brozek, J.L.; Bush, A.; Castro, M.; Sterk, P.J.; Adcock, I.M.; Bateman, E.D.; Bel, E.H.; Bleecker, E.R.; et al. International ERS/ATS guidelines on definition, evaluation and treatment of severe asthma. *Eur. Respir. J.* **2014**, *43*, 343–373. [CrossRef]
2. Israel, E.; Reddel, H.K. Severe and Difficult-to-Treat Asthma in Adults. *N. Engl. J. Med.* **2017**, *377*, 965–976. [CrossRef] [PubMed]
3. Wagener, A.H.; de Nijs, S.B.; Lutter, R.; Sousa, A.R.; Weersink, E.J.; Bel, E.H. Sterk PJ: External validation of blood eosinophils, FE(NO) and serum periostin as surrogates for sputum eosinophils in asthma. *Thorax* **2015**, *70*, 115–120. [CrossRef] [PubMed]
4. Price, D.B.; Rigazio, A.; Campbell, J.D.; Bleecker, E.R.; Corrigan, C.; Thomas, M.; Wenzel, S.; Wilson, A.M.; Small, M.B.; Gopalan, G.; et al. Blood eosinophil count and prospective annual asthma disease burden: A UK cohort study. *Lancet Respir. Med.* **2015**, *3*, 849–858. [CrossRef]
5. Berry, M.A.; Shaw, D.E.; Green, R.H.; Brightling, C.E.; Wardlaw, A.J.; Pavord, I.D. The use of exhaled nitric oxide concentration to identify eosinophilic airway inflammation: An observational study in adults with asthma. *Clin. Exp. Allergy* **2005**, *35*, 1175–1179. [CrossRef] [PubMed]
6. Malinovschi, A.; Janson, C.; Borres, M.; Alving, K. Simultaneously increased fraction of exhaled nitric oxide levels and blood eosinophil counts relate to increased asthma morbidity. *J. Allergy Clin. Immunol.* **2016**, *138*, 1301–1308.e2. [CrossRef] [PubMed]
7. Vatrella, A.; Fabozzi, I.; Calabrese, C.; Maselli, R.; Pelaia, G. Dupilumab: A novel treatment for asthma. *J. Asthma Allergy* **2014**, *7*, 123–130. [CrossRef] [PubMed]
8. Malerba, M.; Ragnoli, B.; Azzolina, D.; Montuschi, P.; Radaeli, A. Predictive Markers of Bronchial Hyperreactivity in a Large Cohort of Young Adults With Cough Variant Asthma. *Front. Pharmacol.* **2021**, *12*, 630334. [CrossRef]
9. Fitzpatrick, A.M.; Teague, W.G.; Meyers, D.A.; Peters, S.P.; Li, X.; Li, H.; Wenzel, S.E.; Aujla, S.J.; Castro, M.; Bacharier, L.B. Heterogeneity of severe asthma in childhood: Confirmation by cluster analysis of children in the National Institutes of Health/National Heart, Lung, and Blood Institute Severe Asthma Research Program. *J. Allergy Clin. Immunol.* **2011**, *127*, 382–389.e13. [CrossRef]
10. Whitsett, J.A.; Alenghat, T. Respiratory epithelial cells orchestrate pulmonary innate immunity. *Nat. Immunol.* **2015**, *16*, 27–35. [CrossRef] [PubMed]
11. Rajavelu, P.; Chen, G.; Xu, Y.; Kitzmiller, J.A.; Korfhagen, T.R.; Whitsett, J.A. Airway epithelial SPDEF integrates goblet cell differentiation and pulmonary Th2 inflammation. *J. Clin. Investig.* **2015**, *125*, 2021–2031. [CrossRef] [PubMed]
12. Doeing, D.C.; Solway, J. Airway smooth muscle in the pathophysiology and treatment of asthma. *J. Appl. Physiol.* **2013**, *114*, 834–843. [CrossRef] [PubMed]

13. Fukushima, K.; Satoh, T.; Sugihara, F.; Sato, Y.; Okamoto, T.; Mitsui, Y.; Yoshio, S.; Li, S.; Nojima, S.; Motooka, D.; et al. Dysregulated Expression of the Nuclear Exosome Targeting Complex Component Rbm7 in Nonhematopoietic Cells Licenses the Development of Fibrosis. *Immunity* **2020**, *52*, 542–556.e13. [CrossRef] [PubMed]
14. Halwani, R.; Al-Muhsen, S.; Al-Jahdali, H.; Hamid, Q. Role of transforming growth factor-beta in airway remodeling in asthma. *Am. J. Respir. Cell Mol. Biol.* **2011**, *44*, 127–133. [CrossRef] [PubMed]
15. Fukushima, K.; Akira, S. Novel insights into the pathogenesis of lung fibrosis: The RBM7-NEAT1-CXCL12-SatM axis at fibrosis onset. *Int. Immunol.* **2021**, *33*, 659–663. [CrossRef]
16. Bergeron, C.; Tulic, M.K.; Hamid, Q. Tools used to measure airway remodelling in research. *Eur. Respir. J.* **2007**, *29*, 596–604. [CrossRef]
17. Berry, A.; Busse, W.W. Biomarkers in asthmatic patients: Has their time come to direct treatment? *J. Allergy Clin. Immunol.* **2016**, *137*, 1317–1324. [CrossRef]
18. Izuhara, K.; Ohta, S.; Ono, J. Using Periostin as a Biomarker in the Treatment of Asthma. *Allergy Asthma Immunol. Res.* **2016**, *8*, 491–498. [CrossRef]
19. Bergeron, C.; Al-Ramli, W.; Hamid, Q. Remodeling in asthma. *Proc. Am. Thorac. Soc.* **2009**, *6*, 301–305. [CrossRef]
20. Marchac, V.; Emond, S.; Mamou-Mani, T.; Le Bihan-Benjamin, C.; Le Bourgeois, M.; De Blic, J.; Scheinmann, P.; Brunelle, F. Thoracic CT in Pediatric Patients with Difficult-to-Treat Asthma. *Am. J. Roentgenol.* **2002**, *179*, 1245–1252. [CrossRef]
21. Bullone, M.; Beauchamp, G.; Godbout, M.; Martin, J.G.; Lavoie, J.-P. Endobronchial Ultrasound Reliably Quantifies Airway Smooth Muscle Remodeling in an Equine Asthma Model. *PLoS ONE* **2015**, *10*, e0136284. [CrossRef] [PubMed]
22. Ichinose, M.; Sugiura, H.; Nagase, H.; Yamaguchi, M.; Inoue, H.; Sagara, H.; Tamaoki, J.; Tohda, Y.; Munakata, M.; Yamauchi, K.; et al. Japanese guidelines for adult asthma 2017. *Allergol. Int.* **2017**, *66*, 163–189. [CrossRef] [PubMed]
23. Manson, M.L.; Säfholm, J.; James, A.; Johnsson, A.-K.; Bergman, P.; Al-Ameri, M.; Orre, A.-C.; Kärrman-Mårdh, C.; Dahlén, S.-E.; Adner, M. IL-13 and IL-4, but not IL-5 nor IL-17A, induce hyperresponsiveness in isolated human small airways. *J. Allergy Clin. Immunol.* **2020**, *145*, 808–817.e2. [CrossRef]
24. Kono, Y.; Soeda, S.; Okada, Y.; Hara, H.; Araki, K.; To, M.; To, Y. A Surrogate Marker of Airway Hyperresponsiveness in Patients with Bronchial Asthma. *Allergol. Int.* **2014**, *63*, 487–488. [CrossRef] [PubMed]
25. Bhatawadekar, S.A.; Keller, G.; Francisco, C.; Inman, M.D.; Fredberg, J.J.; Tarlo, S.; Stanbrook, M.; Lyons, O.D.; Yadollahi, A. Reduced Baseline Airway Caliber Relates to Larger Airway Sensitivity to Rostral Fluid Shift in Asthma. *Front. Physiol.* **2017**, *8*, 1012. [CrossRef] [PubMed]
26. Chang, T.W.; Wu, P.C.; Hsu, C.L.; Hung, A.F. Anti-IgE antibodies for the treatment of IgE-mediated allergic diseases. *Adv. Immunol.* **2007**, *93*, 63–119. [PubMed]
27. Roth, M.; Zhong, J.; Zumkeller, C.; S'Ng, C.T.; Goulet, S.; Tamm, M. The Role of IgE-Receptors in IgE-Dependent Airway Smooth Muscle Cell Remodelling. *PLoS ONE* **2013**, *8*, e56015. [CrossRef]
28. Berger, P.; Scotto-Gomez, E.; Molimard, M.; Marthan, R.; Le Gros, V.; Tunon-De-Lara, J.M. Omalizumab decreases nonspecific airway hyperresponsiveness in vitro. *Allergy* **2007**, *62*, 154–161. [CrossRef]
29. Pelaia, C.; Vatrella, A.; Busceti, M.T.; Gallelli, L.; Terracciano, R.; Savino, R.; Pelaia, G. Severe eosinophilic asthma: From the pathogenic role of interleukin-5 to the therapeutic action of mepolizumab. *Drug Des. Dev. Ther.* **2017**, *11*, 3137–3144. [CrossRef]
30. Cho, J.Y.; Miller, M.; Baek, K.J.; Han, J.W.; Nayar, J.; Lee, S.Y.; McElwain, K.; McElwain, S.; Friedman, S.; Broide, D.H. Inhibition of airway remodeling in IL-5–deficient mice. *J. Clin. Investig.* **2004**, *113*, 551–560. [CrossRef]
31. Pelaia, C.; Vatrella, A.; Bruni, A.; Terracciano, R.; Pelaia, G. Benralizumab in the treatment of severe asthma: Design, development and potential place in therapy. *Drug Des. Dev. Ther.* **2018**, *12*, 619–628. [CrossRef] [PubMed]
32. Pelaia, C.; Calabrese, C.; Vatrella, A.; Busceti, M.T.; Garofalo, E.; Lombardo, N.; Terracciano, R.; Pelaia, G. Benralizumab: From the Basic Mechanism of Action to the Potential Use in the Biological Therapy of Severe Eosinophilic Asthma. *BioMed Res. Int.* **2018**, *2018*, 4839230. [CrossRef] [PubMed]
33. Calzetta, L.; Ritondo, B.L.; Matera, M.G.; Facciolo, F.; Rogliani, P. Targeting IL-5 pathway against airway hyperresponsiveness: A comparison between benralizumab and mepolizumab. *Br. J. Pharmacol.* **2020**, *177*, 4750–4765. [CrossRef] [PubMed]
34. Chachi, L.; Diver, S.; Kaul, H.; Rebelatto, M.C.; Boutrin, A.; Nisa, P.; Newbold, P.; Brightling, C. Computational modelling prediction and clinical validation of impact of benralizumab on airway smooth muscle mass in asthma. *Eur. Respir. J.* **2019**, *54*, 1900930. [CrossRef] [PubMed]
35. Ramalingam, T.R.; Pesce, J.T.; Sheikh, F.; Cheever, A.W.; Mentink-Kane, M.M.; Wilson, M.S.; Stevens, S.; Valenzuela, D.M.; Murphy, A.; Yancopoulos, G.D.; et al. Unique functions of the type II interleukin 4 receptor identified in mice lacking the interleukin 13 receptor α1 chain. *Nat. Immunol.* **2007**, *9*, 25–33. [CrossRef] [PubMed]
36. Pelaia, C.; Vatrella, A.; Gallelli, L.; Terracciano, R.; Navalesi, P.; Maselli, R.; Pelaia, G. Dupilumab for the treatment of asthma. *Expert Opin. Biol. Ther.* **2017**, *17*, 1565–1572. [CrossRef]
37. Harb, H.; Chatila, T.A. Mechanisms of Dupilumab. *Clin. Exp. Allergy* **2020**, *50*, 5–14. [CrossRef]
38. Prieto, L.; Gutiérrez, V.; Colás, C.; Tabar, A.; Pérez-Francés, C.; Bruno, L.; Uixera, S. Effect of Omalizumab on Adenosine 5′-Monophosphate Responsiveness in Subjects with Allergic Asthma. *Int. Arch. Allergy Immunol.* **2006**, *139*, 122–131. [CrossRef]
39. Hanania, N.A.; Alpan, O.; Hamilos, D.L.; Condemi, J.J.; Reyes-Rivera, I.; Zhu, J.; Rosen, K.E.; Eisner, M.D.; Wong, D.A.; Busse, W. Omalizumab in severe allergic asthma inadequately controlled with standard therapy: A randomized trial. *Ann. Intern. Med.* **2011**, *154*, 573–582. [CrossRef]

40. Li, B.; Huang, M.; Huang, S.; Zeng, X.; Yuan, Y.; Peng, X.; Zhao, W.; Ye, Y.; Yu, C.; Liu, L.; et al. Prediction of clinical response to omalizumab in moderate-to-severe asthma patients using the change in total serum IgE level. *J. Thorac. Dis.* **2020**, *12*, 7097–7105. [CrossRef]
41. Hanania, N.A.; Wenzel, S.; Rosen, K.; Hsieh, H.J.; Mosesova, S.; Choy, D.F.; Lal, P.; Arron, J.R.; Harris, J.M.; Busse, W. Exploring the effects of omalizumab in allergic asthma: An analysis of biomarkers in the EXTRA study. *Am. J. Respir. Crit. Care Med.* **2013**, *187*, 804–811. [CrossRef]
42. Normansell, R.; Walker, S.; Milan, S.J.; Walters, E.H.; Nair, P. Omalizumab for asthma in adults and children. *Cochrane Database Syst. Rev.* **2014**, CD003559. [CrossRef] [PubMed]
43. Pelaia, G.; Gallelli, L.; Romeo, P.; Renda, T.; Busceti, M.; Proietto, A.; Grembiale, R.; Marsico, S.; Maselli, R.; Vatrella, A. Omalizumab decreases exacerbation frequency, oral intake of corticosteroids and peripheral blood eosinophils in atopic patients with uncontrolled asthma. *Int. J. Clin. Pharmacol. Ther.* **2011**, *49*, 713–721. [CrossRef]
44. Ortega, H.G.; Liu, M.C.; Pavord, I.D.; Brusselle, G.G.; Fitzgerald, J.M.; Chetta, A.; Humbert, M.; Katz, L.E.; Keene, O.N.; Yancey, S.W.; et al. Mepolizumab Treatment in Patients with Severe Eosinophilic Asthma. *N. Engl. J. Med.* **2014**, *371*, 1198–1207. [CrossRef]
45. Castro, M.; Zangrilli, J.E.; Wechsler, M.E.; Bateman, E.D.; Brusselle, G.G.; Bardin, P.; Murphy, K.; Maspero, J.F.; O'Brien, C.; Korn, S. Reslizumab for inadequately controlled asthma with elevated blood eosinophil counts: Results from two multicentre, parallel, double-blind, randomised, placebo-controlled, phase 3 trials. *Lancet Respir. Med.* **2015**, *3*, 355–366. [CrossRef]
46. Kavanagh, J.E.; D'Ancona, G.; Elstad, M.; Green, L.; Fernandes, M.; Thomson, L.; Roxas, C.; Dhariwal, J.; Nanzer, A.M.; Kent, B.D.; et al. Real-World Effectiveness and the Characteristics of a "Super-Responder" to Mepolizumab in Severe Eosinophilic Asthma. *Chest* **2020**, *158*, 491–500. [CrossRef] [PubMed]
47. Suzukawa, M.; Ohshima, N.; Tashimo, H.; Asari, I.; Kobayashi, N.; Shoji, S.; Tohma, S.; Ohta, K. A Low Serum CCL4/MIP-1β Level May Predict a Severe Asthmatic Responsiveness to Mepolizumab. *Intern. Med.* **2020**, *59*, 2849–2855. [CrossRef]
48. Sposato, B.; Camiciottoli, G.; Bacci, E.; Scalese, M.; Carpagnano, G.E.; Pelaia, C.; Santus, P.; Maniscalco, M.; Masieri, S.; Corsico, A.G.; et al. Mepolizumab effectiveness on small airway obstruction, corticosteroid sparing and maintenance therapy step-down in real life. *Pulm. Pharmacol. Ther.* **2020**, *61*, 101899. [CrossRef]
49. Bleecker, E.R.; FitzGerald, J.M.; Chanez, P.; Papi, A.; Weinstein, S.F.; Barker, P.; Sproule, S.; Gilmartin, G.; Aurivillius, M.; Werkstrom, V.; et al. Efficacy and safety of benralizumab for patients with severe asthma uncontrolled with high-dosage inhaled corticosteroids and long-acting beta2-agonists (SIROCCO): A randomised, multicentre, placebo-controlled phase 3 trial. *Lancet* **2016**, *388*, 2115–2127. [CrossRef]
50. Bleecker, E.R.; Wechsler, M.E.; Fitzgerald, J.M.; Menzies-Gow, A.; Wu, Y.; Hirsch, I.; Goldman, M.; Newbold, P.; Zangrilli, J.G. Baseline patient factors impact on the clinical efficacy of benralizumab for severe asthma. *Eur. Respir. J.* **2018**, *52*, 1800936. [CrossRef] [PubMed]
51. Humbert, M.; Beasley, R.; Ayres, J.; Slavin, R.; Hébert, J.; Bousquet, J.; Beeh, K.-M.; Ramos, S.; Canonica, G.W.; Hedgecock, S.; et al. Benefits of omalizumab as add-on therapy in patients with severe persistent asthma who are inadequately controlled despite best available therapy (GINA 2002 step 4 treatment): INNOVATE. *Allergy* **2005**, *60*, 309–316. [CrossRef]
52. FitzGerald, J.M.; Bleecker, E.R.; Nair, P.; Korn, S.; Ohta, K.; Lommatzsch, M.; Ferguson, G.T.; Busse, W.W.; Barker, P.; Sproule, S.; et al. Benralizumab, an anti-interleukin-5 receptor α monoclonal antibody, as add-on treatment for patients with severe, uncontrolled, eosinophilic asthma (CALIMA): A randomised, double-blind, placebo-controlled phase 3 trial. *Lancet* **2016**, *388*, 2128–2141. [CrossRef]
53. Peters, M.; Mekonnen, Z.; Yuan, S.; Bhakta, N.R.; Woodruff, P.G.; Fahy, J.V. Measures of gene expression in sputum cells can identify TH2-high and TH2-low subtypes of asthma. *J. Allergy Clin. Immunol.* **2014**, *133*, 388–394. [CrossRef] [PubMed]
54. Peters, M.C.; Wenzel, S. Intersection of biology and therapeutics: Type 2 targeted therapeutics for adult asthma. *Lancet* **2020**, *395*, 371–383. [CrossRef]
55. Castro, M.; Corren, J.; Pavord, I.D.; Maspero, J.; Wenzel, S.; Rabe, K.F.; Busse, W.W.; Ford, L.; Sher, L.; Fitzgerald, J.M.; et al. Dupilumab Efficacy and Safety in Moderate-to-Severe Uncontrolled Asthma. *N. Engl. J. Med.* **2018**, *378*, 2486–2496. [CrossRef]
56. Busse, W.W.; Paggiaro, P.; Muñoz, X.; Casale, T.B.; Castro, M.; Canonica, G.W.; Douglass, J.A.; Tohda, Y.; Daizadeh, N.; Ortiz, B.; et al. Impact of baseline patient characteristics on dupilumab efficacy in type 2 asthma. *Eur. Respir. J.* **2021**, *58*, 2004605. [CrossRef]
57. Bachert, C.; Mannent, L.; Naclerio, R.M.; Mullol, J.; Ferguson, B.J.; Gevaert, P.; Hellings, P.; Jiao, L.; Wang, L.; Evans, R.R.; et al. Effect of Subcutaneous Dupilumab on Nasal Polyp Burden in Patients With Chronic Sinusitis and Nasal Polyposis: A Randomized Clinical Trial. *JAMA* **2016**, *315*, 469–479. [CrossRef]
58. Di Bona, D.; Fiorino, I.; Taurino, M.; Frisenda, F.; Minenna, E.; Pasculli, C.; Kourtis, G.; Rucco, A.S.; Nico, A.; Albanesi, M.; et al. Long-term "real-life" safety of omalizumab in patients with severe uncontrolled asthma: A nine-year study. *Respir. Med.* **2017**, *130*, 55–60. [CrossRef]
59. Sposato, B.; Scalese, M.; Latorre, M.; Novelli, F.; Scichilone, N.; Milanese, M.; Olivieri, C.; Perrella, A.; Paggiaro, P. Xolair Italian Study G: Can the response to Omalizumab be influenced by treatment duration? A real-life study. *Pulm. Pharmacol. Ther.* **2017**, *44*, 38–45. [CrossRef] [PubMed]
60. Ledford, D.; Busse, W.; Trzaskoma, B.; Omachi, T.A.; Rosén, K.; Chipps, B.E.; Luskin, A.T.; Solari, P.G. A randomized multicenter study evaluating Xolair persistence of response after long-term therapy. *J. Allergy Clin. Immunol.* **2017**, *140*, 162–169.e2. [CrossRef] [PubMed]

61. Domingo, C.; Pomares, X.; Navarro, A.; Amengual, M.J.; Montón, C.; Sogo, A.; Mirapeix, R.M. A step-down protocol for omalizumab treatment in oral corticosteroid-dependent allergic asthma patients. *Br. J. Clin. Pharmacol.* **2017**, *84*, 339–348. [CrossRef] [PubMed]
62. Vennera, M.D.C.; Sabadell, C.; Picado, C. Duration of the efficacy of omalizumab after treatment discontinuation in 'real life' severe asthma. *Thorax* **2017**, *73*, 782–784. [CrossRef]
63. Chupp, G.L.; Bradford, E.S.; Albers, F.C.; Bratton, D.J.; Wang-Jairaj, J.; Nelsen, L.M.; Trevor, J.L.; Magnan, A.; Brinke, A.T. Efficacy of mepolizumab add-on therapy on health-related quality of life and markers of asthma control in severe eosinophilic asthma (MUSCA): A randomised, double-blind, placebo-controlled, parallel-group, multicentre, phase 3b trial. *Lancet Respir. Med.* **2017**, *5*, 390–400. [CrossRef]
64. Haldar, P.; Brightling, C.; Hargadon, B.; Gupta, S.; Monteiro, W.; Sousa, A.; Marshall, R.P.; Bradding, P.; Green, R.H.; Wardlaw, A.; et al. Mepolizumab and Exacerbations of Refractory Eosinophilic Asthma. *N. Engl. J. Med.* **2009**, *360*, 973–984. [CrossRef] [PubMed]
65. Bjermer, L.; Lemiere, C.; Maspero, J.; Weiss, S.; Zangrilli, J.; Germinaro, M. Reslizumab for Inadequately Controlled Asthma With Elevated Blood Eosinophil Levels: A Randomized Phase 3 Study. *Chest* **2016**, *150*, 789–798. [CrossRef] [PubMed]
66. Corren, J.; Weinstein, S.; Janka, L.; Zangrilli, J.; Garin, M. Phase 3 Study of Reslizumab in Patients With Poorly Controlled Asthma: Effects Across a Broad Range of Eosinophil Counts. *Chest* **2016**, *150*, 799–810. [CrossRef]
67. Wechsler, M.E.; Peters, S.P.; Hill, T.D.; Ariely, R.; DePietro, M.R.; Driessen, M.T.; Terasawa, E.L.; Thomason, D.R.; Panettieri, R.A. Clinical Outcomes and Health-Care Resource Use Associated with Reslizumab Treatment in Adults With Severe Eosinophilic Asthma in Real-World Practice. *Chest* **2021**, *159*, 1734–1746. [CrossRef] [PubMed]
68. Farne, H.A.; Wilson, A.; Powell, C.; Bax, L.; Milan, S.J. Anti-IL5 therapies for asthma. *Cochrane Database Syst. Rev.* **2017**, *9*, CD010834. [CrossRef]
69. Nair, P.; Wenzel, S.; Rabe, K.F.; Bourdin, A.; Lugogo, N.L.; Kuna, P.; Barker, P.; Sproule, S.; Ponnarambil, S.; Goldman, M. Oral Glucocorticoid–Sparing Effect of Benralizumab in Severe Asthma. *N. Engl. J. Med.* **2017**, *376*, 2448–2458. [CrossRef]
70. Kavanagh, J.E.; Hearn, A.P.; Dhariwal, J.; D'Ancona, G.; Douiri, A.; Roxas, C.; Fernandes, M.; Green, L.; Thomson, L.; Nanzer, A.M.; et al. Real-World Effectiveness of Benralizumab in Severe Eosinophilic Asthma. *Chest* **2021**, *159*, 496–506. [CrossRef]
71. Leckie, M.J.; Brinke, A.T.; Khan, J.; Diamant, Z.; O'Connor, B.J.; Walls, C.M.; Mathur, A.; Cowley, H.C.; Chung, K.F.; Djukanovic, R.; et al. Effects of an interleukin-5 blocking monoclonal antibody on eosinophils, airway hyper-responsiveness, and the late asthmatic response. *Lancet* **2000**, *356*, 2144–2148. [CrossRef]
72. Corren, J.; Castro, M.; O'Riordan, T.; Hanania, N.A.; Pavord, I.D.; Quirce, S.; Chipps, B.E.; Wenzel, S.E.; Thangavelu, K.; Rice, M.S.; et al. Dupilumab Efficacy in Patients with Uncontrolled, Moderate-to-Severe Allergic Asthma. *J. Allergy Clin. Immunol. Pract.* **2020**, *8*, 516–526. [CrossRef] [PubMed]
73. Nowsheen, S.; Darveaux, J.I. Real-world efficacy and safety of Dupilumab use in the treatment of asthma. *Ann. Allergy Asthma Immunol.* **2021**, *127*, 147–149. [CrossRef] [PubMed]
74. Campisi, R.; Crimi, C.; Nolasco, S.; Beghè, B.; Antonicelli, L.; Guarnieri, G.; Scichilone, N.; Porto, M.; Macchia, L.; Scioscia, G.; et al. Real-World Experience with Dupilumab in Severe Asthma: One-Year Data from an Italian Named Patient Program. *J. Asthma Allergy* **2021**, *14*, 575–583. [CrossRef] [PubMed]
75. Brusselle, G.; Michils, A.; Louis, R.; Dupont, L.; Van de Maele, B.; Delobbe, A.; Pilette, C.; Lee, C.; Gurdain, S.; Vancayzeele, S.; et al. "Real-life" effectiveness of omalizumab in patients with severe persistent allergic asthma: The PERSIST study. *Respir. Med.* **2009**, *103*, 1633–1642. [CrossRef]
76. Johansson, S.G.O.; Lilja, G.; Hallberg, J.; Nopp, A. A clinical follow-up of omalizumab in routine treatment of allergic asthma monitored by CD-sens. *Immun. Inflamm. Dis.* **2018**, *6*, 382–391. [CrossRef]
77. Amat, F.; Tallon, P.; Foray, A.-P.; Michaud, B.; Lambert, N.; Saint-Pierre, P.; Chatenoud, L.; Just, J. Control of asthma by omalizumab: The role of CD4+Foxp3+regulatory T cells. *Clin. Exp. Allergy J. Br. Soc. Allergy Clin. Immunol.* **2016**, *46*, 1614–1616. [CrossRef]
78. Lemiere, C.; Taillé, C.; Lee, J.K.; Smith, S.G.; Mallett, S.; Albers, F.C.; Bradford, E.S.; Yancey, S.W.; Liu, M.C. Impact of baseline clinical asthma characteristics on the response to mepolizumab: A post hoc meta-analysis of two Phase III trials. *Respir. Res.* **2021**, *22*, 184. [CrossRef] [PubMed]
79. Eger, K.; Kroes, J.A.; Brinke, A.T.; Bel, E.H. Long-Term Therapy Response to Anti–IL-5 Biologics in Severe Asthma—A Real-Life Evaluation. *J. Allergy Clin. Immunol. Pract.* **2021**, *9*, 1194–1200. [CrossRef] [PubMed]
80. Watanabe, S.; Suzukawa, M.; Tashimo, H.; Ohshima, N.; Asari, I.; Imoto, S.; Kobayashi, N.; Tohma, S.; Nagase, T.; Ohta, K. High serum cytokine levels may predict the responsiveness of patients with severe asthma to benralizumab. *J. Asthma* **2021**, *2021*, 1–11. [CrossRef]
81. Cañas, J.; Valverde-Monge, M.; Rodrigo-Muñoz, J.; Sastre, B.; Gil-Martínez, M.; García-Latorre, R.; Rial, M.; Gómez-Cardeñosa, A.; Fernández-Nieto, M.; Pinillos-Robles, E.; et al. Serum microRNAs as Tool to Predict Early Response to Benralizumab in Severe Eosinophilic Asthma. *J. Pers. Med.* **2021**, *11*, 76. [CrossRef]
82. Porsbjerg, C.M.; Sverrild, A.; Lloyd, C.M.; Menzies-Gow, A.N.; Bel, E.H. Anti-alarmins in asthma: Targeting the airway epithelium with next-generation biologics. *Eur. Respir. J.* **2020**, *56*, 2000260. [CrossRef]
83. Gandhi, N.A.; Pirozzi, G. Graham NMH: Commonality of the IL-4/IL-13 pathway in atopic diseases. *Expert Rev. Clin. Immunol.* **2017**, *13*, 425–437. [CrossRef] [PubMed]

84. Soumelis, V.; Reche, P.A.; Kanzler, H.; Yuan, W.; Edward, G.; Homey, B.; Gilliet, M.; Ho, S.; Antonenko, S.; Lauerma, A.; et al. Human epithelial cells trigger dendritic cell–mediated allergic inflammation by producing TSLP. *Nat. Immunol.* **2002**, *3*, 673–680. [CrossRef] [PubMed]
85. Allakhverdi, Z.; Comeau, M.R.; Jessup, H.K.; Yoon, B.-R.P.; Brewer, A.; Chartier, S.; Paquette, N.; Ziegler, S.F.; Sarfati, M.; Delespesse, G. Thymic stromal lymphopoietin is released by human epithelial cells in response to microbes, trauma, or inflammation and potently activates mast cells. *J. Exp. Med.* **2007**, *204*, 253–258. [CrossRef]
86. Camelo, A.; Rosignoli, G.; Ohne, Y.; Stewart, R.A.; Overed-Sayer, C.; Sleeman, M.A.; May, R.D. IL-33, IL-25, and TSLP induce a distinct phenotypic and activation profile in human type 2 innate lymphoid cells. *Blood Adv.* **2017**, *1*, 577–589. [CrossRef]
87. Menzies-Gow, A.; Corren, J.; Bourdin, A.; Chupp, G.; Israel, E.; Wechsler, M.E.; Brightling, C.E.; Griffiths, J.M.; Hellqvist, Å.; Bowen, K.; et al. Tezepelumab in Adults and Adolescents with Severe, Uncontrolled Asthma. *N. Engl. J. Med.* **2021**, *384*, 1800–1809. [CrossRef]
88. Chen, Z.-G.; Zhang, T.-T.; Li, H.-T.; Chen, F.-H.; Zou, X.-L.; Ji, J.-Z.; Chen, H. Neutralization of TSLP Inhibits Airway Remodeling in a Murine Model of Allergic Asthma Induced by Chronic Exposure to House Dust Mite. *PLoS ONE* **2013**, *8*, e51268. [CrossRef]
89. Cao, L.; Liu, F.; Liu, Y.; Liu, T.; Wu, J.; Zhao, J.; Wang, J.; Li, S.; Xu, J.; Dong, L. TSLP promotes asthmatic airway remodeling via p38-STAT3 signaling pathway in human lung fibroblast. *Exp. Lung Res.* **2018**, *44*, 288–301. [CrossRef] [PubMed]
90. Marone, G.; Spadaro, G.; Braile, M.; Poto, R.; Criscuolo, G.; Pahima, H.; Loffredo, S.; Levi-Schaffer, F.; Varricchi, G. Tezepelumab: A novel biological therapy for the treatment of severe uncontrolled asthma. *Expert Opin. Investig. Drugs* **2019**, *28*, 931–940. [CrossRef] [PubMed]
91. Gauvreau, G.M.; O'Byrne, P.M.; Boulet, L.-P.; Wang, Y.; Cockcroft, D.; Bigler, J.; Fitzgerald, J.M.; Boedigheimer, M.; Davis, B.E.; Dias, C.; et al. Effects of an Anti-TSLP Antibody on Allergen-Induced Asthmatic Responses. *N. Engl. J. Med.* **2014**, *370*, 2102–2110. [CrossRef] [PubMed]
92. Corren, J.; Parnes, J.R.; Wang, L.; Mo, M.; Roseti, S.L.; Griffiths, J.M.; van der Merwe, R. Tezepelumab in Adults with Uncontrolled Asthma. *N. Engl. J. Med.* **2017**, *377*, 936–946. [CrossRef]
93. Sverrild, A.; Hansen, S.; Hvidtfeldt, M.; Clausson, C.-M.; Cozzolino, O.; Cerps, S.; Uller, L.; Backer, V.; Erjefält, J.; Porsbjerg, C. The effect of tezepelumab on airway hyperresponsiveness to mannitol in asthma (UPSTREAM). *Eur. Respir. J.* **2021**. [CrossRef] [PubMed]
94. Schmitz, J.; Owyang, A.; Oldham, E.; Song, Y.; Murphy, E.; McClanahan, T.K.; Zurawski, G.; Moshrefi, M.; Qin, J.; Li, X.; et al. IL-33, an Interleukin-1-like Cytokine that Signals via the IL-1 Receptor-Related Protein ST2 and Induces T Helper Type 2-Associated Cytokines. *Immunity* **2005**, *23*, 479–490. [CrossRef] [PubMed]
95. Liew, F.Y.; Girard, J.P.; Turnquist, H.R. Interleukin-33 in health and disease. *Nat. Rev. Immunol.* **2016**, *16*, 676–689. [CrossRef] [PubMed]
96. Barlow, J.L.; Peel, S.; Fox, J.; Panova, V.; Hardman, C.S.; Camelo, A.; Bucks, C.; Wu, X.; Kane, C.M.; Neill, D.; et al. IL-33 is more potent than IL-25 in provoking IL-13–producing nuocytes (type 2 innate lymphoid cells) and airway contraction. *J. Allergy Clin. Immunol.* **2013**, *132*, 933–941. [CrossRef]
97. Kaur, D.; Gomez, E.; Doe, C.; Berair, R.; Woodman, L.; Saunders, R.M.; Hollins, F.; Rose, F.; Amrani, Y.; May, R.; et al. IL-33 drives airway hyper-responsiveness through IL-13-mediated mast cell: Airway smooth muscle crosstalk. *Allergy* **2015**, *70*, 556–567. [CrossRef] [PubMed]
98. Popovic, B.; Breed, J.; Rees, D.G.; Gardener, M.J.; Vinall, L.M.; Kemp, B.; Spooner, J.; Keen, J.; Minter, R.; Uddin, F.; et al. Structural Characterisation Reveals Mechanism of IL-13-Neutralising Monoclonal Antibody Tralokinumab as Inhibition of Binding to IL-13Ralpha1 and IL-13Ralpha2. *J. Mol. Biol.* **2017**, *429*, 208–219. [CrossRef]
99. Maselli, D.J.; Keyt, H.; Rogers, L. Profile of lebrikizumab and its potential in the treatment of asthma. *J. Asthma Allergy* **2015**, *8*, 87–92. [CrossRef]
100. Brightling, C.; Chanez, P.; Leigh, R.; O'Byrne, P.; Korn, S.; She, D.; May, R.; Streicher, K.; Ranade, K.; Piper, E. Efficacy and safety of tralokinumab in patients with severe uncontrolled asthma: A randomised, double-blind, placebo-controlled, phase 2b trial. *Lancet Respir. Med.* **2015**, *3*, 692–701. [CrossRef]
101. Panettieri, R.A.; Jr Sjobring, U.; Peterffy, A.; Wessman, P.; Bowen, K.; Piper, E.; Colice, G.; Brightling, C.E. Tralokinumab for severe, uncontrolled asthma (STRATOS 1 and STRATOS 2): Two randomised, double-blind, placebo-controlled, phase 3 clinical trials. *Lancet Respir. Med.* **2018**, *6*, 511–525. [CrossRef]
102. Hanania, N.A.; Korenblat, P.; Chapman, K.R.; Bateman, E.D.; Kopecky, P.; Paggiaro, P.; Yokoyama, A.; Olsson, J.; Gray, S.; Holweg, C.T.; et al. Efficacy and safety of lebrikizumab in patients with uncontrolled asthma (LAVOLTA I and LAVOLTA II): Replicate, phase 3, randomised, double-blind, placebo-controlled trials. *Lancet Respir. Med.* **2016**, *4*, 781–796. [CrossRef]
103. Busse, W.W.; Brusselle, G.G.; Korn, S.; Kuna, P.; Magnan, A.; Cohen, D.; Bowen, K.; Piechowiak, T.; Wang, M.M.; Colice, G. Tralokinumab did not demonstrate oral corticosteroid-sparing effects in severe asthma. *Eur. Respir. J.* **2019**, *53*, 1800948. [CrossRef]
104. Pelaia, C.; Crimi, C.; Vatrella, A.; Busceti, M.T.; Gaudio, A.; Garofalo, E.; Bruni, A.; Terracciano, R.; Pelaia, G. New treatments for asthma: From the pathogenic role of prostaglandin D2 to the therapeutic effects of fevipiprant. *Pharmacol. Res.* **2020**, *155*, 104490. [CrossRef] [PubMed]
105. Farne, H.; Jackson, D.J.; Johnston, S.L. Are emerging PGD2 antagonists a promising therapy class for treating asthma? *Expert. Opin. Emerg. Drugs* **2016**, *21*, 359–364. [CrossRef] [PubMed]

106. Brightling, C.E.; Gaga, M.; Inoue, H.; Li, J.; Maspero, J.; Wenzel, S.; Maitra, S.; Lawrence, D.; Brockhaus, F.; Lehmann, T.; et al. Effectiveness of fevipiprant in reducing exacerbations in patients with severe asthma (LUSTER-1 and LUSTER-2): Two phase 3 randomised controlled trials. *Lancet Respir. Med.* **2021**, *9*, 43–56. [CrossRef]
107. Larose, M.C.; Chakir, J.; Archambault, A.S.; Joubert, P.; Provost, V.; Laviolette, M.; Flamand, N. Correlation between CCL26 production by human bronchial epithelial cells and airway eosinophils: Involvement in patients with severe eosinophilic asthma. *J. Allergy Clin. Immunol.* **2015**, *136*, 904–913. [CrossRef]
108. Barnes, P.J. The cytokine network in asthma and chronic obstructive pulmonary disease. *J. Clin. Investig.* **2008**, *118*, 3546–3556. [CrossRef] [PubMed]
109. Godar, M.; Deswarte, K.; Vergote, K.; Saunders, M.; de Haard, H.; Hammad, H.; Blanchetot, C.; Lambrecht, B.N. A bispecific antibody strategy to target multiple type 2 cytokines in asthma. *J. Allergy Clin. Immunol.* **2018**, *142*, 1185–1193.e4. [CrossRef]
110. Venkataramani, S.; Low, S.; Weigle, B.; Dutcher, D.; Jerath, K.; Menzenski, M.; Frego, L.; Truncali, K.; Gupta, P.; Kroe-Barrett, R.; et al. Design and characterization of Zweimab and Doppelmab, high affinity dual antagonistic anti-TSLP/IL13 bispecific antibodies. *Biochem. Biophys. Res. Commun.* **2018**, *504*, 19–24. [CrossRef] [PubMed]
111. Staton, T.L.; Peng, K.; Owen, R.; Choy, D.F.; Cabanski, C.R.; Fong, A.; Brunstein, F.; Alatsis, K.R.; Chen, H. A phase I, randomized, observer-blinded, single and multiple ascending-dose study to investigate the safety, pharmacokinetics, and immunogenicity of BITS7201A, a bispecific antibody targeting IL-13 and IL-17, in healthy volunteers. *BMC Pulm. Med.* **2019**, *19*, 5. [CrossRef] [PubMed]
112. Castro, M.; Rubin, A.S.; Laviolette, M.; Fiterman, J.; De Andrade Lima, M.; Shah, P.L.; Fiss, E.; Olivenstein, R.; Thomson, N.C.; Niven, R.M.; et al. Effectiveness and safety of bronchial thermoplasty in the treatment of severe asthma: A multicenter, randomized, double-blind, sham-controlled clinical trial. *Am. J. Respir. Crit. Care Med.* **2010**, *181*, 116–124. [CrossRef] [PubMed]
113. Wechsler, M.E.; Laviolette, M.; Rubin, A.S.; Fiterman, J.; Lapa e Silva, J.R.; Shah, P.L.; Fiss, E.; Olivenstein, R.; Thomson, N.C.; Niven, R.M.; et al. Bronchial thermoplasty: Long-term safety and effectiveness in patients with severe persistent asthma. *J. Allergy Clin. Immunol.* **2013**, *132*, 1295–1302. [CrossRef] [PubMed]
114. Thomson, N.C. Recent Developments in Bronchial Thermoplasty for Severe Asthma. *J. Asthma Allergy* **2019**, *12*, 375–387. [CrossRef]

International Journal of
Molecular Sciences

Review

Targeting Human Papillomavirus-Associated Cancer by Oncoprotein-Specific Recombinant Antibodies

Maria Gabriella Donà [1], Paola Di Bonito [2], Maria Vincenza Chiantore [2], Carla Amici [3,†] and Luisa Accardi [2,*,†]

1 STI/HIV Unit, Istituto Dermatologico San Gallicano IRCCS, 00144 Rome, Italy; mariagabriella.dona@ifo.gov.it
2 Department of Infectious Diseases, Istituto Superiore di Sanità, 00161 Rome, Italy; paola.dibonito@iss.it (P.D.B.); mariavincenza.chiantore@iss.it (M.V.C.)
3 Department of Biology, University of Rome Tor Vergata, 00133 Rome, Italy; carami371@gmail.com
* Correspondence: luisa.accardi@iss.it
† These authors contributed equally.

Abstract: In recent decades, recombinant antibodies against specific antigens have shown great promise for the therapy of infectious diseases and cancer. Human papillomaviruses (HPVs) are involved in the development of around 5% of all human cancers and HPV16 is the high-risk genotype with the highest prevalence worldwide, playing a dominant role in all HPV-associated cancers. Here, we describe the main biological activities of the HPV16 E6, E7, and E5 oncoproteins, which are involved in the subversion of important regulatory pathways directly associated with all known hallmarks of cancer. We then review the state of art of the recombinant antibodies targeted to HPV oncoproteins developed so far in different formats, and outline their mechanisms of action. We describe the advantages of a possible antibody-based therapy against the HPV-associated lesions and discuss the critical issue of delivery to tumour cells, which must be addressed in order to achieve the desired translation of the antibodies from the laboratory to the clinic.

Keywords: antibody therapeutics; recombinant antibodies; intracellular antibodies; single-chain antibody fragment; nanobody; Human papillomaviruses; HPV oncoproteins; HPV-associated cancer; HPV cancer therapy

Citation: Donà, M.G.; Di Bonito, P.; Chiantore, M.V.; Amici, C.; Accardi, L. Targeting Human Papillomavirus-Associated Cancer by Oncoprotein-Specific Recombinant Antibodies. *Int. J. Mol. Sci.* **2021**, *22*, 9143. https://doi.org/10.3390/ijms22179143

Academic Editor: Yong-Seok Heo

Received: 25 May 2021
Accepted: 20 August 2021
Published: 24 August 2021

1. Introduction

In the last decades, because of the huge advances of recombinant DNA technology, recombinant antibodies have found increasing applications in the therapy of many diseases, whether of genetic, infectious, or tumour origin. Several antibodies and antibody-based products are either approved or under investigation in clinical trials and, particularly for tumours, many of them have revolutionized classical chemotherapy based on drugs [1]. Through recombinant antibodies, it is possible to interfere with specific protein functions at DNA, RNA, or protein level. Direct targeting of pathogenic proteins can even be advantageous over the targeting of genomic sequences with an on/off mode, because it allows modulating and tailoring protein activity without affecting genomic sequences.

Currently, thanks to the ability of the mammalian immune system to produce antibodies against virtually any antigen, and to over 30 years of molecular technology studies on antibody manipulation, well-established methods allow the selection of ligands for specific protein epitopes in either intra- or extra-cellular environment. Antibody selection can be performed from recombinant antibody libraries of different kinds, even originating from animals immunized with antigens of interest. Specific antibodies can be delivered directly to the cells as purified proteins or expressed as intracellular antibodies (intrabodies) by recombinant DNA technology. Different antibody formats representing more or less extended regions of an immunoglobulin (Ig) are presently available. The small size formats, i.e., antibodies in single-chain format (scFvs) and single domain antibody or nanobodies (sdAb or Nbs) [2], are the most suitable for expression as intrabodies because they are easily engineerable.

Several monoclonal antibodies (mAbs) in different formats reached the clinical stage or are in different clinical trial stages for the treatment of numerous pathologies including tumours [1,3]. We are principally interested in tumours associated to Human Papillomaviruses (HPVs), which represent a global health problem in terms of morbidity and mortality and for which many therapeutic strategies are under study. Among these, the approach based on recombinant antibodies deserves particular attention because of its potentialities related to safety, precision, and feasibility [3–5].

Here we describe, to the best of our knowledge, the different formats of recombinant antibodies against the HPV oncoproteins of Human Papillomaviruses characterized to date or currently under study and discuss whether and why they show promise for the treatment of pre-neoplastic and neoplastic lesions caused by these viruses.

2. Different Antibody Formats: mAbs, scFvs and Nanobodies

Recombinant antibody technology has undergone tremendous development in recent decades, so to prompt much progress in disease diagnosis and therapy. The use of display technologies allows in vitro selection from non-animal-derived recombinant (naïve or synthetic) repertoires (libraries) of peptides and antibody fragments in different formats such as Fab fragments (Fabs), scFvs, and Nbs. Different platforms are available such as phage display, yeast display, ribosome display, bacterial display, mammalian cell surface display, mRNA display, and DNA display. All of them mimic what occurs in vivo during antibody generation by the immune system as they rely on (1) genotypic diversity, which can be obtained by immune stimulation of a competent organism or by cloning; (2) the link existing between the genotype and phenotype; (3) selective pressure for increasing antibody specificity; and (4) amplification of specific clones originated by selective pressure. The coding sequences of binders specific for a given antigen, identified by the display technology of choice, can be expressed in prokaryotic or eukaryotic systems and tested both in vitro and in vivo for their ability to counteract the target antigen activity.

The possibility to engineer the originally identified antibody sequence represents an added value, since affinity, stability, and expression level can be improved while maintaining the desired antigen-binding properties. Furthermore, it is possible to modify the format so that the antibody could acquire new kinetic properties. Importantly, it is feasible to bypass the risk of immune reactions during clinical use by constructing antibodies from human scaffolds.

A whole IgG molecule (150 kDa) comprises heavy (H) and light (L) chains each consisting of a variable (VH and VL) and a constant (CH and CL) region covalently linked to each other and to oligosaccharides necessary for antibody effector functions and for long serum half-life. The antigen-binding regions responsible for diversity among antibodies are the complementary determining regions (CDRs), three for each VH and VL. The VH and VL joined by a disulphide bond and covalently linked to the first CH domain are obtainable by IgG proteolysis, resulting in a Fab monovalent antibody fragment (55 kDa) (Figure 1).

A few decades ago, it was observed that the N-terminal IgG fragment including the VH and VL retains the same antigen-binding capacity as the whole IgG molecule. The so-called scFvs (27 kDa) lack the constant regions and include only the VH and VL linked by a short peptide consisting of a sequence of glycine and serine residues such as (Gly4Ser)3. This arrangement provides flexibility, hydrophilicity, and resistance to proteases digestion. The linker length can be modified to favour or not the formation of multimers. In fact, shortening the linker to 3–12 amino acids prevents the formation of monomeric forms supporting inter-molecular VH-VL combinations also in different orientations, with spontaneous formation of a scFv dimer called "diabody" (60 kDa), where each of the two antigen-binding sites are formed by the VH of one scFv and the VL of the other one (Figure 1). The linkage of two scFvs in a unique molecule forms a tandem scFv.

Both diabodies and tandem scFvs can have two different binding specificities, and in this case, they are called bispecific (bs). Interestingly, even the VH and VL arrangement in the scFv fusion protein can influence the binding activity, and it is currently possible to predict the best functional structure so as to design scFvs that meet all requirements by molecular modelling using a computer-aided homology method [6,7].

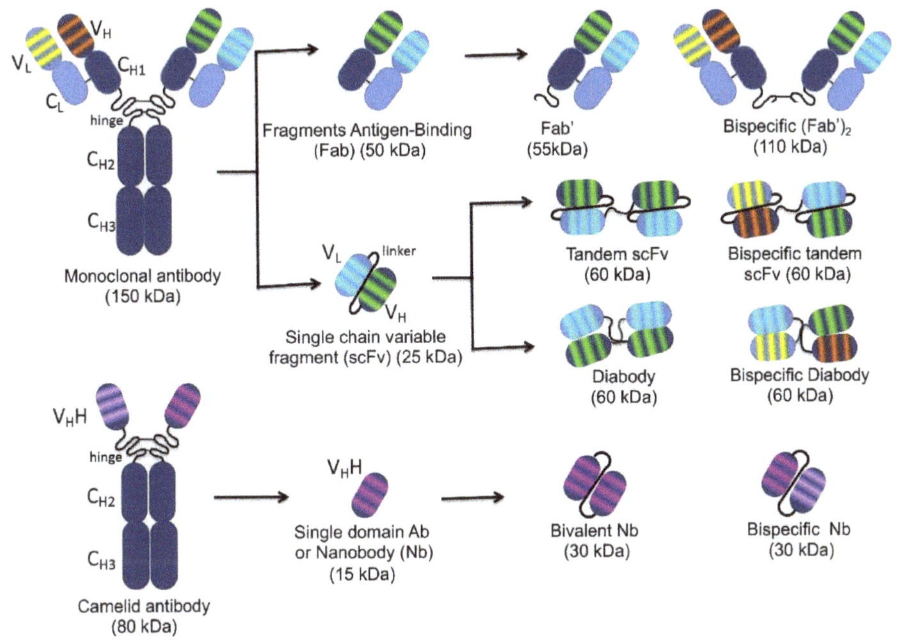

Figure 1. Schematic representation of the structure of conventional and camelidae monoclonal antibodies and of different antibody fragments. On the left, the whole monoclonal antibody (**top**) and camelid antibody (**bottom**) structures are represented. The variable light (VL) and heavy (VH) chains, as well as the constant light (CL) and heavy (CH1, CH2, CH3) chains are indicated. The complementarity determining regions responsible for antigen binding, three for each VL and each VH, are represented by stripes highlighted in different colours according to the different antigen specificity. Arrows indicate different monospecific and bispecific antibody fragments derived from the original antibody molecules with their nomenclature and molecular weight. The VH and VL in the different arrangements are connected by peptide linkers of 3–12 amino acids represented by black curved lines.

The CDRs of a scFv are embedded in an amino acid scaffold of either human or animal origin, according to the library utilized for selection. Of note, CDRs with specific binding activities can be isolated and grafted onto different scaffolds suitable for the purposes of interest. Both scFv and Fab fragments can be engineered into stable oligomers to increase binding avidity and widen antigen specificity. Specific applications of these formats are the recruitment of T-cells to tumours in immunotherapy, viral retargeting in gene therapy, and targeting of multiple antigens for a synergic/additive effect. All the mentioned antibody formats, having a size of 15–80 kDa (Figure 1), show an easy tumour penetration and are cleared from the bloodstream flow more quickly with respect to the full size IgGs (150 kDa, Figure 1). Furthermore, their genes can be easily manipulated to modify their stability, specificity, and affinity for the antigens.

Antibody engineering also allows cloning of scFv sequences into eukaryotic vectors equipped with intracellular localization signals, for the scFv expression in specific cell compartments as intrabodies. These can reach and recognize target antigens in the cellular compartments where they are located, with outcomes ranging from direct antigen blockade to indirect impairment of its activity through delocalization, to its targeted degradation [8,9].

The discovery of the smallest format of antibody fragments, the Nbs, expanded the possibilities of targeting intracellular antigens through biotechnology. Nbs derive from Camelidae species (e.g., llamas, dromedaries and camels), which in their antibody repertoire have IgG lacking both light chains and CH1 domains (heavy-chain-only antibodies: HCAbs) [10]. The variable domains of these HCAbs are named VHHs and can be isolated as single-domain antibodies (sdAbs), which are small-sized (~15 kDa) but retain the antigen-binding capability of the full-size antibody. Thanks to the small size, VHHs can easily penetrate tissues and access cryptic epitopes [11,12]. They are more soluble and capable of efficient folding with respect to conventional mAbs, which renders them suitable for high-yield production in *E. coli* and even for delivery to or expression in infected cells as intrabodies. Nbs can resist a wide pH range and high temperatures, and some of them tolerate the presence of organic compounds. Despite the non-human origin, VHHs are rarely immunogenic due to the small size and high sequence homology to the human VH3 gene family, which avoids the necessity of humanization for translation into clinic [13]. The small size also favours rapid renal clearance and facilitates the in vivo application in diagnosis rather than therapy, as the latter use requires prolongation of their half-life, which is approximately 2 h. Nevertheless, VHHs targeting haematological, oncological, infectious, inflammatory/auto-immune, bone and neurological diseases are already being evaluated in clinical trials, while the humanized VHH Caplacizumab (CabliviTM) was recently approved in Europe and USA for the treatment of acquired thrombotic thrombocytopenic purpura [14–16].

3. HPV-Associated Lesions and Current Therapies

HPVs are small, non-enveloped viruses, with a circular dsDNA genome of about 8 Kbp. The icosahedral capsid is composed of the major L1 protein and the minor L2 protein. Following infection of the epithelium basal cells, the E1 and E2 early proteins play key roles in viral DNA replication and amplification, as well as in regulating viral transcription. When actively expressed, the viral genome is maintained as an episome. Viral genome amplification, late gene expression, and viral progeny assembly are limited to terminally differentiated layers of the epithelium. Since terminally differentiated keratinocytes undergo growth arrest, HPV genomes have evolved, as a replication strategy, the expression of E6, E7, and E5 proteins, which are able to keep the infected cells in a competent state for DNA synthesis. Most HPV infections usually clear within 1–2 years but, in some cases, the virus may persist and occasional integration of its genome in the host's genome may occur. Consequently, the infected cells overexpress E6 and E7 due to the loss of the E2 transcriptional repressor coding sequence.

HPV infections are among the most common sexually-transmitted diseases and cause annually around 5% of all cancers worldwide [17–19]. However, only some genotypes are responsible for morbidity and mortality related to cancer, mostly of the cervix (CC) but also of the anogenital area and of the oropharynx, whose number is constantly increasing. According to the different oncogenic potential, HPVs are defined as high-risk (HR) types, which may cause the development of high-grade squamous intraepithelial (H-SIL) and cancer lesions, and low risk (LR) types, mainly causing anogenital warts. Worldwide, the HR HPV16 and HPV18 cause 71% of CC, with the remaining genotypes causing the residual HPV-associated cases [20,21].

Since more than 10 years, a bivalent vaccine against HPV16 and HPV18, and a quadrivalent vaccine that also targets the LR HPV6 and HPV11, responsible for genital warts, have been available. Recently, a nonvalent vaccine that offers protection against the five other most common HR genotypes (HPV 31, 33, 45, 52, and 58) and prevents about 90% of CC cases was developed [22]. The vaccines consist of DNA-free virus-like particles (VLPs) obtained by the only expression of the viral L1 protein through recombinant technology, and are administered with proper adjuvants. Nevertheless, effective prevention of the

HPV-associated pathologies is expected only in the long-term if HPV vaccination is able to reach a significant percentage of the target population worldwide [22–24]. The three HPV vaccines (bivalent, tetravalent, and nonavalent) have been licensed as prophylactic vaccines, but currently only 8% of low- and middle-income nations have introduced HPV vaccination programs in their health policies. In addition, in recent years many trials were performed to investigate the efficacy of these vaccines in preventing HPV disease recurrence after the treatment of high-grade cervical or anal lesions and condylomatosis, showing some promising results [24].

Of note, the 73rd World Health Assembly, held on August 2020, strongly encouraged the acceleration of actions aimed at eliminating cervical cancer as a public health problem. This should be pursued through "the inclusion of HPV vaccine into national immunization programs" and the "improvement of availability, affordability, accessibility, utilization and quality of screening, vaccines, diagnostics, and treatment and care of pre- and invasive cervical cancer" [23].

Treatment of HPV-associated lesions varies widely, mainly depending on lesion grade (high-grade lesions versus invasive cancer), lesion localization (lower genital tract, uterine cervix or head and neck), and tumour stage. In general, current therapeutic approaches aim at eliminating abnormal/malignant cells. This can mainly be achieved through surgery, chemotherapy, radiotherapy, targeted therapy, or immunotherapy. These approaches can be used alone or, in some cases, in combination.

In HPV-associated malignancies, E6 and E7 oncoproteins represent tumour-associated antigens, which are ideal targets for the development of vaccines stimulating specific cytotoxic T lymphocytes (CTLs). In HPV natural infection, E6- and E7-specific CD4 and CD8 immune responses are associated with the regression of HPV-cervical lesions. However, therapeutic vaccines are not yet available for clinical practice in spite of the numerous clinical experimentations carried out during the last 25 years, which used E6 and E7 through different platforms to raise specific immunity. The poor efficacy of these vaccines, due the lack of specific adjuvants of T-cell responses, has led to the interruption of many clinical trials in the early stages. Only recently, an improvement in efficacy was achieved by combining E6-E7 therapeutic vaccines with the use of radio- and chemotherapy (Cisplatin, Carboplatin, Paclitaxel), immune check-point inhibitors (anti-PD-1, anti-PDL1, anti-CTL4), cytokines (IFNalpha and IL-12), angiogenesis inhibitors (anti-VEGF), and modulators of tumour microenvironment (TME, Histone Deacetylase Inhibitors). Several new clinical trials are currently underway and the time for any authorizations has been further lengthened [24,25].

This context accounts for the huge bulk of research, particularly in the field of immunotherapy, still underway on therapeutic approaches against HPV lesions [26]. One of the promising treatments is undoubtedly that involving the use of intrabodies to block viral oncoproteins activities, and will be described below.

4. Molecular Mechanisms of HPV-Induced Carcinogenesis

HPV-associated carcinogenesis is known to be driven by the expression, in the transcription order, of the non-structural E6, E7, and E5 oncoproteins encoded by early genes [27].

The activity of E5, E6, and E7 has not been conclusively characterized and new functions are constantly being discovered. The following sections will briefly describe those molecular targets and biological activities that, causing the subversion of important regulatory pathways, are associated with the hallmarks of cancer as outlined by Hanahan and Weinberg [28]. In some instances, the role of the oncoproteins in determining a specific hallmark is well characterized, while in other cases, the precise activity connected with a hallmark has yet to be fully elucidated and the available lines of evidence provide only hints on the link between HPV oncoproteins and some hallmarks. A schematic representation of the HPV oncoprotein role in determining the hallmarks of cancer is shown in Figure 2.

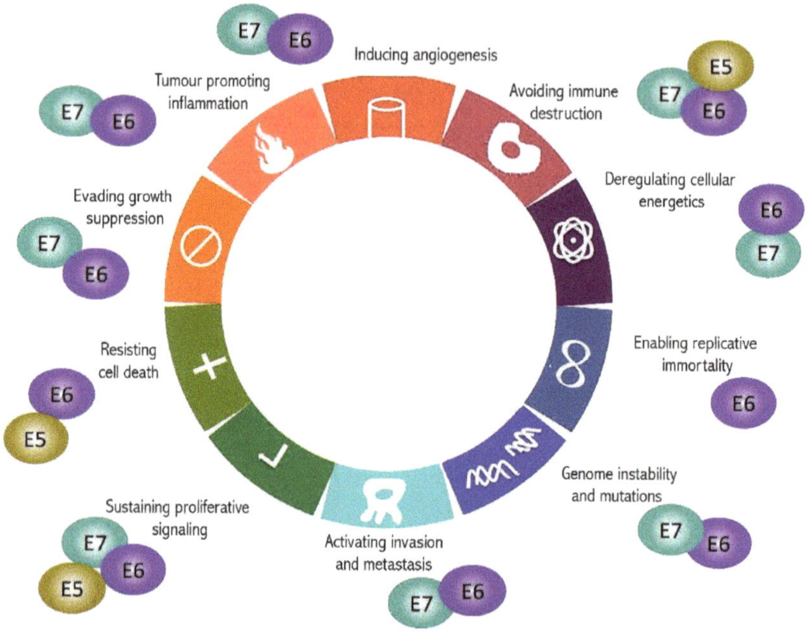

Figure 2. Involvement of HPV oncoproteins in cancer hallmarks. Dysregulation of cell pathways ascribable to E6, E7, and E5 oncoproteins of HR HPVs is responsible for the entire spectrum of hallmarks of Human Papillomavirus (HPV)-related cancer (see text for details). In the figure, the involvement of each oncoprotein in the different hallmarks is reported.

4.1. Cell Cycle Deregulation and Sustaining of Proliferative Signalling

Deregulation of cell proliferation is one of the most characteristic traits of malignant cells. E7 oncoprotein targets key cellular mediators leading to uncontrolled cell proliferation. In particular, it establishes well-characterized interactions with the members of the "pocket proteins" family, represented by pRB, p107, and p130, and promotes their degradation [29]. This, in turns, allows the release of the E2F transcription factor, with the consequent expression of S-phase genes as well as of the p16INK4A cyclin-dependent kinase inhibitor. S-phase entry is also induced by E7 through the direct inactivation of essential regulators of G1-to-S-phase transition, such as p21 and p27 cyclin inhibitors. Sustained proliferation of HPV-infected cells is also induced by E5 oncoprotein, which increases the Epidermal Growth Factor Receptor (EGFR) signalling activity by forming an activating complex with it and impairing its degradation [30].

4.2. Resistance to Cell Death

Escape from cell death is one of the most important hallmarks of cancer, allowing cells with genomic defects to survive and continue to proliferate [31]. E6 interferes with several cell death pathways. It can abrogate apoptosis by promoting proteasomal degradation of p53 tumour suppressor, which controls the expression of pro-apoptotic genes [32]. E6 further promotes cell survival by impairing cell response to tumour necrosis factor (TNF), protecting the infected cells from Fas-induced apoptosis [33] and transactivating survivin gene promoter [34]. E5 oncoprotein also supports antiapoptotic activity during the first steps of the oncogenic process through downregulation of Fas-Ligand (Fas-L) on the cell membrane [33] and increased degradation of Bax [35].

4.3. Avoiding Immune Destruction

HPVs have developed mechanisms to counter the destruction of infected cells by the host's immune system. In this context, E5 plays an important role by promoting MHC class I retention in the Golgi apparatus, resulting in impaired viral antigen recognition [36]. Recently, E5 was found to be also involved in the increased expression of PD-L1 and inhibition of effector T cells, events that facilitate the immune evasion of HPV-infected cells [37]. E6 plays a direct role in modulating the immune response against HPV antigens by impairing Interferon (IFN)-mediated host defence in different and interrelated ways [38,39]. E7 also interferes with IFN signalling [40] and inhibits the Toll-like receptor-9 (TLR9) recognition in cooperation with E6 [41].

4.4. Replicative Immortality

To ensure the unlimited cell proliferation associated with carcinogenesis, E6 induces overexpression of human telomerase reverse transcriptase (hTERT), the catalytic unit of the human telomerase [42]. This occurs through both direct promoter activation and proteasomal degradation of its transcriptional repressor NFX1-91 through the E6/E6AP complex [43]. Constitutive expression of hTERT is also established through epigenetic mechanisms depending on alteration of the activity of histone methylases and demethylases [44], with E6 representing the main player.

4.5. Induction of Angiogenesis

HPV-infected cells derive sustenance and oxygen from the surrounding tissues thanks to the ability of the viral oncoproteins to induce angiogenesis. E6 and E7 regulate several angiogenesis modulators, including both inducers and inhibitors of this process. Both E6 and E7 are able to trigger the angiogenic switch by upregulating the expression of Vascular Endothelial Growth Factor (VEGF) respectively through direct [45] or E2F1-mediated [46] transcriptional activation of the angiogenetic factor gene [47]. In response to E6 and E7 expression, Interleukin-8 (IL-8), a major angiogenesis inducer, is also promoted [48]. On the other hand, expression of the thrombospondin-1 and maspin inhibitors of angiogenesis is indirectly perturbed by E6 as a result of E6-mediated degradation of p53, which positively regulates these inhibitors [48].

4.6. Deregulation of Cellular Energetics

Alterations of cell metabolism are among the earliest changes observed in cancer cells. Both the E6 and E7 oncoproteins contribute to the switch from oxidative to glycolytic cell metabolism, known as Warburg effect. Mechanisms by which HPV oncoproteins induce reprogramming of cell metabolism are reviewed in detail elsewhere [49]. E6 interferes with the expression of genes involved in the control of glycolytic metabolism through its interactions with p53 and c-Myc, while E7 promotes the glycolytic pathway by upregulating the expression of different glycolytic enzymes, such as hexokinase, involved in the first step of glucose metabolism, and by direct binding and activation of M2-pyruvate kinase. In addition, HPV16 E5 does not directly regulate glycolytic enzymes but contributes to the metabolic switch by activating the EGFR pathway that, in turn, promotes an enhancement of the glycolytic metabolic program [49].

4.7. Invasiveness and Metastasis Induction

The E6 encoded by HR HPVs plays a pivotal role in this cancer hallmark as it down-regulates proteins modulating cell polarity and motility such as the scribbled planar cell polarity protein (SCRIB) involved in cell polarization and differentiation, and the membrane-associated guanylate kinases 1, 2, and 3 (MAGI-1, 2 and 3) [50]. Furthermore, E6-mediated functional modulation or degradation of adhesion effectors allows matrix-independent cell growth [51], resulting in enhanced motility and invasion of HPV-positive cells. E6/E7 contribute to the metastatic and invasive behavior of HPV-positive tumours by increasing the expression of different matrix metalloproteinases (MMPs) [52]. Both E6 and

E7 are involved in the epithelial–mesenchymal transition (EMT), crucial process for invasion and metastasis, by regulation of E-cadherin [53,54] and N-cadherin [55]. HPV-induced invasive cancer behavior has recently been correlated with E5 activity as well [56]. E5 is in fact able to upregulate the growth factor receptor MET, critical for tumour cell invasion, motility, and cancer metastasis, at both protein and mRNA level. Through this activity, E5 contributes to increase motility of the HPV-positive keratinocytes, and may thus promote metastasis of HPV-associated malignancies.

4.8. Genome Instability

The uncontrolled cell proliferation promoted by HPV oncoproteins facilitates the accumulation of genetic aberrations and genomic instability. E7 plays a central role in this process by inducing centrosome aberrations [57]. By increasing the activity of the cyclin-dependent kinase 2 (CDK2), E7 further leads to an augmented risk of genomic instability [58]. Concomitantly, a higher mutation rate is caused by E6 [59]. Altogether, E6 and E7 interfere with almost all the main actors of the cellular DNA repair pathway, thus reducing and delaying the removal of damages from the host cell genetic material. Another important hallmark associated with the expression of E6 and E7 is the interference with effectors of epigenetic modifications (e.g., DNA methyltransferases and histone modification enzymes). By influencing their activity, HPV oncoproteins may cause either the activation of oncogenes or the silencing of tumour suppressor genes [60].

4.9. Tumour-Promoting Inflammation

Through various mechanisms, E5, E6, and E7 are all involved in the development of chronic inflammation, a major cofactor of malignant transformation. In fact, the expression of genes involved in the inflammatory response increases due to E6/E7 activity. Persistent expression of oncoproteins leads to changes in the release of several pro-inflammatory cytokines (e.g., IL-6 and IL-18) and chemokines with a well-characterized role in inflammation and carcinogenesis. By acting in an autocrine manner, cytokines affect keratinocyte differentiation, proliferation, and secretion of other soluble mediators while, in a paracrine manner, they lead to the increase of infiltrating inflammatory cells. This tumour microenvironment contributes to tumour growth, angiogenesis, resistance to apoptosis, and local immune surveillance [61]. In addition, HPV oncoproteins stimulate cyclo-oxygenase-2 (COX-2) production with the consequent activation of the COX-prostaglandin (PG) pathway, which is considered the main cause of HPV-induced inflammation [62].

5. Therapeutic Recombinant Antibodies Targeting HPV Oncoproteins

Safe and non-invasive interventions without side effects would be desirable for the treatment of HPV-related lesions. In order to be effective also in immunodeficient patients, therapeutic strategies possibly not involving the individual immune response would be recommended.

An effective and timely treatment of pre-neoplastic lesions could avoid their progression toward invasive cancer. At the same time, a well-timed and effective therapy for already established tumours could ameliorate patient prognosis. Another important therapeutic area of intervention could be the prevention of metastases deriving from surgically removed HPV tumours.

Much progress has been made in the last years to develop therapeutic vaccines against HPV-associated tumours. The main platforms include peptide- and protein-based vaccines; DNA virus- and RNA virus-based vectors; bacterial vectors; cell-based, DNA-based, and RNA-based vaccines; and vaccines combining two of the mentioned platforms. Other lines of research involve the combined use of therapeutic vaccines with other treatment modalities such as PD-1/PD-L1 axis inhibitors or other checkpoint inhibitors, HDAC inhibitors or other treatments. Many clinical trials are ongoing, with some having even reached Phase II. They are reviewed in detail elsewhere [25]. Nevertheless, critical issues remain to be solved such as anti-vector immunity, HLA-restriction of peptides, or the difficulty of identifying valid outcomes to compare the efficacy of these strategies.

In view of their crucial role in the onset and progression of HPV-driven tumours [63], E5, E6, and E7 proteins represent ideal targets for alternative anti-tumour therapeutic approaches based on protein knock out or knock down methods. In this context, recombinant antibodies seem to represent a valid therapeutic opportunity. Currently, a number of recombinant antibodies against the HPV oncoproteins are available in different formats. In recent years, such antibodies have been tested for their therapeutic potential against HPV-associated disease. They are summarized here referring to their targets.

5.1. E6-Specific Recombinant Antibodies

Many studies demonstrated that E6 protein, with its multiple direct and indirect interactions, is an undiscussed druggable target [64]. Since its X-ray structure in complex with E6-associated protein (E6AP), the ubiquitin ligase involved in p53 polyubiquitination, and p53 has been resolved, the possibility of inhibiting this complex has been increasingly investigated through several methods among which those based on specific recombinant antibodies appear promising.

5.1.1. ScFvs and mAbs

The 1F1 and 6F4 (F4) scFvs, derived from mAbs obtained by mice immunization with the GST-HPV16E6 fusion protein and targeting the E6 N-terminus, were able to hamper p53 degradation in vitro by inhibiting the formation of the E6/p53 complex [65]. Lagrange et al. characterized three further anti-16E6 mAbs (1F5, 3B8, 3F8) targeting the 16ZD2 zinc-binding domain, which were able to bind E6 through a shared 16 amino acid sequence. By comparing the activity of these mAbs to that of scFv F4, they found opposite effects, with the mAbs being unable to affect the E6AP-dependent and able to affect the E6AP-independent binding of p53, possibly as a consequence of an antibody-induced conformational change at the E6AP-binding site of E6 [66]. The capacity of intracellular folding and cytosolic stability/solubility of scFvF4 was improved by mutagenesis, obtaining the IF4-P41L scFv [66]. Such scFv expressed by adenoviral system was able to cause specific apoptosis of HPV16-positive cells in a way proportional to the scFv solubility and not related to p53 rescue, showing not to depend on the block of p53 degradation [67] (Figure 3).

Courtête et al. delivered the anti-16E6 4C6 mAb to HPV16- and HPV18-positive cells and found a specific p53 accumulation in the nucleus of HPV16-positive cells, which was favoured in the presence of a network of scFv peptide dimers linked through COOH-terminal Cysteine residues (Figure 3). Interestingly, cell proliferation was hampered but apoptosis was not restored, and a synergistic effect was obtained by co-delivery of silencing RNA targeting E6 [68].

GTE6-1, a 16E6 binder selected from a scFv library constructed by Griffin et al., was able to bind to the first zinc finger of E6 with high affinity. GTE6-1 was able to recognize specifically both partially denatured and native E6 and to inhibit E6-mediated degradation of p53 in vitro [69] (Figure 3). To evaluate the capability of antibodies in different formats to hamper the E6 activity, Griffin et al. expressed the GTE6-1 scFv also as a diabody and a triabody in a number of cell lines whose proliferation depends on E6 and E7, and compared such capability to that of peptides containing the E6-binding motif ELLG. Only the scFv format induced significant nuclear apoptosis and p53 rescue in HPV16-positive cells. The reason for the poor biological effect of diabody and triabody probably relies on the size-dependent inability to diffuse through nuclear pores. The ELLG-containing peptides exhibited high target avidity but were not effective as inhibitors of E6 function.

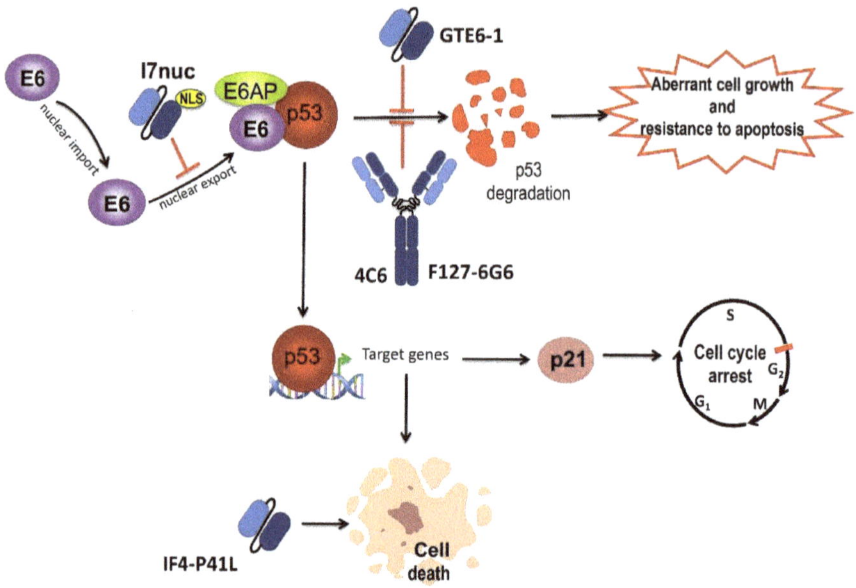

Figure 3. Schematic representation of the known effects of anti-E6 intrabodies expressed in HPV-positive cells. The effects of the intracellular expression of specific single-chain antibody fragments (scFvs) (GTE6-1 and IF4-P41L) and monoclonal antibodies (mAbs) (4C6 and F127-6G6) are shown. The binding of I7nuc to E6 inhibits its nuclear export and the subsequent cytoplasmic degradation of p53. Similarly, E6 binding by the GTE6-1 scFv or 4C6 and F127-6G6 mAbs inhibits p53 degradation, preventing the resistance to apoptosis and leading to the uncontrolled cell proliferation characteristic of HPV-positive cells. The rescue of nuclear p53 levels activates the transcription of genes involved in the induction of apoptosis and in the control of cell proliferation. The pro-apoptotic effect of IF4-P41L scFv, apparently p53-independent, is also shown.

By delivering the 16E6-targeting F127-6G6mAb to HPV16-positive cells by sonoporation, Togtema et al. were able to reduce the E6-mediated p53 degradation but not to induce apoptosis [70] (Figure 3). Nevertheless, the effect was transient probably due to the inability of molecules as large as mAbs to penetrate the cell nucleus, and the outcome was different in the two HPV16-positive cell lines utilized, suggesting that different treatment plans might be necessary for in vivo tumour therapy. No mAb effect was observed in HPV-negative cells, confirming the safety of a mAb-based treatment, effective only in tumour cells.

Direct selection of scFvs as intrabodies is appropriate to identify stable binders able to recognize intracellular antigens such as E6 and E7. Indeed, scFvs unstable in reducing the intracellular environment will spontaneously exclude themselves from selection. In our studies, we selected from the SPLINT library [71] the anti-16E6 scFvI7 intrabody by Intracellular Antibody Capture Technology (IACT), which allows performing selection in the intracellular environment. In the light of E6 activity in the cell nucleus, we provided scFvI7 with a signal for nuclear localization (NLS), and tested the I7nuc effect in HPV16-positive cells. When co-transfecting the same cells with I7nuc and the recombinant E6, we observed I7nuc/E6 co-localization in cell nucleus. I7nuc caused a partial rescue of p53, which accumulated in cell nucleus and was able to markedly hamper cell proliferation and induce apoptosis and necrosis of SiHa cells [71] (Figure 3).

We then investigated the I7nuc antitumour activity in mouse models for HPV tumours based on the injection of HPV16-positive tumour cells in C57BL6 mice. The scFv capability to either prevent cancer development from scFv-expressing tumour cells, or to hinder cancer progression by delivery to already established tumours, was evaluated [71,72]

(Figure 4). We observed a clear impairment of tumour growth in all mice injected with TC-1 tumour cells expressing I7nuc by retroviral transduction before inoculation into mice, with 60% of them completely protected from tumour onset for the 4 months of observation time [71]. In a different experimental setting, we delivered the scFvI7-expressing plasmids by electroporation to newly implanted tumours. Even in this case, it was possible to hamper tumour growth, providing the proof of principle for a scFv-based early treatment of cancer. The result was confirmed using two different HPV16-positive tumour cells, namely C3 and TC-1 cells, and also by employing higher amounts of TC-1 cells to mimic tumours that are more aggressive. Through histology and immunohistochemistry, we showed that the antitumour activity is based on the induction of tumour cell death by apoptosis [72].

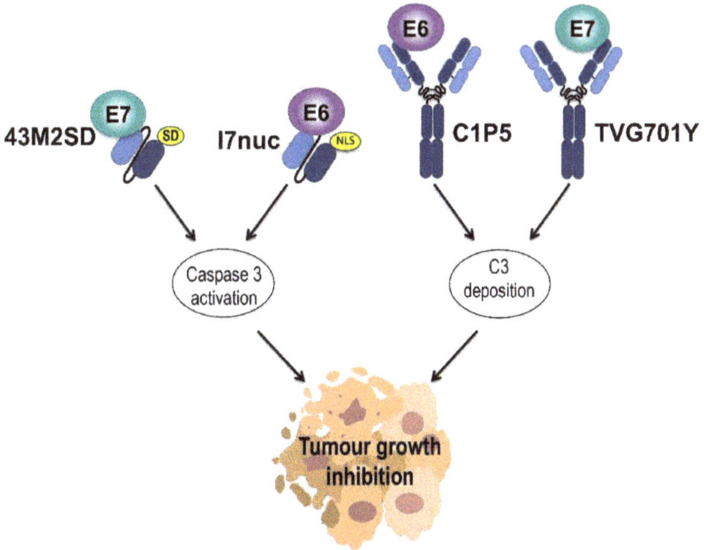

Figure 4. Antitumour effect of anti-E6 and anti-E7 recombinant antibodies in vivo. The effect of the anti-16E7 (43M2SD with localization in the endoplasmic reticulum, ER) and anti-16E6 scFvs (I7nuc with localization in the cell nucleus) in HPV-driven tumour mouse models is shown on the left. Mice tumours were electroporated after injection of scFv-expressing plasmids, resulting in the induction of apoptosis and large necrotic areas in the tumour mass due to caspase 3 activation. The effect of intratumour injection of anti-16E6 anti-16E7 mAbs in HPV16-positive tumour-bearing mice is shown on the right. The significant inhibition of tumour growth by C1P5 and TVG701Y might be due to the complement C3 deposition.

In view of a possible direct use of antibodies in protein format for therapeutic purposes, we expressed the anti-16E6 scFv coding sequences, provided or not with the NLS, in prokaryotes. We tested the stability, reactivity, and specificity towards 16E6, of I7 and I7nuc proteins purified from *E. coli* in soluble form. The scFvs in protein format delivered to HPV16-positive cell lines were able to recognize the endogenous monomeric E6 in the cell nucleus and hampered the proliferation of these cells. These results could have interesting implications for therapy also in consideration of the high safety of scFv proteins, even though a prolonged administration over time would be necessary as the proteins are subject to degradation [73].

A recent study by Jiang et al. utilized anti-16 E6 and -16 E7 mAbs in an experimental murine model based on HPV16-positive CaSki cells implanted in Balb/c nude mice. Two different doses of the anti-16E6 C1P5 and anti-16E7 TVG701Y mAbs were delivered via intraperitoneal or intratumour injections and both showed significant ability to specifically inhibit tumour growth at an extent comparable to the Cisplatin chemotherapeutic agent. Inhibition of tumour growth was virus-specific and suggested that the mechanism underlying the mAb activity consists of a specific effect causing complement deposition and a non-specific effect on macrophage polarization [74] (Figure 4). Accumulation of complement in tumour tissue facilitates the elimination of cancer cells due to opsonisation, and significantly activates complementary pathways, thus promoting surveillance by the immune system.

5.1.2. Nanobodies

Nanobodies represent the new generation of anti-HPV recombinant antibodies (Figure 1). In view of the preferential localization of 16E6 protein in the cell nucleus [75], and of their advantageous properties of thermal and chemical stability, VHHs are increasingly attracting interest for the targeting of E6. Indeed, they can penetrate into the nucleus through nuclear pores and interact with epitopes inaccessible to conventional mAbs. Three VHHs binding to the recombinant E6 with nanomolar affinities were identified from two llama, immune VHH phage display libraries by Togtema et al. [76]. The capacity of the selected VHHs to bind the native E6 derived from HPV16-positive biological samples had not yet been determined at the time of the study, nor had the bound E6 epitopes been characterized.

More recently, a different 16E6-targeting nanobody was isolated and characterized [77]. Zhang et al. advocated the possible therapeutic use of such nanobody to counteract HPV-induced tumours given its capacity to inhibit both the proliferation of HPV16 -positive cells in vitro and the growth of xenograft tumours in nude mice.

Celegato et al. explored a different approach also based on nanobodies and equally aimed at neutralizing the E6 ability to degrade p53. VHHs against the degradation-binding domain (DBD) of p53 were developed and shown to stabilise nuclear p53 in HeLa cells, which harbour the HPV18 genome, with a specific effect for HPV-positive cells. Nevertheless, the VHHs were unable to rescue the p53 tumour-suppressive functions. The authors hypothesized that this was due to inhibition of p53 transactivation associated with an increased cell proliferation and viability, and highlighted that anti-p53 DBD VHHs were able to modulate protein properties even if not reaching the desired antiproliferative effect [78].

5.2. E7-Specific Recombinant Antibodies

The E7 protein of HR HPVs cooperates with E6 protein to drive oncogenesis mainly through deregulation of growth suppressors, which leads to uncontrolled cell proliferation as above detailed. Therefore, E7 is widely studied as a therapeutic target, and the now in-depth knowledge of its functions suggests that specific recombinant antibodies may be a useful tool to fulfil the anticancer purposes [79].

5.2.1. ScFvs and mAbs

The first scFvs selected against 16E7 oncoprotein were constructed directly from murine spleen cells, and then provided with signals for subcellular localization by cloning [80]. When the scFv-expressing plasmids were transfected in HPV16-positive cells, the scFv with SEKDEL signal for localization in the endoplasmic reticulum (ER) was effective in decreasing E7 expression in a manner inversely related to the amount of plasmid used for cell transfection. Interestingly, when trying to generate cells stably expressing the anti-E7 scFvs, the researchers observed that stable expression of these antibodies was not compatible with clonal outgrowth of E7-expressing tumour cells. In fact, the expression of anti-16E7 scFvs, and of that with localization in the ER in particular, successfully and specifically inhibited the proliferation of HPV16-positive CaSki and SiHa cells (Figure 5). Wang-Johanning et al. concluded that the alteration obtained was due to the interaction between the scFv and E7 [80].

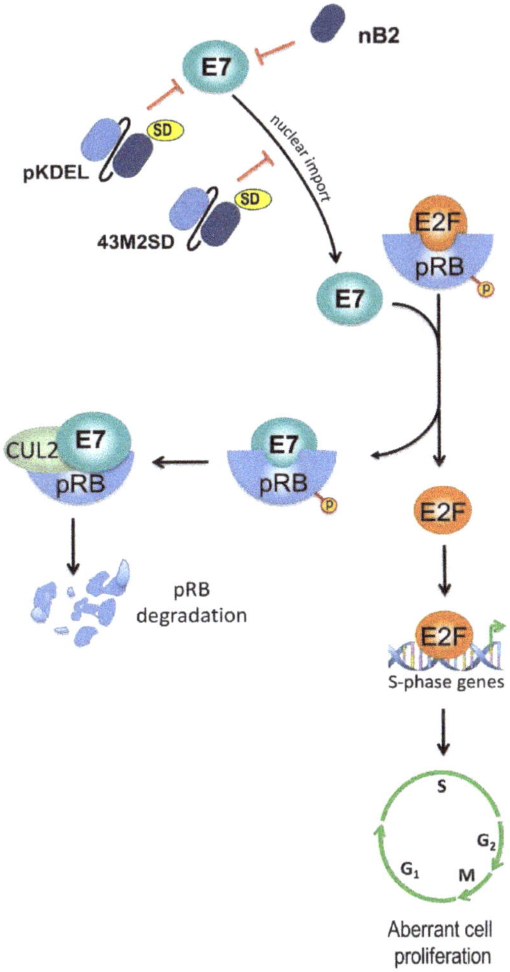

Figure 5. Schematic representation of the known effects of anti-E7 intrabodies expressed in HPV-positive cells. The effects of the intracellular expression of specific scFvs (pKDEL and 43M2SD) with localization in the ER are shown in the figure. pKDEL reduces the intracellular levels of E7, thus hampering its effect on cell proliferation. The binding of 43M2SD to E7 inhibits the translocation of the oncoprotein to the cell nucleus. This, in turn, hampers E7-mediated inactivation of Retinoblastoma (pRB), which regulates E2F activity on S-phase genes. The binding of 43M2SD and pKDEL can also inhibit the proteosomal pRB degradation mediated by the Cullin 2-RING ubiquitin ligase complex (CUL2). The effect of intracellular expression of the nB2 nanobody, which inhibits cell proliferation with a mechanism not yet investigated, is also shown in the figure.

More recently, our group selected from a Phage library of human recombinant antibodies, three different scFvs against the 16E7, provided them with signals for localization in the cell nucleus or ER by cloning in eukaryotic vectors, and evidenced their specific and significant antiproliferative effect in HPV16-positive cells in vitro [81]. We also characterized the scFv-binding regions by epitope mapping using immunoassays based on GST-tagged E7 proteins carrying deletions or aminoacid variations. This allowed deciphering E7 regions targeted by scFvs, and revealed that different regions known to be directly involved in transforming activities of E7 are bound by the scFvs. This suggested that different scFvs may be used to target diverse E7 activities [82,83]. We were able to improve the half-life and thermal stability of the most reactive of the anti-16E7 scFvs, scFv43, by site-directed mutagenesis, confirming that small variations in the amino acid sequence can modify the antibody biophysical characteristics [84]. We then provided the modified scFv, namely scFv43M2, with the SEKDEL signal (SD) for localization in the ER and thereafter tested the resulting scFv43M2SD for its ability to counteract the 16E7 activity. In SiHa cells, the intrabody was able to subtract E7 from the usual localization and cause it to accumulate in the ER. In addition, the scFv43M2SD intracellular expression was able to inhibit significantly and specifically the proliferation of different HPV16-positive cell lines [85]. The scFv43M2 was then tested in vivo in mouse HPV tumour models, demonstrating the ability to counteract tumour progression both when administered to tumour cells before their injection into mice and when administered to already implanted tumours [72,85] (Figure 4).

The anti-tumour activity of the anti-16E7 TVG701Y mAb has been described together with the anti-16E6 C1P5 mAb in the previous paragraph, as the two mAbs were utilized in the same study [74] (Figure 4).

5.2.2. Nanobodies

Li et al. selected four VHHs with high affinity for 16E7 from llama libraries by Phage display, and one of these was chosen for further analyses because of lacking Cysteine residues potentially able to form intra-molecular disulphide bonds. The nanobody was expressed in prokaryotic system as a protein, and its ability to bind to the recombinant E7 in vitro was confirmed in immunological assays. Furthermore, the nanobody was able to detect the endogenous E7 protein in Western blotting and, most importantly, induced a specific inhibition of the proliferation of HPV16-positive cells when these cells were transfected with a recombinant eukaryotic plasmid [86] (Figure 5).

5.3. E5-Specific scFvs

In light of the recognized tumourigenic role in the early phases of HPV-induced carcinogenesis and in immunoevasion, E5 protein can be also considered a suitable target for therapeutic purposes, possibly in combination with the main E6 and E7 oncoproteins. Nevertheless, the first and currently only scFv anti-HPV16 E5 (16E5) was developed with the purpose of investigating the E5 functions [87]. Monjarás-Ávila et al. selected this antibody by Phage display technology against the recombinant 16E5 fused to Maltose-binding protein to bypass difficulties due to the E5 hydrophobicity (Figure 6). They then tested this E5-specific scFv in W12 cells, with immortalized keratinocytes carrying up to a maximum of 1000 episomal copies of the HPV16 genome at a low number of passages [88]. The scFv was able to recognize E5 in W12 cells and to reveal its co-localization with EGFR. Therefore, it deserves further investigations to explore its possible application in the therapeutic field.

5.4. E6 and E7-Specific Affibodies

Although they are not properly recombinant antibodies, a mention is deserved by affibodies, a new class of single-domain protein scaffolds based on non-Ig Z domain derived from the staphylococcal protein A. Affibodies are very small molecules (6 kDa) that can be selected against any protein target, and are attracting the attention of the scientific community for biotechnological applications, in particular for in vivo imaging but also for anticancer therapy. Some anti-16E6, -16E7, -18E6, and -18-E7 affibodies were selected and tested successfully both in diagnostic and therapeutic applications [89–91], either as bs affibodies [92] or as fusion with toxins (affitoxins) [93,94].

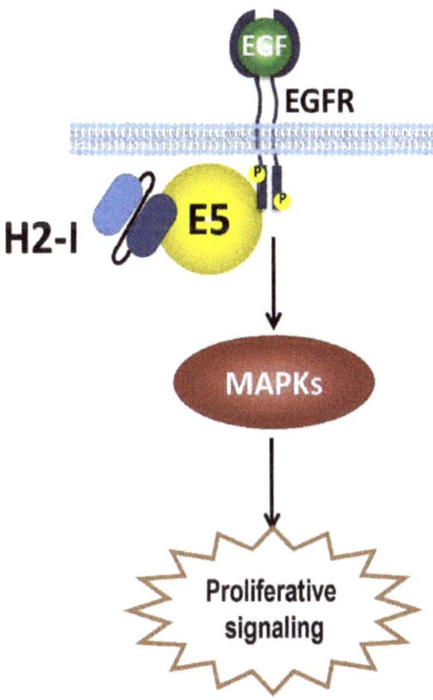

Figure 6. Representation of binding of the H2-I intrabody to E5. The scFv H2-I, when expressed within HPV-positive cells, colocalizes with E5 and its target, the Epidermal Growth Factor Receptor (EGFR), able to activate the mitogen-activated protein kinase (MAPK) signalling cascade, leading to DNA synthesis and cell proliferation.

6. Intracellular Delivery Methods for Recombinant Antibodies against HPV Oncoproteins

In the various experimental contexts described above, recombinant antibodies showed to be effective in hindering the action of the HPV E6 and E7 oncoproteins, thus interfering with the main cancer hallmarks in which they are involved. Despite the safety and benefits of what would be a recombinant antibody-based therapy for HPV-associated lesions, still a low number of Nbs, scFvs, and mAbs against HPV oncoproteins have been developed, and none of them has reached the clinical stage so far. One of the reasons behind this essentially lies in the difficulty of identifying a delivery method that allows recombinant antibodies to cross biological barriers while maintaining biological activity, particularly when the targets are intracellular. In fact, when the target antigens are on the cell plasma membrane, the therapeutic antibodies diffuse in the extracellular environment from the bloodstream to the body tissues until they reach the target. In the case of intracellular targets, the delivery must be made first to the tumour cells, and secondly to the intracellular environment. Several studies are underway to address this criticality and permit translation to humans. In general, recombinant antibodies for intracellular targets can be either expressed within cells from DNA plasmids or delivered directly to cells as purified proteins. This is achievable by physical methods, transfection, electroporation, or fusion with a peptide transduction domain (PTD) or nanocarriers. Delivery as proteins guarantees high safety but implies the need for large quantities of Good Manufacturing Practices (GMP)-grade purified products. Without wishing to be exhaustive since the topic of "delivery" is addressed in more detail elsewhere [95], here we will mention potentially useful methods for the in vivo delivery of therapeutic antibodies against HPV E6, E7, and E5, some of which implement or are alternatives to those already explored for in vitro and in vivo use (Figure 7).

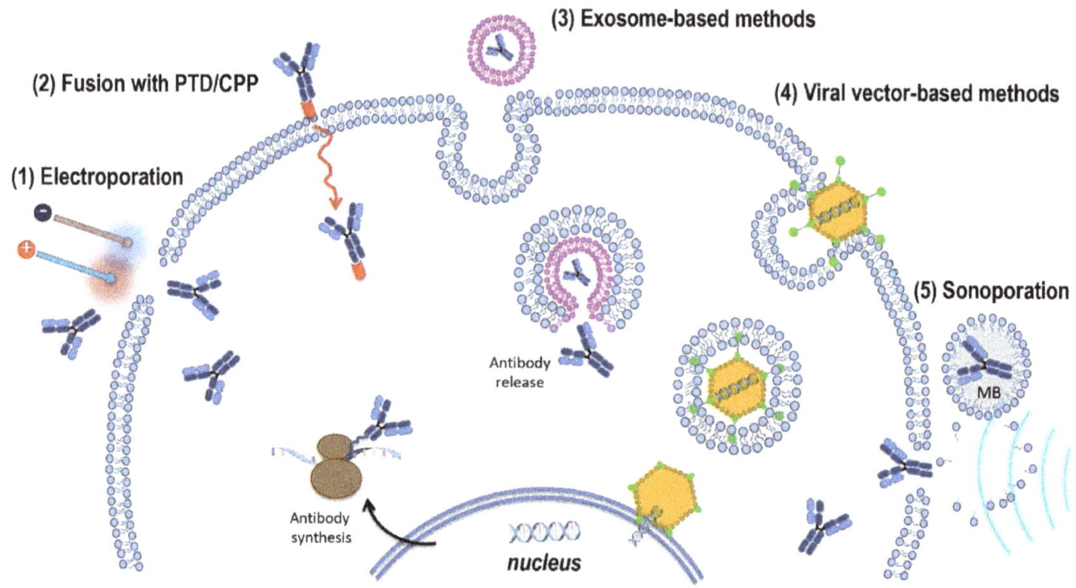

Figure 7. Schematic representation of delivery systems for recombinant antibodies. Some delivery systems already in use or potentially usable for the delivery to cells of mAbs and antibody fragments are illustrated. The mechanisms of cell entry are schematized for: (1) Electroporation; (2) Fusion with protein transduction domains (PTD)/Cell-penetrating peptides (CPP), shown with a red tail; (3) Exosome-based methods (entry by endocytosis is depicted as an example); (4) Viral vector-based methods; and (5). Ultrasound-based methods (sonoporation). MB, microbubbles.

6.1. Electrotransfer/Electroporation

EP applies voltage pulses to generate an electric field between two electrodes, which interrupts the integrity of cell membranes with the formation of pores allowing cell uptake of nucleic acids as well as proteins. EP is therefore a safe method for intracellular protein expression since it avoids insertional mutagenesis and immunogenicity problems inherent in other methods. As such, it can be exploited in a wide range of applications, particularly in immunotherapy [96]. One of the studies reported here used EP to achieve efficient expression of therapeutic scFvs injected as DNA plasmids in HPV-driven tumours [72]. Nevertheless, the methodology could even be used to deliver scFvs as proteins or mRNAs. Indeed, RNA electroporation of hematopoietic cells has been used successfully for two decades [97].

6.2. Fusion with Protein Transduction Domain

PTDs or cell penetrating peptides (CPPs) are cationic and/or hydrophobic 10–30 amino acid long peptides that can be conjugated or fused to antibodies to make them able to penetrate the cell membrane via different mechanisms [98]. However, for effective translation in the clinic, the CPP-based delivery has some limitations to circumvent, mainly due to low in vivo stability and reduced binding capability.

6.3. Exosome-Based Methods

In our laboratories, an exosome-based strategy was recently investigated in vitro for the delivery of one anti-16E7 scFv previously studied, showing promise for translation to humans [99]. The approach relies on the property of a functional defective Nef protein of HIV-1 (Nefmut), acting as an exosome-anchoring protein for proteins fused to its C-terminus. The scFv43M2 delivered to HPV16-positive cells by engineered extracellular vesicles (EVs) carrying the Nefmut/43M2s chimeric product, was able to reproduce the already observed antiproliferative effect of scFv43M2. The proliferation of HPV16-positive cells was hindered also when they were co-cultured in transwells with cells producing EVs uploading the Nefmut/43M2scFv fusion. This result confirmed the ability of therapeutic exosomes to be released and reach other cells, with interesting implications for in vivo translation. The established proof-of-concept that the EV-mediated delivery of scFvs can target intracellular antigens renders it feasible the development of this system for in vivo use. In addition, the possibility to obtain recombinant exosomes from the host following the administration of a genetic construct as a vaccine, suggests a feasible translation to humans of this delivery system for anti-E6 and E7 intrabodies [100]. This would also take advantage of the capacity of the recipient organism to produce the exosomes. Once the technology is optimized, the intramuscular injection of DNA plasmids expressing antibody constructs followed or not by electroporation, will permit the exosome-loaded antibodies to reach several body districts. As the antibodies are specific for the HPV oncoproteins, such broad distribution will not result in off-target effects while potentially affecting any metastatic cells derived from the primary tumour. Of course, further experiments are necessary to clarify the route followed by exosomes loaded with a therapeutic cargo in the recipient organism, and to establish dosages and timing of administration.

6.4. Viral Vector-Based Methods

In the last 30 years, several clinical trials used viral vectors for gene transfer. Gamma-retroviral and lentiviral vectors for haematological cancers; adenoviral vectors for prostate, ovarian and bladder cancer; and adenovirus-associated vectors for pathologies other than cancer were employed with more or less success, and are still the object of preclinical and clinical proof-of-concept studies [101]. Therefore, on the basis of the effective antibody expression achievable in vitro through the transduction of tumour cells with recombinant retroviruses [71,85], and of the advanced state of clinical studies, we believe that viral vectors can be considered a valid resource in addition to the non-viral systems for in vivo antibody delivery. Noteworthy, HPV-associated lesions have a confined localization that renders them accessible to topical therapy whatever the delivery system chosen. Furthermore, the expression of the target oncoproteins being limited to cancer cells represents an additional advantage for the safety of a therapy designed to inhibit protein–protein interactions such as that based on recombinant antibodies.

6.5. Ultrasound-Based Methods

The Ultrasound-mediated targeted delivery (UMTD) is a non-invasive method that is attracting increasing interest for many biochemical applications including immunotherapy of tumours. UMTD combined with microbubbles allows delivery of therapeutic molecules precisely in the tumour site. In fact, oscillation and cavitation of microbubbles under the influence of the acoustic beam causes the reversible formation of localized pores of about 100 nm in diameter in the cell membrane [102]. This phenomenon, known as sonoporation, allows the passive release of therapeutic molecules into target cells. The feasibility and specificity of sonoporation for anti-16E6 mAb delivery to cervical carcinoma cell lines were assessed in the in vitro study outlined above, although the effect obtained was transient and incomplete as it affected p53 levels but did not induce apoptosis [70]. However, the issue of delivery to nucleus, which probably underlies the observed partial efficacy, could be addressed using smaller antibody formats provided with NLS. Sonoporation is increasingly explored for both passive and active immunotherapy in vivo. For example, dendritic cells (DC) sonoporated with antigen mRNA and immunomodulating TriMix mRNA were successful in inhibiting tumour growth in mice [103]. Ultrasound in combination with microbubbles even allowed the Herceptin mAb (trastuzumab) to cross the blood-brain barrier in mice, thus opening up the possibility of treating brain metastases of breast cancer [104]. However, translation of the methodology to human therapy requires further investigation on the possible elicitation of immune response by microbubbles, the exact mechanism of the therapeutic material release, the size-based microbubble capacity of penetrating cell membranes, and the excretion of microbubbles from the body.

7. Conclusions and Perspectives

Currently, recombinant antibodies for targeting antigens involved in the pathogenesis of a variety of diseases are obtainable by robust methodologies of immunization and in vitro screening. Nevertheless, their use as therapeutics may require optimization of crucial characteristics such as binding specificity and affinity, solubility, and pharmacokinetics, as well as setting up an appropriate delivery system. The possibility of designing bs antibodies that combine binding domains from different parental antibodies can expand the binding capacity of a single molecule. Bs antibodies could target at the same time multiple antigens such as E6 and E7, or multiple epitopes on the same antigen (such as DBD and E6AP binding domain on E6) but their solubility and stability may be affected and require corrections [105].

The implementation of therapeutic antibodies is an exciting challenge that can now make use of refined computational methods, allowing to design antibodies with the highest affinity towards antigens of interest [106], to predict the biochemical and biophysical characteristics of specific sequences, and to determine whether they conform well to antibodies that have already reached clinical stage [83]. Given that the global burden of HPV-associated cancers is unacceptably high, major efforts are required for the effective prevention and treatment of these tumours. A therapy for HPV-associated lesions relying on antibodies would present some advantages over more conventional systems of immunization such as, for example, those based on triggering tumour rejection. Specificity is among the main merits, due to the possibility of inhibiting the activity of oncoproteins that are expressed only in tumour cells. A further benefit is that such a therapy, not based on the need to elicit the host immune response, can also be effective in subjects immunosuppressed by natural or induced causes as co-infections or pharmacological treatments. The extraordinary potential of anti-HPV recombinant antibodies makes them key tools in the global strategy of fighting HPV-associated cancers.

Author Contributions: Conceptualization, L.A. and C.A.; methodology, C.A. and L.A.; validation, L.A., C.A., P.D.B. and M.G.D.; formal analysis, C.A.; data curation, L.A., C.A.; writing—original draft preparation, L.A.; writing—review and editing, L.A., C.A., M.G.D., P.D.B., M.V.C.; visualization, C.A.; supervision, L.A. All authors have read and agreed to the published version of the manuscript.

Funding: This research received no external funding.

Conflicts of Interest: The authors declare no conflict of interest.

References

1. Antibody Therapeutics Approved or in Regulatory Review in the EU or US—The Antibody Society. Available online: https://www.antibodysociety.org/resources/approved-antibodies/ (accessed on 7 May 2021).
2. Lu, R.-M.; Hwang, Y.-C.; Liu, I.-J.; Lee, C.-C.; Tsai, H.-Z.; Li, H.-J.; Wu, H.-C. Development of therapeutic antibodies for the treatment of diseases. *J. Biomed. Sci.* **2020**, *27*, 40. [CrossRef]
3. Kaplon, H.; Reichert, J.M. Antibodies to watch in 2021. *MAbs* **2021**, *13*, 1860476. [CrossRef] [PubMed]
4. Arlotta, K.J.; Owen, S.C. Antibody and antibody derivatives as cancer therapeutics. *Wiley Interdiscip. Rev. Nanomed. Nanobiotechnol.* **2019**, *11*, e1556. [CrossRef] [PubMed]
5. Ahamadi-Fesharaki, R.; Fateh, A.; Vaziri, F.; Solgi, G.; Siadat, S.D.; Mahboudi, F.; Rahimi-Jamnani, F. Single-Chain Variable Fragment-Based Bispecific Antibodies: Hitting Two Targets with One Sophisticated Arrow. *Mol. Ther. Oncolytics* **2019**, *14*, 38–56. [CrossRef] [PubMed]
6. Sawant, M.S.; Streu, C.N.; Wu, L.; Tessier, P.M. Toward drug-like multispecific antibodies by design. *Int. J. Mol. Sci.* **2020**, *21*, 7496. [CrossRef] [PubMed]
7. Tiller, K.E.; Tessier, P.M. Advances in Antibody Design. *Annu. Rev. Biomed. Eng.* **2015**, *17*, 191–216. [CrossRef]
8. Visintin, M.; Quondam, M.; Cattaneo, A. The intracellular antibody capture technology: Towards the high-throughput selection of functional intracellular antibodies for target validation. *Methods* **2004**, *34*, 200–214. [CrossRef]
9. Zhang, C.; Ötjengerdes, R.M.; Roewe, J.; Mejias, R.; Marschall, A.L.J. Applying Antibodies Inside Cells: Principles and Recent Advances in Neurobiology, Virology and Oncology. *BioDrugs* **2020**, *34*, 435–462. [CrossRef] [PubMed]

10. Hamers-Casterman, C.T.; Atarhouch, T.; Muyldermans, S.A.; Robinson, G.; Hammers, C.; Songa, E.B.; Bendahman, N.; Hammers, R. Naturally occurring antibodies devoid of light chains. *Nature* **1993**, *363*, 446–448. [CrossRef]
11. Harmsen, M.M.; De Haard, H.J. Properties, production, and applications of camelid single-domain antibody fragments. *Appl. Microbiol. Biotechnol.* **2007**, *77*, 13–22. [CrossRef]
12. Steeland, S.; Vandenbroucke, R.E.; Libert, C. Nanobodies as therapeutics: Big opportunities for small antibodies. *Drug Discov. Today* **2016**, *21*, 1076–1113. [CrossRef]
13. Ackaert, C.; Smiejkowska, N.; Xavier, C.; Sterckx, Y.G.J.; Denies, S.; Stijlemans, B.; Elkrim, Y.; Devoogdt, N.; Caveliers, V.; Lahoutte, T.; et al. Immunogenicity Risk Profile of Nanobodies. *Front. Immunol.* **2021**, *12*, 632687. [CrossRef]
14. Chanier, T.; Chames, P. Nanobody Engineering: Toward Next Generation Immunotherapies and Immunoimaging of Cancer. *Antibodies* **2019**, *8*, 13. [CrossRef]
15. Duggan, S. Caplacizumab: First Global Approval. *Drugs* **2018**, *78*, 1639–1642. [CrossRef]
16. Duggan, S. Correction to: Caplacizumab: First Global Approval. *Drugs* **2018**, *78*, 1955. [CrossRef]
17. De Martel, C.; Plummer, M.; Vignat, J.; Franceschi, S. Worldwide burden of cancer attributable to HPV by site, country and HPV type. *Int. J. Cancer* **2017**, *141*, 664–670. [CrossRef]
18. De Sanjosé, S.; Brotons, M.; Pavón, M.A. The natural history of human papillomavirus infection. *Best Pract. Res. Clin. Obstet. Gynaecol.* **2018**, *47*, 2–13. [CrossRef]
19. De Martel, C.; Georges, D.; Bray, F.; Ferlay, J.; Clifford, G.M. Global burden of cancer attributable to infections in 2018: A worldwide incidence analysis. *Lancet Glob. Health* **2020**, *8*, e180–e190. [CrossRef]
20. Zur Hausen, H. Papillomaviruses in the causation of human cancers—a brief historical account. *Virology* **2009**, *384*, 260–265. [CrossRef] [PubMed]
21. De Sanjose, S.; Quint, W.G.; Alemany, L.; Geraets, D.T.; Klaustermeier, J.E.; Lloveras, B.; Tous, S.; Felix, A.; Bravo, L.E.; Shin, H.R.; et al. Human papillomavirus genotype attribution in invasive cervical cancer: A retrospective cross-sectional worldwide study. *Lancet Oncol.* **2010**, *11*, 1048–1056. [CrossRef]
22. Burger, E.A.; Portnoy, A.; Campos, N.G.; Sy, S.; Regan, C.; Kim, J.J. Choosing the optimal HPV vaccine: The health impact and economic value of the nonavalent and bivalent HPV vaccines in 48 Gavi-eligible countries. *Int. J. Cancer* **2021**, *148*, 932–940. [CrossRef]
23. 73rd World Health Assembly Decisions. Available online: https://www.who.int/news-room/feature-stories/detail/73rd-world-health-assembly-decisions (accessed on 21 May 2021).
24. Garbuglia, A.R.; Lapa, D.; Sias, C.; Capobianchi, M.R.; Del Porto, P. The Use of both Therapeutic and Prophylactic Vaccines in the Therapy of Papillomavirus Disease. *Front. Immunol.* **2020**, *11*, 188. [CrossRef]
25. Rumfield, C.S.; Roller, N.; Pellom, S.T.; Schlom, J.; Jochems, C. Therapeutic Vaccines for HPV-Associated Malignancies. *Immunotargets Ther.* **2020**, *9*, 167–200. [CrossRef]
26. Attademo, L.; Tuninetti, V.; Pisano, C.; Cecere, S.C.; Di Napoli, M.; Tambaro, R.; Valabrega, G.; Musacchio, L.; Setola, S.V.; Piccirillo, P.; et al. Immunotherapy in cervix cancer. *Cancer Treat. Rev.* **2020**, *90*, 102088. [CrossRef] [PubMed]
27. Burley, M.; Roberts, S.; Parish, J.L. Epigenetic regulation of human papillomavirus transcription in the productive virus life cycle. *Semin. Immunopathol.* **2020**, *42*, 159–171. [CrossRef]
28. Hanahan, D.; Weinberg, R.A. Hallmarks of cancer: The next generation. *Cell* **2011**, *144*, 646–674. [CrossRef] [PubMed]
29. Songock, W.K.; Kim, S.M.; Bodily, J.M. The human papillomavirus E7 oncoprotein as a regulator of transcription. *Virus Res.* **2017**, *231*, 56–75. [CrossRef]
30. Ilahi, N.E.; Bhatti, A. Impact of HPV E5 on viral life cycle via EGFR signaling. *Microb. Pathog.* **2020**, *139*, 103923. [CrossRef]
31. Demény, M.A.; Virág, L. The PARP Enzyme Family and the Hallmarks of Cancer Part 1. Cell Intrinsic Hallmarks. *Cancers* **2021**, *13*, 2042. [CrossRef] [PubMed]
32. Martinez-Zapien, D.; Ruiz, F.X.; Poirson, J.; Mitschler, A.; Ramirez, J.; Forster, A.; Cousido-Siah, A.; Masson, M.; Pol, S.V.; Podjarny, A.; et al. Structure of the E6/E6AP/p53 complex required for HPV-mediated degradation of p53. *Nature* **2016**, *529*, 541–545. [CrossRef] [PubMed]
33. Filippova, M.; Parkhurst, L.; Duerksen-Hughes, P.J. The human papillomavirus 16 E6 protein binds to Fas-associated death domain and protects cells from Fas-triggered apoptosis. *J. Biol. Chem.* **2004**, *279*, 25729–25744. [CrossRef] [PubMed]
34. Branca, M.; Giorgi, C.; Santini, D.; Di Bonito, L.; Ciotti, M.; Costa, S.; Benedetto, A.; Casolati, E.A.; Favalli, C.; Paba, P.; et al. Survivin as a marker of cervical intraepithelial neoplasia and high-risk human papillomavirus and a predictor of virus clearance and prognosis in cervical cancer. *Am. J. Clin. Pathol.* **2005**, *124*, 113–121. [CrossRef] [PubMed]
35. Oh, J.M.; Kim, S.H.; Cho, E.A.; Song, Y.S.; Kim, W.H.; Juhnn, Y.S. Human papillomavirus type 16 E5 protein inhibits hydrogen peroxide-induced apoptosis by stimulating ubiquitin-proteasome-mediated degradation of Bax in human cervical cancer cells. *Carcinogenesis* **2010**, *31*, 402–410. [CrossRef] [PubMed]
36. Ashrafi, G.H.; Brown, D.R.; Fife, K.H.; Campo, M.S. Down-regulation of MHC class I is a property common to papillomavirus E5 proteins. *Virus Res.* **2006**, *120*, 208–211. [CrossRef] [PubMed]
37. Yang, W.; Song, Y.; Lu, Y.L.; Sun, J.Z.; Wang, H.W. Increased expression of programmed death (PD)-1 and its ligand PD-L1 correlates with impaired cell-mediated immunity in high-risk human papillomavirus-related cervical intraepithelial neoplasia. *Immunology* **2013**, *139*, 513–522. [CrossRef] [PubMed]

38. Ronco, L.V.; Karpova, A.Y.; Vidal, M.; Howley, P.M. Human papillomavirus 16 E6 oncoprotein binds to interferon regulatory factor-3 and inhibits its transcriptional activity. *Genes Dev.* **1998**, *12*, 2061–2072. [CrossRef]
39. Li, S.; Labrecque, S.; Gauzzi, M.C.; Cuddihy, A.R.; Wong, A.H.; Pellegrini, S.; Matlashewski, G.J.; Koromilas, A.E. The human papilloma virus (HPV)-18 E6 oncoprotein physically associates with Tyk2 and impairs Jak-STAT activation by interferon-α. *Oncogene* **1999**, *18*, 5727–5737. [CrossRef]
40. Park, J.S.; Kim, E.-J.; Kwon, H.-J.; Hwang, E.-S.; Namkoong, S.-E.; Um, S.-J. Inactivation of Interferon Regulatory Factor-1 Tumour Suppressor Protein by HPV E7 Oncoprotein. Implication for the E7-mediated immune evasion mechanism in cervical carcinogenesis. *J. Biol. Chem.* **2000**, *275*, 6764–6769. [CrossRef]
41. Hasan, U.A.; Bates, E.; Takeshita, F.; Biliato, A.; Accardi, R.; Bouvard, V.; Mansour, M.; Vincent, I.; Gissmann, L.; Iftner, T.; et al. TLR9 Expression and Function Is Abolished by the Cervical Cancer-Associated Human Papillomavirus Type 16. *J. Immunol.* **2007**, *178*, 3186–3197. [CrossRef]
42. Klingelhutz, A.J.; Foster, S.A.; McDougall, J.K. Telomerase activation by the E6 gene product of human papillomavirus type 16. *Nature* **1996**, *380*, 79–82. [CrossRef]
43. Gewin, L.; Myers, H.; Kiyono, T.; Galloway, D.A. Identification of a novel telomerase repressor that interacts with the human papillomavirus type-16 E6/E6-AP complex. *Genes Dev.* **2004**, *18*, 2269–2282. [CrossRef]
44. Zhang, Y.; Dakic, A.; Chen, R.; Dai, Y.; Schlegel, R.; Liu, X. Direct HPV E6/Myc Interactions Induce Histone Modifications, Pol II Phosphorylation, and HTERT Promoter Activation. *Oncotarget* **2017**, *8*, 96323–96339. [CrossRef]
45. López-Ocejo, O.; Viloria-Petit, A.; Bequet-Romero, M.; Mukhopadhyay, D.; Rak, J.; Kerbel, R.S. Oncogenes and tumour angiogenesis: The HPV-16 E6 oncoprotein activates the vascular endothelial growth factor (VEGF) gene promoter in a p53 independent manner. *Oncogene* **2000**, *19*, 4611–4620. [CrossRef]
46. Stanelle, J.; Stiewe, T.; Theseling, C.C.; Peter, M.; Pützer, B.M. Gene expression changes in response to E2F1 activation. *Nucleic Acids Res.* **2002**, *30*, 1859–1867. [CrossRef]
47. Schaal, C.; Pillai, S.; Chellappan, S.P. The Rb-E2F transcriptional regulatory pathway in tumour angiogenesis and metastasis. In *Advances in Cancer Research*; Academic Press Inc.: San Diego, CA, USA, 2014; Volume 121, pp. 147–182. [CrossRef]
48. Toussaint-Smith, E.; Donner, D.B.; Roman, A. Expression of Human Papillomavirus Type 16 E6 and E7 Oncoproteins in Primary Foreskin Keratinocytes Is Sufficient to Alter the Expression of Angiogenic Factors. *Oncogene* **2004**, *23*, 2988–2995. [CrossRef]
49. Martínez-Ramírez, I.; Carrillo-García, A.; Contreras-Paredes, A.; Ortiz-Sánchez, E.; Cruz-Gregorio, A.; Lizano, M. Regulation of cellular metabolism by high-risk human papillomaviruses. *Int. J. Mol. Sci.* **2018**, *19*, 1839. [CrossRef]
50. Vande Pol, S.B.; Klingelhutz, A.J. Papillomavirus E6 oncoproteins. *Virology* **2013**, *445*, 115–137. [CrossRef] [PubMed]
51. Ganti, K.; Broniarczyk, J.; Manoubi, W.; Massimi, P.; Mittal, S.; Pim, D.; Szalmas, A.; Thatte, J.; Thomas, M.; Tomaić, V.; et al. The Human papillomaviruses and the specificity of PDZ domain targeting. *Viruses* **2015**, *7*, 3530–3537. [CrossRef] [PubMed]
52. Zhu, D.; Ye, M.; Zhang, W. E6/E7 oncoproteins of high risk HPV-16 upregulate MT1-MMP, MMP-2 and MMP-9 and promote the migration of cervical cancer cells. *Int. J. Clin. Exp. Pathol.* **2015**, *8*, 4981–4989. [PubMed]
53. D'Costa, Z.J.; Jolly, C.; Androphy, E.J.; Mercer, A.; Matthews, C.M.; Hibma, M.H. Transcriptional Repression of E-Cadherin by Human Papillomavirus Type 16 E6. *PLoS ONE* **2012**, *7*, e48954. [CrossRef]
54. Laurson, J.; Khan, S.; Chung, R.; Cross, K.; Raj, K. Epigenetic repression of E-cadherin by human papillomavirus 16 E7 protein. *Carcinogenesis* **2010**, *31*, 918–926. [CrossRef]
55. Cheng, Y.M.; Chou, C.Y.; Hsu, Y.C.; Chen, M.J.; Wing, L.Y.C. The role of human papillomavirus type 16 E6/E7 oncoproteins in cervical epithelial-mesenchymal transition and carcinogenesis. *Oncol. Lett.* **2012**, *3*, 667–671. [CrossRef]
56. Scott, M.L.; Coleman, D.T.; Kelly, K.C.; Carroll, J.L.; Woodby, B.; Songock, W.K.; Cardelli, J.A.; Bodily, J.M. Human papillomavirus type 16 E5-mediated upregulation of Met in human keratinocytes. *Virology* **2018**, *519*, 1–11. [CrossRef] [PubMed]
57. Nguyen, C.L.; Eichwald, C.; Nibert, M.L.; Münger, K. Human Papillomavirus Type 16 E7 Oncoprotein Associates with the Centrosomal Component γ-Tubulin. *J. Virol.* **2007**, *81*, 13533–13543. [CrossRef] [PubMed]
58. Duensing, A.; Spardy, N.; Chatterjee, P.; Zheng, L.; Parry, J.; Cuevas, R.; Korzeniewski, N.; Duensing, S. Centrosome overduplication, chromosomal instability, and human papillomavirus oncoproteins. *Environ. Mol. Mutagen.* **2009**, *50*, 741–747. [CrossRef]
59. Vieira, V.C.; Leonard, B.; White, E.A.; Starrett, G.J.; Temiz, N.A.; Lorenz, L.D.; Lee, D.; Soares, M.A.; Lambert, P.F.; Howley, P.; et al. Human papillomavirus E6 triggers upregulation of the antiviral and cancer genomic DNA deaminase APOBEC3B. *MBio* **2014**, *5*, e02234-14. [CrossRef]
60. Durzynska, J.; Lesniewicz, K.; Poreba, E. Human papillomaviruses in epigenetic regulations. *Mutat. Res. Rev. Mutat. Res.* **2017**, *772*, 36–50. [CrossRef]
61. Boccardo, E.; Lepique, A.P.; Villa, L.L. The role of inflammation in HPV carcinogenesis. *Carcinogenesis* **2010**, *31*, 1905–1912. [CrossRef] [PubMed]
62. Hemmat, N.; Bannazadeh Baghi, H. Association of Human Papillomavirus Infection and Inflammation in Cervical Cancer. *Pathog. Dis.* **2019**, *77*, ftz048. [CrossRef] [PubMed]
63. Estêvão, D.; Costa, N.R.; Gil da Costa, R.M.; Medeiros, R. Hallmarks of HPV carcinogenesis: The role of E6, E7 and E5 oncoproteins in cellular malignancy. *Biochim. Biophys. Acta Gene Regul. Mech.* **2019**, *1862*, 153–162. [CrossRef]
64. Kumar, A.; Rathi, E.; Hariharapura, R.C.; Kini, S.G. Is viral E6 oncoprotein a viable target? A critical analysis in the context of cervical cancer. *Med. Res. Rev.* **2020**, *40*, 2019–2048. [CrossRef]

65. Giovane, C.; Travé, G.; Briones, A.; Lutz, Y.; Wasylyk, B.; Weiss, E. Targetting of the N-terminal domain of the human papillomavirus type 16 E6 oncoprotein with monomeric ScFvs blocks the E6-mediated degradation of cellular p53. *J. Mol. Recognit.* **1999**, *12*, 141–152. [CrossRef]
66. Lagrange, M.; Charbonnier, S.; Orfanoudakis, G.; Robinson, P.; Zanier, K.; Masson, M.; Lutz, Y.; Trave, G.; Weiss, E.; De Ryckere, F. Binding of human papillomavirus 16 E6 to p53 and E6AP is impaired by monoclonal antibodies directed against the second zinc-binding domain of E6. *J. Gen. Virol.* **2005**, *86*, 1001–1007. [CrossRef] [PubMed]
67. Lagrange, M.; Boulade-Ladame, C.; Mailly, L.; Weiss, E.; Orfanoudakis, G.; DeRyckere, F. Intracellular scFvs against the viral E6 oncoprotein provoke apoptosis in human papillomavirus-positive cancer cells. *Biochem. Biophys. Res. Commun.* **2007**, *361*, 487–492. [CrossRef] [PubMed]
68. Courtête, J.; Sibler, A.-P.; Zeder-Lutz, G.; Dalkara, D.; Oulad-Abdelghani, M.; Zuber, G.; Weiss, E. Suppression of cervical carcinoma cell growth by intracytoplasmic codelivery of anti-oncoprotein E6 antibody and small interfering RNA. *Mol. Cancer Ther.* **2007**, *6*, 1728–1735. [CrossRef] [PubMed]
69. Griffin, H.; Elston, R.; Jackson, D.; Ansell, K.; Coleman, M.; Winter, G.; Doorbar, J. Inhibition of papillomavirus protein function in cervical cancer cells by intrabody targeting. *J. Mol. Biol.* **2006**, *355*, 360–378. [CrossRef] [PubMed]
70. Togtema, M.; Pichardo, S.; Jackson, R.; Lambert, P.F.; Curiel, L.; Zehbe, I. Sonoporation Delivery of Monoclonal Antibodies against Human Papillomavirus 16 E6 Restores p53 Expression in Transformed Cervical Keratinocytes. *PLoS ONE* **2012**, *7*, e50730. [CrossRef]
71. Amici, C.; Visintin, M.; Verachi, F.; Paolini, F.; Percario, Z.; Di Bonito, P.; Mandarino, A.; Affabris, E.; Venuti, A.; Accardi, L. A novel intracellular antibody against the E6 oncoprotein impairs growth of human papillomavirus 16-positive tumour cells in mouse models. *Oncotarget* **2016**, *7*, 15539–15553. [CrossRef]
72. Paolini, F.; Amici, C.; Carosi, M.; Bonomo, C.; Di Bonito, P.; Venuti, A.; Accardi, L. Intrabodies targeting human papillomavirus 16 E6 and E7 oncoproteins for therapy of established HPV-associated tumours. *J. Exp. Clin. Cancer Res.* **2021**, *40*, 37. [CrossRef]
73. Verachi, F.; Percario, Z.; Di Bonito, P.; Affabris, E.; Amici, C.; Accardi, L. Purification and Characterization of Antibodies in Single-Chain Format against the E6 Oncoprotein of Human Papillomavirus Type 16. *Biomed. Res. Int.* **2018**, *2018*, 6583852. [CrossRef]
74. Jiang, Z.; Albanese, J.; Kesterson, J.; Warrick, J.; Karabakhtsian, R.; Dadachova, E.; Phaëton, R. Monoclonal Antibodies Against Human Papillomavirus E6 and E7 Oncoproteins Inhibit Tumour Growth in Experimental Cervical Cancer. *Transl. Oncol.* **2019**, *12*, 1289–1295. [CrossRef] [PubMed]
75. Masson, M.; Hindelang, C.; Sibler, A.P.; Schwalbach, G.; Travé, G.; Weiss, E. Preferential nuclear localization of the human papillomavirus type 16 E6 oncoprotein in cervical carcinoma cells. *J. Gen. Virol.* **2003**, *84*, 2099–2104. [CrossRef] [PubMed]
76. Togtema, M.; Hussack, G.; Dayer, G.; Teghtmeyer, M.R.; Raphael, S.; Tanha, J.; Zehbe, I. Single-domain antibodies represent novel alternatives to monoclonal antibodies as targeting agents against the human papillomavirus 16 E6 protein. *Int. J. Mol. Sci.* **2019**, *20*, 2088. [CrossRef]
77. Zhang, W.; Shan, H.; Jiang, K.; Huang, W.; Li, S. A novel intracellular nanobody against HPV16 E6 oncoprotein. *Clin. Immunol.* **2021**, *225*, 108684. [CrossRef] [PubMed]
78. Celegato, M.; Messa, L.; Goracci, L.; Mercorelli, B.; Bertagnin, C.; Spyrakis, F.; Suarez, I.; Cousido-Siah, A.; Travé, G.; Banks, L.; et al. A novel small-molecule inhibitor of the human papillomavirus E6-p53 interaction that reactivates p53 function and blocks cancer cells growth. *Cancer Lett.* **2020**, *470*, 115–125. [CrossRef]
79. Pal, A.; Kundu, R. Human Papillomavirus E6 and E7: The Cervical Cancer Hallmarks and Targets for Therapy. *Front. Microbiol.* **2020**, *10*, 3116. [CrossRef]
80. Wang-Johanning, F.; Gillespie, G.Y.; Grim, J.; Rancourt, C.; Alvarez, R.D.; Siegal, G.P.; Curiel, D.T. Intracellular Expression of a Single-Chain Antibody Directed against Human Papillomavirus Type 16 E7 Oncoprotein Achieves Targeted Antineoplastic Effects. *Cancer Res.* **1998**, *58*, 1893–1900.
81. Accardi, L.; Donà, M.G.; Di Bonito, P.; Giorgi, C. Intracellular anti-E7 human antibodies in single-chain format inhibit proliferation of HPV16-positive cervical carcinoma cells. *Int. J. Cancer* **2005**, *116*, 564–570. [CrossRef]
82. Accardi, L.; Donà, M.G.; Mileo, A.M.; Paggi, M.G.; Federico, A.; Torreri, P.; Petrucci, T.C.; Accardi, R.; Pim, D.; Tommasino, M.; et al. Retinoblastoma-independent antiproliferative activity of novel intracellular antibodies against the E7 oncoprotein in HPV 16-positive cells. *BMC Cancer* **2011**, *11*, 17. [CrossRef]
83. Amici, C.; Donà, M.G.; Chirullo, B.; Di Bonito, P.; Accardi, L. Epitope Mapping and Computational Analysis of Anti-HPV16 E6 and E7 Antibodies in Single-Chain Format for Clinical Development as Antitumour Drugs. *Cancers* **2020**, *12*, 1803. [CrossRef]
84. Donà, M.G.; Giorgi, C.; Accardi, L. Characterization of antibodies in single-chain format against the E7 oncoprotein of the Human papillomavirus type 16 and their improvement by mutagenesis. *BMC Cancer* **2007**, *7*, 25. [CrossRef] [PubMed]
85. Accardi, L.; Paolini, F.; Mandarino, A.; Percario, Z.; Di Bonito, P.; Di Carlo, V.; Affabris, E.; Giorgi, C.; Amici, C.; Venuti, A. In vivo antitumour effect of an intracellular single-chain antibody fragment against the E7 oncoprotein of human papillomavirus 16. *Int. J. Cancer* **2014**, *134*, 2472–2477. [CrossRef] [PubMed]
86. Li, S.; Zhang, W.; Jiang, K.; Shan, H.; Shi, M.; Chen, B.; Hua, Z. Nanobody against the E7 oncoprotein of human papillomavirus 16. *Mol. Immunol.* **2019**, *109*, 12–19. [CrossRef] [PubMed]
87. Monjarás-Ávila, C.; Bernal-Silva, S.; Bach, H. Development of Novel Single-Chain Antibodies against the Hydrophobic HPV-16 E5 Protein. *Biomed. Res. Int.* **2018**, *2018*, 5809028. [CrossRef]

88. Stanley, M.A.; Browne, H.M.; Appleby, M.; Minson, A.C. Properties of a non-tumourigenic human cervical keratinocyte cell line. *Int. J. Cancer* **1989**, *43*, 672–676. [CrossRef]
89. Xue, X.; Wang, B.; Du, W.; Zhang, C.; Song, Y.; Cai, Y.; Cen, D.; Wang, L.; Xiong, Y.; Jiang, P.; et al. Generation of affibody molecules specific for HPV16 E7 recognition. *Oncotarget* **2016**, *7*, 73995–74005. [CrossRef]
90. Wang, L.; Du, W.; Zhu, S.; Jiang, P.; Zhang, L. A high-risk papillomavirus 18 E7 affibody-enabled in vivo imaging and targeted therapy of cervical cancer. *Appl. Microbiol. Biotechnol.* **2019**, *103*, 3049–3059. [CrossRef]
91. Zhu, J.; Kamara, S.; Wang, Q.; Guo, Y.; Li, Q.; Wang, L.; Chen, J.; Du, Q.; Du, W.; Chen, S.; et al. Novel affibody molecules targeting the HPV16 E6 oncoprotein inhibited the proliferation of cervical cancer cells. *Front. Cell Dev. Biol.* **2021**, *9*, 1150. [CrossRef] [PubMed]
92. Zhu, S.; Zhu, J.; Song, Y.; Chen, J.; Wang, L.; Zhou, M.; Jiang, P.; Li, W.; Xue, X.; Zhao, K.-N.; et al. Bispecific affibody molecule targeting HPV16 and HPV18E7 oncoproteins for enhanced molecular imaging of cervical cancer. *Appl. Microbiol. Biotechnol.* **2018**, *102*, 7429–7439. [CrossRef]
93. Jiang, P.; Wang, L.; Hou, B.; Zhu, J.; Zhou, M.; Jiang, J.; Wang, L.; Chen, S.; Zhu, S.; Chen, J.; et al. A novel HPV16 E7-affitoxin for targeted therapy of HPV16-induced human cervical cancer. *Theranostics* **2018**, *8*, 3544–3558. [CrossRef]
94. Wang, W.; Tan, X.; Jiang, J.; Cai, Y.; Feng, F.; Zhang, L.; Li, W. Targeted biological effect of an affitoxin composed of an HPV16E7 affibody fused with granzyme B (ZHPV16E7-GrB) against cervical cancer in vitro and in vivo. *Curr. Cancer Drug Targets* **2020**, *21*, 232–243. [CrossRef]
95. Slastnikova, T.A.; Ulasov, A.V.; Rosenkranz, A.A.; Sobolev, A.S. Targeted intracellular delivery of antibodies: The state of the art. *Front. Pharmacol.* **2018**, *9*, 1208. [CrossRef]
96. Meijerink, M.R.; Scheffer, H.J.; Naranayan, G. *Irreversible Electroporation in Clinical Practice*; Springer International Publishing: New York, NY, USA, 2017. [CrossRef]
97. Van Tendeloo, V.; Ponsaerts, P.; Lardon, F.; Nijs, G.; Lenjou, M.; Van Broeckhoven, C.; Van Bockstaele, D.R.; Berneman, Z.N. Highly efficient gene delivery by mRNA electroporation in human hematopoietic cells: Superiority to lipofection and passive pulsing of mRNA and to electroporation of plasmid cDNA for tumour antigen loading of dendritic cells. *Blood* **2001**, *98*, 49–56. [CrossRef]
98. Kardani, K.; Milani, A.; Shabani, S.H.; Bolhassani, A. Cell penetrating peptides: The potent multi-cargo intracellular carriers. *Expert Opin. Drug Deliv.* **2019**, *16*, 1227–1258. [CrossRef] [PubMed]
99. Ferrantelli, F.; Arenaccio, C.; Manfredi, F.; Olivetta, E.; Chiozzini, C.; Leone, P.; Percario, Z.; Ascione, A.; Flego, M.; Di Bonito, P.; et al. The intracellular delivery of anti-HPV16 E7 scFvs through engineered extracellular vesicles inhibits the proliferation of HPV-infected cells. *Int. J. Nanomed.* **2019**, *14*, 8755–8768. [CrossRef] [PubMed]
100. Di Bonito, P.; Chiozzini, C.; Arenaccio, C.; Anticoli, S.; Manfredi, F.; Olivetta, E.; Ferrantelli, F.; Falcone, E.; Ruggieri, A.; Federico, M. Antitumour HPV E7-specific CTL activity elicited by in vivo engineered exosomes produced through DNA inoculation. *Int. J. Nanomed.* **2017**, *12*, 4579–4591. [CrossRef] [PubMed]
101. Keeler, A.M.; ElMallah, M.K.; Flotte, T.R. Gene Therapy 2017: Progress and Future Directions. *Clin. Transl. Sci.* **2017**, *10*, 242–248. [CrossRef]
102. Tian, Y.; Liu, Z.; Tan, H.; Hou, J.; Wen, X.; Yang, F.; Cheng, W. New aspects of ultrasound-mediated targeted delivery and therapy for cancer. *Int. J. Nanomed.* **2020**, *15*, 401–418. [CrossRef]
103. Dewitte, H.; Van Lint, S.; Heirman, C.; Thielemans, K.; De Smedt, S.; Breckpot, K.; Lentacker, I. The potential of antigen and TriMix sonoporation using mRNA-loaded microbubbles for ultrasound-triggered cancer immunotherapy. *J. Control. Release* **2014**, *194*, 28–36. [CrossRef]
104. Kinoshita, M.; McDannold, N.; Jolesz, F.A.; Hynynen, K. Noninvasive localized delivery of Herceptin to the mouse brain by MRI-guided focused ultrasound-induced blood-brain barrier disruption. *Proc. Natl. Acad. Sci. USA* **2006**, *103*, 11719–11723. [CrossRef]
105. Chen, S.; Li, L.; Zhang, F.; Wang, Y.; Hu, Y.; Zhao, L. Immunoglobulin Gamma-Like Therapeutic Bispecific Antibody Formats for Tumour Therapy. *J. Immunol. Res.* **2019**, *2019*, 4516041. [CrossRef] [PubMed]
106. Adolf-Bryfogle, J.; Kalyuzhniy, O.; Kubitz, M.; Weitzner, B.D.; Hu, X.; Adachi, Y.; Schief, W.; Dunbrack, R.L., Jr. RosettaAntibodyDesign (RAbD): A general framework for computational antibody design. *PLoS Comput. Biol.* **2018**, *14*, e1006112. [CrossRef] [PubMed]

International Journal of
Molecular Sciences

MDPI

Review

Brain Disposition of Antibody-Based Therapeutics: Dogma, Approaches and Perspectives

Aida Kouhi, Vyshnavi Pachipulusu, Talya Kapenstein, Peisheng Hu, Alan L. Epstein and Leslie A. Khawli *

Department of Pathology, Keck School of Medicine of University of Southern California,
Los Angeles, CA 90033, USA; kouhi@usc.edu (A.K.); pachipul@usc.edu (V.P.); talya.kapenstein@gmail.com (T.K.); peisheng@usc.edu (P.H.); aepstein@usc.edu (A.L.E.)
* Correspondence: lkhawli@usc.edu

Abstract: Due to their high specificity, monoclonal antibodies have been widely investigated for their application in drug delivery to the central nervous system (CNS) for the treatment of neurological diseases such as stroke, Alzheimer's, and Parkinson's disease. Research in the past few decades has revealed that one of the biggest challenges in the development of antibodies for drug delivery to the CNS is the presence of blood–brain barrier (BBB), which acts to restrict drug delivery and contributes to the limited uptake (0.1–0.2% of injected dose) of circulating antibodies into the brain. This article reviews the various methods currently used for antibody delivery to the CNS at the preclinical stage of development and the underlying mechanisms of BBB penetration. It also describes efforts to improve or modulate the physicochemical and biochemical properties of antibodies (e.g., charge, Fc receptor binding affinity, and target affinity), to adapt their pharmacokinetics (PK), and to influence their distribution and disposition into the brain. Finally, a distinction is made between approaches that seek to modify BBB permeability and those that use a physiological approach or antibody engineering to increase uptake in the CNS. Although there are currently inherent difficulties in developing safe and efficacious antibodies that will cross the BBB, the future prospects of brain-targeted delivery of antibody-based agents are believed to be excellent.

Keywords: blood–brain barrier; antibody; pharmacokinetics; disposition; biochemical and physicochemical properties; Fc binding; receptor-mediated transcytosis; brain shuttle; molecular Trojan horse; transferrin

Citation: Kouhi, A.; Pachipulusu, V.; Kapenstein, T.; Hu, P.; Epstein, A.L.; Khawli, L.A. Brain Disposition of Antibody-Based Therapeutics: Dogma, Approaches and Perspectives. *Int. J. Mol. Sci.* **2021**, *22*, 6442. https://doi.org/10.3390/ijms22126442

Academic Editor: Yong-Seok Heo

Received: 18 May 2021
Accepted: 11 June 2021
Published: 16 June 2021

1. Introduction

Drug uptake into the brain is quite challenging, although not impossible [1]. Since the brain is located in a non-expandable vault (cranium) and is very sensitive to pressure and the environment, cerebrospinal fluid (CSF) flow in and out of the brain is highly regulated and controls the selective uptake of key nutrients and fluid to maintain normal brain function. This regulation also includes the passage of large molecules such as immunoglobulin thereby accounting for the observed difficulties of targeting the central nervous system (CNS) with therapeutic proteins and reagents. Many potentially useful drugs, which, because of their low entrance into the CNS, are not being used to treat brain disease. This lack of access to the brain has been described as a major hurdle in the development of large biomolecules and a reason given for their comparatively long development times and high failure rate [2]. As a consequence, several approaches are currently being investigated to enhance the CNS delivery of various types of large biomolecules, such as antibodies, recombinant proteins, gene vectors, liposomes, and nanoparticles (Table 1). To evaluate CNS delivery, quantitative measurements are used to understand better and potentially even improve upon methods for the targeted delivery of antibody-based therapeutics across the BBB. In particular, scientific and technological advancements that focus on evaluating methods for altering antibody penetration and distribution in the brain have not yet been developed adequately to treat neurological diseases. Moreover, even if candidate antibodies for the therapy of CNS diseases may be already available, they cannot currently be utilized because of their poor blood-to-brain penetration due to the presence of the tight-junctioned BBB preventing the passage of antibodies [3]. Thus, increased attention is being placed on novel antibodies capable of successfully enhancing brain tissue concentration as well as targeting specific disease regions within the CNS [4,5]. If proven safe and effective, these new technologies could represent the future of antibody therapy in the treatment of neurologic diseases.

Table 1. Overview of large biomolecules in current preclinical development for enhanced delivery across the BBB. Part of this table is reproduced from Tucker (2011) with permission of the copyright owner [1].

	Key Classes and Functions of Biomolecules
1.	Single-domain brain-targeting antibody fragments derived from llama antibodies; led to discovery of TMEM30A, a selective BBB receptor [6,7]
2.	RMT delivery of decoy receptor antibodies facilitated by fusion with an antibody to any BBB receptor leading to an elevation of drug concentration in the brain [8]
3.	Bidirectional vectors, comprising one part for entry into brain by RMT and a second part to exit the brain via a second receptor-mediated BBB transport system [8]
4.	Fusion antibodies for bi-directional transport across the BBB [8]
5.	Delivery of a drug to the brain via a drug-loaded liposome decorated with appropriate vectors [7]
6.	Synthetic low-density lipoprotein (LDL) containing cloned apolipoprotein (Apo E), for delivery of a drug across the BBB [9]
7.	Liposome and poly(lactic-co-glycolic acid) (PLGA) nanoparticles coated with specified surfactants and loaded with drug for delivery across the BBB [9]
8.	Nanoparticles with covalently coupled Apo E for delivery across the BBB [9]
9.	A combination product comprising drug and apolipoprotein for delivery of drug to the brain and where the drug and lipoprotein can be delivered simultaneously, separately, or sequentially by intravenous injection [10]
10.	Conjugates of drug with specified polypeptides derived from aprotinin, designed to increase the potency or modify the pharmacokinetics of the drug [11]
11.	Conjugates of nucleic molecules and specified polypeptides from aprotinin for delivery across the BBB [11,12]
12.	Specified peptides from the rabies virus glycoprotein (RVG) linked to a carrier that contains the drug for delivery across the BBB [6,13]
13.	A conjugate comprising an antiviral agent with a CRM197 ligand for a receptor [7,14]

Here, we review some of the most important principles and multiple strategies for enhancing antibody delivery to the brain and discuss how they can be applied to the pre-clinical development of CNS therapeutics. The guiding principles and knowledge gained from preclinical evaluation of these different strategies for CNS-targeting antibodies that are currently under development are also discussed, with a particular emphasis on pharmacokinetic (PK) and disposition properties. In addition, this review includes a brief description of the physicochemical and biochemical interactions between antibodies and biological matrices. As such, focus is given to defining the general properties of antibodies, their similarities and differences with regard to charge, neonatal Fc receptor (FcRn) binding, and target affinity. These types of studies provide scientists with the knowledge necessary to select the appropriate antibody characteristics to maximize brain exposure, which in turn, could provide better efficacy of their product. Finally, an improved understanding of the effects of these critical characteristics may allow for the better design of novel antibody therapeutics with unique and useful properties that conceptually are able to efficiently cross the BBB [5]. Hence, the objective of this review was to describe the progress of antibody-based drugs and highlight the principles and existing approaches for enhancing their entrance into the brain to achieve a desirable concentration range for the therapy of CNS disease.

2. Delivery of Antibodies into the Brain: Mechanism of Delivery

Diseases of the CNS are in need of effective biotherapeutics. However, the CNS has been considered off-limits to antibody therapeutics because of the presence of the BBB, which separates the circulating blood from the brain and extracellular fluid in the CNS to prevent brain uptake of most large molecules [11,15]. Recent advances in preclinical and clinical drug development suggest that antibodies can cross the BBB in limited quantities and act centrally to mediate their effects [4]. In particular, immunotherapy studies of AD have shown that targeting beta amyloid with antibodies can reduce disease pathology in both mouse models and patients, with strong evidence supporting a central mechanism of action.

2.1. Physiology and Barriers of the CNS

The arrangement of cells at the interface between the blood and the CNS restricts both the paracellular and transcellular diffusion of hydrophilic and hydrophobic substances into the CNS [16]. The blood–brain barrier (BBB) is used to describe the barrier between the blood and the brain and spinal cord parenchyma proper. At this interface, cerebral microvessels, lined with endothelial cells, limit the passage of small molecules from the blood into the brain or spinal cord [11]. Microvascular endothelial cells make up a large portion of the brain's surface area, which helps account for its ability to restrict the flow of substances into the brain [17]. A second barrier, referred to as the blood–CSF barrier, exists between the blood and the ventricular CSF. Formed by CSF producing tight-junctioned epithelium of the choroid plexuses, this epithelial cell barrier accounts for a significant surface area of exchange [16]. Additionally, the blood flow rate within the choroid plexuses is higher than any other brain structures, and therefore, the blood flow through these areas significantly contributes to exchanges between the blood and the CNS. A third barrier to the CNS is the arachoid membrane, which completely encircles the CNS and separates the subarachnoid CSF from the bones and *dura mater* extracellular fluids [16,18]. These three barriers to the CNS work to manage the traffic of small and large molecules from the blood into the brain.

2.2. BBB Structure

As described above, the BBB consists of the network of cells that communicate and associate together to form a barrier between the interstitial fluid of the brain and circulating blood. A thin monolayer of brain microvascular endothelial cells (BMECs) joined together by tight junction forms the physical BBB. The BMECs are supported by the capillary basement membrane, pericytes, astrocytes, and microglial cells. It is the interaction of the BMECs with these other cell types that creates the specific brain microvascular network. The tight junctions are responsible for the selective permeability of the BBB, as they seal the apical region of the endothelial cells together and restrict the entrance of hydrophilic drugs into the brain. Additionally, actin filaments, such as cadherins and catenins, arranged below the tight junctions, link together to form a band of adherence junctions. These adherence junctions contribute to the brain barrier, and also, among other roles, they promote BMECs adhesions, cell polarity, and control paracellular permeability regulations. It is the dynamic interaction between the tight junctions and the adhesion junctions and the other cellular components of the BBB via signaling pathways that regulate the BBB's permeability. The arrangement of cells that form the BBB allow it to have uniform thickness, a negative surface charge, little pinocytotic activity, and no fenestrae [19].

2.3. Pharmacokinetics and CNS Distribution of Antibodies

The PK properties of therapeutic antibodies are an essential factor that determine their in vivo efficacy by impacting their biodistribution and have been extensively studied in recent years [20]. The processes that govern the biodistribution of therapeutic antibodies depends on the species they are administered to and on the properties of the antibody itself. While physiological conditions are frequently constant, various properties of a therapeutic antibody such as its charge or size can be modified during development in order to optimize its PK behavior. Structural modifications such as glycosylation can also impact the biodistribution of an antibody. Of particular importance, however, is the role of FcRn on PK properties of an antibody, which must be considered in designing therapeutic antibodies for neurological disorders. FcRn is a receptor that is highly expressed in various tissues and prolongs an IgG antibody's half-life by protecting it from lysosomal degradation. It has been reported that the receptor contributes to the efflux of IgG therapeutic antibodies at the BBB and can reduce brain uptake following administration despite prolonging its half-life. The crucial role of FcRn on the CNS distribution behavior of antibodies is further discussed in Section 4.

2.4. Mechanisms of Antibody Passage Across the BBB

In the past few decades, various transport mechanisms have been identified as major pathways for macromolecules to cross the BBB. Generally, approximately 0.1% of circulating antibodies enter the brain. Mechanisms in play include: i) Adsorptive-mediated endocytosis; (ii) Carrier-mediated transport; and (iii) Receptor-mediated transcytosis.

(i) Adsorptive-mediated endocytosis (AMT) is a mechanism of BBB transport that relies on an electrostatic interaction between a cationic molecule in the circulation and the negatively charged cell membrane at the BBB, which will in turn trigger internalization of the positively charged molecule [3]. Cationic modification of proteins such as albumin and IgGs have been used to enhance their uptake into the brain. Studies have demonstrated that cationization of antibodies by covalently linking primary amine groups to their surface enhances their uptake into the brain by AMT. The capacity of AMT is high, but this mechanism is low in affinity and therefore has poor specificity. This is because cationized molecules can interact with negatively charged cell membranes of peripheral organs so that uptake in the brain does not increase proportionally [4,21]. The non-specificity of AMT mechanism should be considered in designing therapeutic antibodies that are targeted to the brain [6].

(ii) Carrier-mediated transport (CMT) is a mechanism by which small molecules such as glucose, amino acids, vitamins, hormones, and other nutrients rapidly cross the BBB [4]. This is a saturable mechanism due to the engagement of carriers and maintains homeostasis in the CNS by transporting these molecules bidirectionally [3]. Carrier-mediated transporters include CLUT1, which mediates transport of glucose and mannose and LTA1, which mediates transport of large neutral amino acids [21]. In principle, molecules can enter the brain using the CMT if they are conjugated to either endogenous ligands of the carriers or their analogues. However, this process has proved to be challenging for transport of antibodies because these carriers transport small molecules and are highly stereoselective.

(iii) Receptor-mediated transcytosis (RMT) is one of the most promising approaches for delivering antibodies to the brain [4]. There are three categories of receptors that mediate RMT: iron transporters such as transferrin receptors (TfR); insulin transporters such as insulin receptor (IR); and lipid transporters such as low-density lipoprotein receptor- related protein 1 (LRP1). This process entails binding of the ligand to the receptor, internalization of the ligand–receptor complex, and exocytosis on the abluminal side of the cell [3]. It is important to keep in mind, however, that high-affinity antibodies toward receptors that mediate RMT will follow the lysosomal pathway when internalized, which results in their degradation [22]. While this phenomenon creates a challenge in using the RMT mechanism, optimizing the affinity of the ligand that is targeting these receptors has proved to be an effective strategy [22].

3. Current In Vitro and In Vivo Methodologies for Measuring Brain Access of Antibodies: Advantages and Limitations

Implementation of in vitro models of the BBB that correlate with in vivo studies would provide desirable preclinical tools for the mechanistic understanding of drug transport via brain endothelial cells and uptake into the CNS monitored by the BBB. Use of these as a screening tool are of critical importance for the determination of drug permeability, PK, and distribution to brain tissues and cells.

3.1. In Vitro Methods

To aid in our understanding of the role of the BBB in protecting the brain microenvironment, different types of in vitro models of the BBB have been developed, which are classified into either static or dynamic BBB models [19,23]. Static BBB models are commonly used, but they do not imitate the shear stress, which is usually generated in vivo due to the blood flow. Static BBB models are further divided into monolayer and co-culture models, based on type of cells involved in the BBB design. While the brain microvessel endothelial cell culture model presents many differences compared with the in vivo system, monolayer cultures in a trans-well system allow a simple method for drug screening and permeability studies. The co-culture BBB model, however, is used to mimic the anatomic structure of BBB in vivo, in which BMECs are co-cultured with other CNS cells that directly contribute to the barrier properties of the BBB. As none of these in vitro models can entirely imitate the in vivo conditions, there is no perfect in vitro model of the BBB. Therefore, it is important to choose the in vitro model according to the requirement of the study. More details about the advantages and disadvantages of the different in vitro BBB models are currently covered in a thorough review article by Bagchi et al. (2019) [19].

3.2. In Vivo Methods

In contrast to in vitro methods, various in vivo methods have been employed to determine the kinetics of drug transport across the BBB. These include intravenous injection, in situ brain perfusion, microdialysis, quantitative whole-body autoradiography (QWBA), and molecular imaging such as single-photon emission computed tomography (SPECT), positron emission tomography (PET), and optical imaging. Brain perfusion is the most widely used technique for obtaining in vivo permeability values for drugs [24,25]. As such, brain perfusion allows injection of a solute into the brain vasculature at higher flow rates and solute concentrations than can be achieved by systemic circulation and hence allows a wider range of solute permeabilities to be measured at a fixed perfusate concentration. Direct injection of the solute into the brain minimizes metabolic loss and plasma protein binding. In this technique, the common carotid artery is cannulated and connected to a perfusion system. Immediately after the animal's heart is stopped, the molecule of interest dissolved in a physiological solution is infused into the brain typically for 5–300 s. Subsequently, the brain is removed, and the ipsilateral hemisphere is dissected, weighed, and the solute concentration determined by chromatography (LC-MS, HPLC, GC) or by radioactive counting methods (gamma or liquid scintillation counting) if the drug is radiolabeled.

In vivo microdialysis is another well-established quantitative technique in neuroscience for measuring small molecule concentrations in brain interstitial fluid (ISF) and CSF with minimal invasion into live animals. This technique essentially began with the push–pull method, which examined the possibility of using a semi-permeable membrane to sample free amino acids and other electrolytes in neuronal extracellular fluid. The technique was further improved by the development of the dialysis bag as a means of collecting the dialysate [26]. Since multiple microdialyis probes can be implanted in the brain, the disposition of drug within different regions of the brain can be simultaneously characterized. The use of this technique to measure macromolecule concentrations in brain, however, has been very limited. This is mainly due to the lack of availability until recently of large molecular weight cutoff (MWCO) probes and the need for a complicated push–pull system to perform microdialysis with large pore probes [27]. Although the push–pull microdialysis procedure for antibodies is challenging and requires extensive training, recent studies have shown that it can provide direct in vivo measurement of free antibody concentration in selected regions of the brain in freely moving animals [28,29]. This technique can avoid the detection of bound antibodies to the brain capillary endothelial cells and the neurons, and readouts of free antibody concentration in the brain interstitial ISF tend to better represent the required therapeutic concentration at the site-of-action in the brain. The theory and underlying general principles of in vivo microdialysis in general and brain microdialysis in particular are discussed in a review by Darvesh et al. [26].

On the other hand, to evaluate the in vivo PK and tissue distribution of antibodies, intravenous injection of radiolabeled antibody followed by collection of blood and tissue samples from the CNS at different time points ("cut and count") can be used as assays for sensitive uptake analysis [30]. Such an approach, however, is tedious and requires a large number of animals to ensure the reproducibility and reliability of the results. Today, QWBA, which relies on the use of X-ray film and phosphor imaging technology or radioluminography, is another standard method for conducting tissue distribution studies throughout the body of laboratory animals. These studies suggest that QWBA helps study the spatial and regional differences in areas as fine as 50–100 μm and is a good method for studying the targeted delivery of therapeutic proteins across the BBB [31,32]. The main advantage of QWBA is the minimal sample processing at true tissue-level (as opposed to organ-level) concentrations from an in situ preparation.

Furthermore, the continuing development of high-resolution PET and SPECT scanners and the availability of suitable radionuclides (e.g., Cu-64, Zr-89, In-111, I-131, I-124) are providing a non-invasive in vivo alternative that simplifies considerably the visualization and measurement of the whole body and organ PK, as well as brain uptake of antibodies. In this way, real-time dynamics can be obtained on whole body biodistribution of radiolabeled antibodies in the same animal or patient. The major advantages of these radionuclide-based molecular imaging techniques (SPECT and PET) are that they are very sensitive (down to the picomolar level), quantitative, and there is no tissue penetration limit. As a result, new applications of brain molecular imaging in animals are continually being established, which show a correlation between brain uptake of radiolabeled antibodies and brain target levels [33–36]. Another advantage is that molecular imaging methods have good spatial resolution (0.35–1.5 mm), allowing differentiation of tracer uptake on the suborgan level. Accordingly, the importance of spatial resolution in understanding therapeutic protein distribution within the brain has been the subject of several studies in which differences in brain penetration and distribution related to drug format are characterized [30,37,38].

Thus, significant effort has been made to radiolabel protein drugs with radionuclides, which in turn provides a method for tracking the location and quantifying the total radioactivity in tissues. However, the main limitation, which is shared by all these in vivo studies (e.g., "cut and count", QWBA, and molecular imaging) that rely on the usage of a radiolabeled compound, is that these technologies provide data on total radioactivity only and not specifically of the parent compound. In other words, the concentration of radioactivity does not always equate with the identity of the original compound that was radiolabeled, and it may also include radioactivity associated with metabolites and/or degradation products. The reader is referred to a comprehensive review by Tibbitts et al. (2016) of the different radiolabeling methods and the different in vivo technologies and approaches in order to gain a better mechanistic understanding of PK and protein distribution as a way to drive forward the selection of successful drug candidates [31].

In summary, in vitro BBB model selection parameters using human derived cells are critical for predicting drug transport because the disease in question may affect the barrier properties. Although many in vivo experiments have been traditionally performed, drug permeability tests are now carried mostly by in vitro BBB models due to ethical problems, differences between species, and expensive in vivo experiments. Nevertheless, a combinatorial approach of in vitro BBB models and in vivo tests will be the key to the development of CNS therapeutics with improved PK properties and better BBB penetrability [19,39].

4. Approaches to Optimize BBB Internalization and Uptake of Antibodies

Research has revealed that the BBB is not only a substantial barrier for drug delivery to the CNS but also a complex, dynamic interface that adapts to the needs of the

CNS and responds to physiological changes [40]. Optimization of drug delivery across the BBB could be achieved by several approaches: (a) pharmacologically, to increase the passage of drugs through the BBB by optimizing the specific biochemical properties of a compound [11]; (b) by BBB modulation, which includes transient osmotic opening of the BBB; and (c) physiologically, exploiting the various transport mechanisms present at the BBB. Many biomolecules (e.g., antibodies, recombinant fusion proteins, and nanoparticles), however, cannot get through the BBB unless the permeability of the BBB is altered using modulation of the tight junctions of the cerebral endothelial cells, which can result in some serious complications [11]. Research has shown that BBB internalization and trans-barrier transport of biomolecules can be manipulated on the basis of their physicochemical characteristics [41]. As a result, it is evident that various biomolecules with different parameters and characteristics are able to transverse biological barriers dictated by the barrier's set of limitations and specific criteria for internalization. Hence, it is expected that at some point the BBB physiology and physicochemical characteristics of antibodies will allow for the control of the rate and extent of cellular uptake, as well as the delivery of the antibody intracellularly, which is imperative for drugs that require a specific cellular level to exert their effects at the targeted site in vivo. Designing antibodies that can overcome this BBB protection system and achieve optimal concentration at the desired therapeutic target in the brain is a specific and major challenge for scientists working in CNS discovery [42]. In recent years, some progress has been made in terms of enabling the development of pharmacokinetic and pharmacodynamic (PK/PD) relationships for antibodies as therapeutic agents as well as in understanding how these relationships are influenced by target antigens and molecular properties.

In order to enhance antibody delivery to the brain, the following strategies for delivery optimization have been explored: (i) development of BBB-crossing bispecific antibodies, which have been engineered to incorporate one specificity against a BBB RMT receptor (Table 2) and the second specificity against a CNS therapeutic target to produce a pharmacological effect; and (ii) protein engineering efforts, which allow for the customized design of antibody constructs with physicochemical, molecular, and binding properties better optimized for successful transport across the BBB. Notably, antibody uptake is highly influenced by factors such as their size, surface charge, structure, hydrophobicity, affinity, antigen internalization, and dual targeting with bispecific antibodies [40,41,43–45]. The previous sections discussed the different transport mechanisms for the internalization of antibodies. Taken together, this section discusses the ideal antibody characteristics when employing transport mechanisms to achieve optimal cellular uptake (i.e., achieve desirable concentration range) at the BBB. Thus, this section focuses on examining the physicochemical and functional parameters of antibodies in regard to their relations and interactions with the physiology of the BBB and how those relations and interactions both facilitate their development as outstanding therapeutics.

Table 2. Receptor-mediated targets (RMT) for transport at the blood–brain barrier. Part of this table is reproduced from Gao (2016) with permission of the copyright owner [9].

	Receptors
1.	Transferrin receptor (TfR) [12]
2.	Insulin receptor (IR) [46,47]
3.	Low-density lipoprotein receptor–related protein (LRP) [12]
4.	Nicotinic acetylcholine receptor [9]
5.	Insulin-like growth factor receptor [9,48]
6.	Diphtheria toxin receptor [7,14]
7.	Scavenger receptor call B type [48]
8.	Leptin receptor [13,49]
9.	Neonatal Fc receptor (FcRn) [50]

4.1. Modification of BBB Permeability

The BBB is the first barrier that restricts the transportation of drugs from the blood to the brain. Because of this, researchers have developed various strategies to overcome or bypass the BBB, including penetration of the BBB by temporarily enlarging the BBB pore size, which could allow molecules such as antibodies to diffuse directly into brain [9]. In essence, modulating the efficacy of the tight junctions between cerebral endothelial cells so that the paracellular route of access to the brain is accessible is an applicable approach that has been utilized to permeabilize the BBB to drugs and enhance brain uptake. For instance, Neuwelt et al. (1981) discovered that mannitol, a hypertonic solution, can be administered simultaneously with drugs to enhance their delivery to brain tumors [51]. Currently, researchers are still using this strategy to deliver drugs to the CNS. Hypertonic solutions are thought to osmotically remove water from the endothelial cells, causing the cell to shrink, which may cause cellular changes that can affect the tight junctions [11]. This method is transitory, as the barrier closes within 10–20 min following BBB disruption. Unfortunately, this method is not selective for a specific drug and may increase uptake of other blood-borne molecules, such as neurotransmitters, which could be potentially harmful. Similarly, solvents such as high dose ethanol or dimethylsulfide, alkylating agents such as etoposide, alkylglycerols, and vasoactive agents such as bradykinin and histamine, have all been used to open the BBB and facilitate the delivery of drugs to the brain [52]. Since these compounds must be of a certain concentration to open the BBB, the BBB returns to its intact status when the blood concentration of these compounds falls lower than the threshold. Therefore, the dose and administration schedule must be optimized. The opening of the BBB is again presumably nonselective; thus, the use of these agents to affect BBB permeability can be highly traumatic, and could potentially cause serious side effects, such as seizures, permanent neurological disorders, and brain edema [9,11].

To circumvent these problems, focused ultrasound (FUS) and MRI are being employed as modulators of BBB function [53]. FUS has been used to enhance the delivery of various drugs to the brain, and it has been shown that the concentration of drugs in the brain hemisphere treated with FUS was approximately 3.5 times higher than the control hemisphere [53]. Combining FUS with other targeting methods could further elevate the accumulation of drugs in the brain. As an example, combining FUS with MRI targeting could improve the brain accumulation of drugs by 16-fold [54]. Although the toxicity of FUS on the brain is considered minor, and neurotoxicity was not observed, the clinical application of this method still should be viewed cautiously [55]. An advantage of these methods is that they can be focused with some precision to a particular region of the brain, thus modulating the BBB at a preferred site in order to release the drug locally. These modifications in BBB function and integrity appear to be transient and reversible, increasing the apparent safety of this method.

4.2. Physiological Approach to Transport Antibodies Across the BBB

Although the BBB is intact, mechanisms described in detail in Section 2 can be used to overcome this barrier. These strategies have been explored extensively over the past several decades when designing therapeutic antibodies for neurological disorders. Many of these strategies rely on receptors and carriers that are overexpressed on the BBB (Table 2), which can mediate the transport of specific ligands and their cargo.

Large molecules necessary for the brain's normal function are delivered to the brain by specific receptors that are highly expressed on the endothelial cells that form the BBB. This mechanism is described in the previous section as receptor-mediated transport (RMT). Additionally, the intercapillary distance in the brain is very small (on average 40 μm), and every neuron is virtually perfused by its own blood vessel, making these receptors abundant at the BBB [33]. Antibodies can be modified to be able to passage the BBB by conjugation to ligands that recognize receptors expressed at the BBB. This strategy in fact is the most effective way of delivering antibodies through the BBB and into the brain. This physiological approach targets IR, TfR, LRP-1 and 2, and other receptors.

Overall, therapeutic compounds are able to cross the BBB after association with these specific ligands, forming "molecular Trojan horses" (Table 3). Proof of concept studies have demonstrated that TfR-specific antibodies bind to the receptor on the endothelial cells and allow the associated therapeutic agent to cross the BBB via receptor-mediated transcytosis, making TfR particularly promising in brain-targeted delivery [56]. Modifications are still being made in the use of TfR as a delivery system after studies showed that antibodies bound to the TfR were retained in the brain endothelium and did not penetrate into the CNS. To address this problem, a "brain shuttle" approach has been developed that fuses the C-terminus of a monoclonal antibody against Aβ, the peptide that accumulates in the brain of AD patients, to an anti-TfR Fab, which facilitates the BBB transcytosis of an attached immunoglobulin [57]. This differs from current approaches where the TfR antibody carries a therapeutic cargo or a bispecific antibody with optimized binding to TfR that targets the enzyme β-secretase (BACE1) associated with AD [58,59]. Compared with the monospecific anti-BACE1 antibody, the bispecific antibody had increased accumulation in the brain and led to an increased reduction in Aβ levels [60].

Table 3. Selected new peptides and antibodies with specific ability to cross the blood–brain barrier.

	Biomolecules
1.	Angiopep-2, a peptide ligand of low-density lipoprotein receptor-related protein 1 (LRP1), with high permeability across the BBB [12,61,62]
2.	Angiopep-2-conjugated systems by conjugating the therapeutic peptides and proteins to Angiopep-2 for efficient brain delivery [12,63]
3.	Two single-domain antibodies (sdAb), FC5 and FC44, were cloned using a phage-display library of llama single-domain antibodies. Owing to specific and high permeability across the BBB, FC5 and FC44 could be developed as the vectors for brain delivery [12,64,65].
4.	Molecular Trojan horse: fusion of the therapeutic proteins to the monoclonal antibodies against human insulin receptor (IR) or transferrin receptor (TfR) [8,12,47]

Multiple studies have extensively documented the use of the insulin receptor (IR) for the targeted delivery of drugs to the brain using specific antibodies directed against IR [46,66]. Animal studies have shown that total brain uptake of the anti-human IR is 4% of injected dose at 3 h post injection and confirmed that it is able to transport an associated molecule across the BBB. Furthermore, applications of the TfR and IR antibodies to a molecular Trojan horse for the delivery of therapeutics have been documented where different forms of conjugated and fusion proteins have been generated [33]. LRP-1 and 2 expressed on neuronal cells have also been exploited to deliver drugs to the brain in a similar fashion as TfR and IR [67]. For now, these receptor antibodies described above may not be the only answer to the biologics brain targeting question [68]. Regardless, the substantial research performed with these available antibodies has provided invaluable insight on the mechanisms of action of receptors at the BBB and has also helped to highlight protein engineering issues that must be addressed (as presented below) in order to develop a successful approach for transporting therapeutic antibodies across the BBB.

4.3. Antibody Engineering Approaches to Increase Trans-BBB Transport

A serious limitation to the use of many antibodies in the design of improved biotherapeutics is their non-optimal behavior in the organism, including their poor PK parameters, non-optimal distribution, inhibition of binding with FcRn, and toxicity [69]. At the same time, one of the main problems is their frequent administration at a large dosage, which increases the risk of immunogenicity and side effects and reduces patient tolerance for the antibody. As such, one should note that antibody production is a continual design process that involves the generation and optimization of antibodies to enhance their clinical potential [70]. Moreover, much of the development and clinical experience that is gained from the generation and optimization of one antibody is applicable to other antibodies, thereby streamlining certain activities and decreasing some of the risks that are intrinsic to drug development. For example, to optimize the properties of an antibody for a particular indication, it would be preferable to improve or even delete particular characteristics. As an example, one major goal in developing therapeutic antibodies in neurological diseases is to improve the clinical utility of these reagents with respect to antigen targeting and better brain uptake (i.e., better brain-to-blood ratio) to encourage effective disease therapy. Achieving this goal depends not only upon a thorough understanding of molecular properties underlying antibody behavior and function but also upon the development of techniques to manipulate these properties in such a way that enhances their therapeutic potential [43]. For instance, PD response is often directly proportional to brain exposure and, thus, plasma half-life. As such, a typical goal in biotherapeutic development is to identify a candidate molecule having desirable PK properties or, alternatively, to manipulate a molecule's properties to improve its PK while preserving antigen recognition. PKPD properties of antibodies are governed by both molecule-dependent and species-dependent parameters. Biological processes such as antigen binding and receptor binding are important determinants in antibody PK. Since the field of therapeutic monoclonal antibodies has become extremely competitive, especially against validated antigens, it is necessary to develop highly optimized antibodies, above and beyond humanization [70]. A highly optimized humanized antibody would have superior pharmacological properties important for clinical efficacy, such as high antigen-binding activity and long half-life, as well as biophysical properties important for commercial development of the therapeutic antibody, including stability and expression yield in host cells. In order to generate such highly optimized antibodies, it is necessary to consider these pharmacological and biophysical properties during the process of humanization and manufacture. This section describes the critical properties of therapeutic antibodies that should be sufficiently qualified, including Fc and antigen binding affinity, and physiochemical properties and PK.

Fortunately, antibody fragments, such as single-chain Fv, diabody, triabody, Fab, F(ab′)2, and full length antibodies, ranging in size from 30 to 150 kDa and valence from one to three binding sites can be also derived via molecular engineering [71]. The single chain Fv (scFv, 30 kDa) is one of smallest forms of antibody that consists of variable light and heavy domains connected by a flexible peptide linker of approximately 15 amino acids generating one binding site. Diabodies (60 kDa) consist of two single chains joined by a very short linker, while triabodies (90 kDa) do not have a linker, thereby forcing trimerization. For example, the ability of these fragments to bind to tumor lies in a fine balance between their ability to penetrate tumor tissues due to their small size and their fast clearance from the body by the kidneys [72]. While retaining their antigen-binding capabilities, these fragments not only cleared faster but were also shown to have much higher tumor/organ ratios compared with their larger counterparts [72]. These antibody fragments are also used in neuroimaging agents in various diseases [35,73]. In this aspect, these studies showed that a diabody and a triabody penetrate the brain parenchyma more rapidly than the full length antibody, which in turn enables in vivo imaging of Aβ pathology at an earlier time point after administration [73].

4.3.1. Role of Fc Receptors

Receptors on the blood–brain barrier bind ligands to facilitate their transport to the CNS. Therefore, it is hypothesized that by targeting these receptors, therapeutic macromolecules (e.g., nanoparticles, antibodies) can be delivered to the CNS [74]. In this regard, FcRn, LRP, TfR, and IR receptors play an important role in regulating the endocytosis and transcytosis of IgGs, peptides, and proteins across the BBB (Table 2) [12]. The function and mechanism of FcRn in regulating IgG recycling have been well characterized. Because of the protective effects of FcRn against lysosomal degradation of IgG, generating Fc fusion proteins and modulating the pH dependent affinity between Fc and FcRn has been utilized to improve the PK of therapeutic antibodies [74]. In vitro studies have shown that FcRn regulates the transport of IgGs in both directions across the endothelial barriers of blood vessels, including those in brain, intestine, and placenta [75]. Importantly, studies using immortalized rat brain endothelial cells suggested that the human Fc fragment transports faster in the brain-to-blood direction than in the opposite direction [76]. These studies showed that while FcRn mediated the transport of IgGs across peripheral vascular cells in both directions, FcRn only mediated transport across BBB in the brain-to-blood direction. Modulating the interaction between Fc and FcRn through protein engineering has been applied to improve the PK of the therapeutic antibodies. Various studies have shown that the prolonged half-life and exposures of therapeutic antibodies can be achieved by increasing the pH-dependent binding affinity between Fc and FcRn [74].

There have been controversial studies on the role of FcRn in regulating the efflux of IgG from the brain and whether FcRn behaves as an efflux receptor that can transport antibodies across the blood–brain barrier back into the systemic circulation. One study in rats suggested that BBB FcRn mediates the efflux of IgG from the brain to the blood [77]. This study showed this efflux mechanism can be avoided when using antibody fragments devoid of Fc regions (Fab, $F(ab')_2$ and scFv fragments). Subsequently, another study investigated the mechanism of Aβ immunotherapy in the clearance of Aβ amyloid peptide in APPsw mice, a model that develops Alzheimer's disease-like amyloid pathology [76]. The study showed that anti-Aβ IgG-assisted efflux of Aβ amyloid peptide from the brain to the blood in wild-type mice was inhibited when the FcRn gene was knocked out. Taken together, these data suggest that FcRn at the BBB may play a role in regulating IgG-assisted Aβ amyloid peptide removal from the aging brain.

Unfortunately, other studies have shown that brain distribution and disposition of IgG is not regulated by FcRn and FcγR [78,79]. In these studies, IgG was injected intravenously to FcRn knockout and control mice [78]. As anticipated, the plasma clearance of IgG was increased by about 10 times, and the plasma exposures decreased by 4–5 times in FcRn deficient mice when compared with the controls. The brain exposure of IgG, however, was also reduced to a similar extent, and as a result, the brain-to-plasma ratios of IgG were not significantly different between the FcRn deficient and the controls. In another study, the role of FcRn in regulating brain IgG disposition was further investigated in the FcRn knockout, FcγR knockout, and control mice [79]. Compared with controls, the plasma and brain exposures from FcγR knockout mice were not significantly different, and the plasma and brain exposures from FcRn knockout mice decreased by 3–4 times as anticipated. However, similar to what was observed in the previous study, the brain-to-blood exposure ratio was not significantly different among the knockout and control mice. Together, these two studies indicate that FcRn and FcγR do not contribute to the "BBB" that limits IgG uptake into the brain. Similar to what was reported by Garg et al. and Abuqayyas and Balthasar, recent results from other groups showed that there was no IgG uptake difference between FcRn knockout and wild-type mice in the brain, which suggested that FcRn has little effect on the distribution of IgG in the brain [80]. In support of these findings, a more current study evaluating IgG uptake in tissues for FcRn wild type and $FcRn^-$ constructs indicates that FcRn does not contribute significantly to the brain for IgG in mice [81]. This study also demonstrates that FcRn does not play a protective role in the brain. These data are not consistent with previous studies that showed higher brain uptake for the engineered high-IgG FcRn binder relative to the wild type [82]. As postulated above, higher brain concentrations of the IgG variant with enhanced binding to FcRn could result from a role in efflux of IgG, as opposed to influx [76,77]. Further evidence toward this notion is the fact that the brain expression of FcRn is co-localized with the glucose transporter 1 (Glut1) in the capillary endothelium, suggesting that FcRn is expressed in the proper location to potentially mediate reverse transcytosis of IgG from the brain to the blood [83]. In summary, there is no consensus on the role of FcRn in influencing the blood-to-brain transcytosis of IgG across the brain endothelial cells (BECs) despite several notable studies. Indirect evidence of potential FcRn-mediated recycling was provided by recent studies demonstrating that IgG transcytosis across an in vitro BBB exhibits a non-saturable and nonspecific mechanism and supports the use of RMT approaches or modifications of biophysical properties, such as pI, to achieve improved brain uptake of therapeutic IgGs [7,84].

4.3.2. Role of Antigen Binding

Trans-BBB delivery methods that use targeting antibodies are often hampered by limited flux through the BBB. A solution to this problem lies in the rational engineering of BBB-targeting antibodies. Leveraging knowledge of intracellular trafficking, researchers have begun to tune selected binding properties of the antibody–antigen receptor interaction. Engineered binding affinity, avidity, and pH sensitivity have been shown to affect binding, intracellular sorting, and release, ultimately leading to increased brain uptake of the targeting antibody and its associated cargo [7]. The first successful attempts for chimeric proteins targeting cell receptors initially relied on cationized albumin, which lacked brain selectivity, and then later IgGs directed against IR or TfR receptors [85]. However, the success of these initial antibodies was limited by their high affinity, which hindered an efficient release and penetration into the brain parenchyma [58]. A variety of protein shuttles have been investigated; most of them are ligands of receptors on the brain endothelium that compete with their endogeneous proteins (e.g., apolipoproteins A and E, receptor-associated protein, transferrin, lactotransferrin, melanotransferrin, and leptin). Although a few non-endogenous proteins have been used (e.g., wheat germ agglutinin, non-toxic mutant of diphtheria toxin), they also have shown moderate efficacy and selectivity [13]. Recent efforts have leveraged antibody engineering strategies to increase trans-BBB transport and have highlighted the importance of the antigen-binding and trafficking issues. As shown in Tables 1 and 2, each targeted receptor may exhibit differential responses to engineered binding properties, illustrating the need to better understand antibody–antigen receptor interactions and trafficking dynamics.

Regarding the above, well-designed experiments have engineered the binding properties of anti-transferrin (anti-TfR) antibodies to study their trafficking and delivery in vitro and in vivo. First, antibody affinity and avidity for TfR were evaluated, and it was shown that higher brain uptake of anti-TfR antibodies can be accomplished by lowering antibody affinity [58]. Intravenous administration of antibodies having a range of affinity to TfR (Kd = 6.9–111 nM) indicated that at trace doses, mouse brain uptake directly correlated with affinity, suggesting that receptor engagement at the blood side of the BBB was the key parameter governing uptake (Figure 1). This figure shows the diagram taken from Goulatis and Shusta (2017) to illustrate that high-affinity monovalent and bivalent anti-TfR antibodies internalize readily into the early endosomes but then direct the antibody–receptor complex toward lysosomal degradation, possibly by crosslinking the TfR and altering its intracellular trafficking [7]. While high-affinity monovalent anti-TfR antibodies can transcytose the BBB, they remain bound to the receptor on the abluminal side, limiting the dose to the brain. In contrast, low-affinity anti-TfR antibodies decrease antibody-TfR sorting to the lysosome and can either be recycled back to the luminal side or get transcytosed to the abluminal side where they dissociate from TfR, leading to increased brain accumulation. Further, pH-sensitive TfR-binding antibodies that can dissociate from TfR in the acidic endosome led to increased transcytosis compared with pH-insensitive antibodies. In the case of the single-domain antibody FC5 (Table 3), increased affinity toward the receptor leads to an increase in the amount of transcytosed antibody, highlighting the fact that antibodies utilizing different trafficking machinery may require customized optimization (Figure 1). However, at therapeutic dosing (20 mg/kg), an inverse correlation was observed, where the lowered affinity antibody demonstrated greater brain accumulation (up to 0.6% ID/ g) (Figure 2). These data demonstrate that lowered affinity allows for antibody release from the TfR at the abluminal membrane, while higher-affinity variants remain bound to the TfR. Further studies provided the evidence that affinity-derived effects on brain uptake of anti-TfR antibodies were at least in part caused by altered intracellular trafficking and lysosomal degradation [37]. The high-affinity anti-TfR antibody was found to be more prominently trafficked to the lysosome and degraded, resulting in reduced cortical TfR levels. Thus, productive trans-BBB anti-TfR antibody trafficking could be increased by lowering antibody affinity.

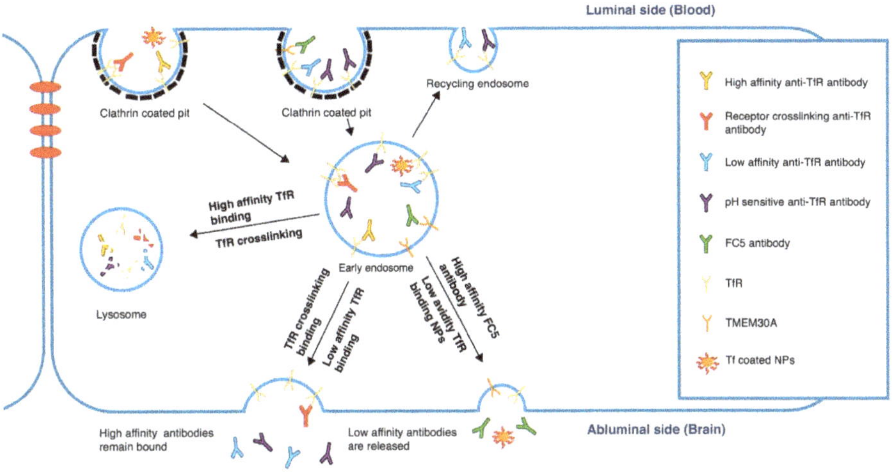

Figure 1. A schematic depiction of the various engineering optimization strategies for increased transcytosis of antibodies and nanoparticles (NPs) across the BBB. High-affinity monovalent and bivalent anti-TfR antibodies internalize readily into the early endosome (EE) but then direct the antibody–receptor complex toward lysosomal degradation, possibly by crosslinking the TfR and altering its intracellular trafficking. While high-affinity monovalent anti-TfR antibodies can transcytose the BBB, they remain bound to the receptor on the abluminal side, limiting the dose to the brain. In contrast, low-affinity anti-TfR antibodies decrease antibody-TfR sorting to the lysosome and can either be recycled back to the luminal side or are transcytosed to the abluminal side where they dissociate from TfR, leading to increased brain accumulation. Similarly, Tf-coated nanoparticles show a higher transcytosis capability when lowering the Tf coating content, resulting in reduced avidity. Further, pH-sensitive TfR-binding antibodies that can dissociate from TfR in the acidic EE lead to increased transcytosis compared with pH-insensitive antibodies. In the case of the single domain antibody FC5, increased affinity toward the receptor leads to an increase in the amount of transcytosed antibody, highlighting the fact that vectors utilizing different trafficking machinery may require customized optimization. This figure is reproduced from Goulatis and Shusta (2017) with permission of the copyright owner [7].

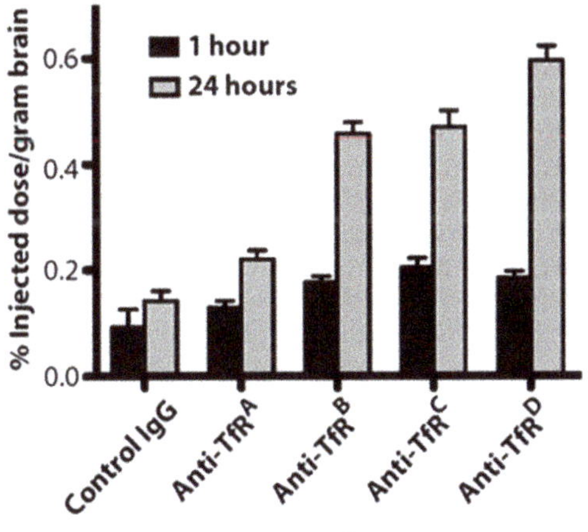

Figure 2. Lower-affinity anti-TfR^D antibodies (A > D) at therapeutic doses show increased brain uptake. This figure is reproduced from Yu et al. (2013) with permission of the copyright owner [58].

In addition to studies of TfR antibody-binding affinity, the role of avidity has also been explored with similar conclusions. In order to investigate avidity effects on trans- BBB transport, a Fab fragment targeting the TfR was fused to the carboxy-terminus of an anti-BACE1 (β-amyloid cleaving enzyme-1) antibody in a bivalent (dFab) or monovalent (sFab) format [57]. Monovalent binding of an anti-TfR antibody allowed for preferential transcellular transport in brain endothelia, while bivalent binding led to diversion of trafficking toward the lysosome. The results of this study strongly suggest that differences in TfR-binding mode led to major differences in intracellular trafficking, which ultimately allows sFab-associated cargos to cross the BBB. Similarly, another in vitro study has investigated whether or not pH-insensitive TfR binding could be an additional engineering approach for regulating anti-TfR antibody trafficking and increasing trans-BBB transport [86]. These data demonstrated that attenuated binding of an anti-TfR antibody at endosomal pH can lead to differential intracellular trafficking, ultimately enhancing transcytosis across the BBB.

4.3.3. Role of Biophysical Properties

The majority of small drugs that are used to treat CNS disease have a molecular weight between 150 and 500 Da [11]. This does not indicate that drugs with a molecular weight less than 150 or greater than 500 Da are unable to cross. Characteristics that reduce the ability of small molecules to cross the BBB include a polar surface area in excess of 80 A ° and a high potential for hydrogen bond formation. Additionally, increased number of positive charges and increased flexibility contribute to BBB crossing. Lipid solubility is a clear indicator of small drugs that can pass through the BBB [87]. Rules for proteins have some similarities and some apparent differences from those for small drugs [11]. Most proteins are poorly soluble in lipids and so would not be expected to penetrate the BBB very well by trans-endothelial diffusion. However, lipid solubility was a predictor of BBB penetration for one series of peptides and proteins that had molecular weights ranging from 486 to 6000 Da. The largest substance found to cross the BBB using transmembrane diffusion thus far is cytokine-induced neutrophilchemoattractant-1, which has a molecular weight of 7800 Da [88]. This is thought to represent a direct correlation between BBB penetration and the ability of a drug to deliver cargoes across the cell membrane. One of the primary factors in determining whether a protein will cross the BBB is its lipophilicity. A strategy for enhancing the ability of a peptide to cross the BBB is increasing its lipophilicity. There are a number of techniques able to do this, including alteration of the protein structure, methylation, halogenation, or acylation. Structural changes, for example covalently binding the drug to lipidic moieties, such as long chain fatty acids, will increase the lipophilicity of a peptide [89]. Peptides with a high number of hydroxyl groups tend to promote hydrogen bonding with water, which leads to a decrease in membrane permeability. Decreasing hydrogen bonding therefore increases membrane permeability. Ideally, there should be potential for the formation of fewer than eight hydrogen bonds when developing new drugs. Methylation is one method used to reduce hydrogen bonding. This illustrates an important point for protein modifications: that the location and type of modification play a significant role in improving BBB transport of your peptide of interest [11]. Halogenation of peptides and proteins can also lead to increased lipophilicity and BBB permeability. The increase in BBB transport of peptides was dependent on which halogen was utilized; chloro and bromo additions increased BBB transport, while fluoro and iodo additions had no effect [90]. An alternative approach is acylation of the N-terminal amino acid, which can increase the lipophilicity of peptides and proteins. For example, acylation of insulin improved its ability to cross the BBB while maintaining its pharmacological effects. Another approach involves glycosylation and hyperglycosylation of therapeutic proteins [91]. In this case, the in vivo results showed that glycosylation is required to maintain protein exposure in blood and proved to increase protein uptake into the CNS [92].

Along these lines, the large change in biophysical properties induced by therapeutic cargoes and the distinct location of the targets of these drugs inside the brain has limited the universal aspiration of most BBB shuttles [13]. Hence, in general, each protein shuttle is prominent in the delivery of a particular family of cargoes. There are many receptors and carriers that are overexpressed on the BBB (Table 2), which can mediate the transport of specific ligands and their cargoes. Additionally, the membrane of the BBB is negatively-charged and shows high affinity with positively charged compounds, which could also trigger the internalization by cells [9]. Thus, these kinds of ligands could mediate the penetration of macromolecules through the BBB. Efficient transport of macromolecules across the BBB through endocytic mechanisms involves both specific (receptor-mediated transcytosis) and/or nonspecific (adsorptive-mediated transcytosis) interactions with proteins and receptors expressed on the brain endothelial cell surfaces. In adsorptive-mediated transcytosis, endocytosis is generally promoted by the interaction of the often positively charged molecule with membrane phospholipids and the glycocalyx [13]. The most common approach relies on enhancing positive charge, in order to mediate interaction with the anionic glycocalyx. However, this approach leads to higher unspecific uptake in many other tissues, often resulting in off-target effects, which in addition requires a high degree of tailoring for certain small molecules that are rarely applicable to biotherapeutics. Another approach for drug delivery to the CNS, as shown in the previous section, focuses on BBB shuttles that allow the transport of a wide range of molecules, comprising small molecules, proteins, nanoparticles, and IgGs across the BBB. Substrates of natural carriers such as glucose and neutral amino acids have been applied to transport small molecules through their natural carriers on the BBB, while for biomolecules the focus has been set on receptor ligand proteins (Table 2) since endocytic pathways tolerate a high cargo load [13].

A common goal for therapeutic antibodies is to extend plasma half-life as a means to increase exposure, often expressed in terms of the area under the plasma concentration-time curve [74]. In contrast, cationization tends to shorten plasma half-life due to an enhancement in both the rate and the magnitude of tissue distribution. However, cationization might prove to be a useful strategy in specific applications in which prolonged antibody exposure may be sacrificed for the sake of rapid, enhanced tissue uptake (e.g., targeting antibodies to efficiently cross the BBB) [93]. Cationization of antibodies has also been explored as a means to encourage extravasation, antigen binding, and receptor-mediated endocytosis of antibodies into target cells [94]. In contrast to native Abs, which are generally excluded from cell membranes in the absence of receptor-mediated endocytosis, cationized Abs are better able to reach the intracellular space via absorptive-mediated transcytosis (AMT). Electrostatic interactions between positively charged proteins and negatively charged cell membranes could permit cell entry via nonspecific membrane flow and have been implicated in the mechanism by which cationized antibodies are rapidly endocytosed by cells in vitro. A similar phenomenon is suggested to induce absorptive-mediated transcytosis across microvascular endothelial barriers in vivo [94]. This interaction also occurs further with sialic acid moieties on the luminal surface and heparin sulfate group on the abluminal surface. AMT of cationized albumin is triggered by this electrostatic interaction and results in the transport of the moiety across the BBB [93]. The use of cationized albumin for the transport of β-endorphin, a very large molecule that cannot cross the BBB, has been reported in rats [95]. After conjugation with cationized albumin brain uptake of β-endorphin was increased. When the isoelectric point of antibodies is raised from neutral to highly alkaline, cationized antibodies are formed. These antibodies are used mainly as neuroimaging agents in various diseases, including brain tumors, AD, and stroke [96]. Mechanisms governing the passage and partitioning of small molecule drugs and antibodies across the BBB have also been the subject of several reviews and modeling studies [29,97,98]. While the distribution of small molecules is influenced by multiple factors, including drug liposolubility, free vs bound concentrations in blood and brain fluids, and their (bidirectional) transport via BBB carriers and efflux pumps, some of these processes may not be important in the case of some biologic molecules [61]. For example, antibodies (including VHHs) are not substrates of efflux pumps and their "bound" concentration in body fluids can be considered negligible in most cases. Their paracellular "filtration" across the BBB is essentially completely restricted by tight junctions of brain endothelium and choroid plexus epithelium, respectively. In the absence of specific transport mechanisms such as the RMT, they therefore can access the brain only via a low-rate nonspecific adsorptive endocytosis. To discover new antigen–ligand systems for transvascular brain delivery, a recent study developed a method for functional selection of brain microvascular endothelial cell-specific internalizing and transmigrating antibodies [62] from a phage-display llama single-domain antibody (sdAb) library (Table 3). sdAbs are the VHH fragments of the heavy-chain IgGs, which occur naturally in camelid species and lack light chain, and are half the size (15 kDa) of a single-chain antibody (scFv) [99]. These sdAbs have been shown to internalize into the brain's endothelial cell and transmigrate in an in vitro BBB model via a saturable, energy-dependent and charge-independent process; pretreatment of cells with highly cationic protamine sulfate did not affect sdAb transcytosis [100]. Similarly, two positively charged control antibodies, showed minimal "passive" transcytosis in an in vitro BBB model. As such, it can be assumed that CSF levels of control sdAb, which does not bind any known receptor in mammals, are representative of nonspecific passive uptake processes (macropinocytosis; adsorptive endocytosis) of large, hydrophilic, and positively charged biologic molecules at the BBB.

Nevertheless, as discussed above, other antibodies and single-chain antibody fragments have also been developed as "Trojan horse" bispecific antibodies for delivery of therapeutics via RMT, including IR and TfR receptor antibodies; the extensive literature on these antibodies reports a range of their serum/brain partitions (from 0.1% to 4% ID/g vs 0.06% ID/g for IgG) [58]. Due to a lack of comparative studies using the same experimental and analytical methods as well as vast differences in size and pharmacokinetics, the direct comparison between known antibody "Trojan horses" with unmodified single-domain antibodies (sdAbs) remains difficult. These sdAbs will require further engineering for improvement of their plasma half-life and potentially their binding properties before their comparative assessment with similar antibody RMT technologies can be properly performed [61].

5. Conclusions and Outlook

This review focuses mainly on the historic trends and current practices of research and development activities involving the BBB as a complex interface between the blood and the CNS, essentially for the targeted delivery of antibodies to treat neurodegenerative diseases. It is well established that nearly 0.1% of circulating biotherapeutics, i.e., recombinant proteins or gene-based medicines, cross the BBB [42,45]. Hence, improving brain exposure for at least some of these molecules is the ultimate goal of the brain delivery systems. It has been proposed that CNS diseases can be initiated by several mechanisms, including decreased cerebral blood flow, perturbation of transporters, BBB disruption, deformations of capillaries, and secretion of neurotoxic substances by the BBB. Thus, the BBB may have a fundamental role in brain diseases [40,98]. Nonetheless, the BBB is intimately involved in crosstalk with the rest of the CNS and peripheral tissues and is crucial for normal brain pressure and functioning, and therefore, perturbation of its function might have physiologic consequences. As shown in Tables 2 and 3, different physiological approaches are used to deliver biotherapeutics in the brain parenchyma. Generally, the techniques used involve direct injection or infusion of therapeutic compounds into the brain or the cerebro-ventricles or the CSF. All these approaches, however, are severely limited by poor distribution into brain parenchyma [14]. In fact, the most promising new technology uses a physiological approach to take advantage of endogenous receptors highly expressed at the BBB (e.g., TfR and IR). Fundamentally, this latter approach has been employed by cells of the BBB to enhance the delivery of antibodies across the BBB by receptor-mediated transcytosis. While the physiological approach has the potential to achieve improved brain delivery and to play a significant role in the treatment of CNS disease, in vivo preclinical studies quantifying antibody levels systematically and determining antibody activity relationship in the brain is difficult [56,101]. Despite these challenges, however, current efforts are focused on developing newer generations of antibody therapeutics that can cross or otherwise interact with the BBB for optimal in vivo benefit. For now, exploiting TfR receptors for delivering antibodies across the BBB may not be the answer to the brain targeting question [68]. However, the research performed with the available anti-TfR antibodies has provided invaluable insight into the mechanisms of action of receptors at the BBB and has also helped to highlight protein engineering issues that must be addressed in order for a successful BBB shuttle to be developed. Additionally, perhaps the most challenging aspect of moving anti-TfR antibodies to the clinic is the lack of species cross reactivity observed in the available antibodies. To solve this problem, antibodies are being engineered for use in each species under investigation, or transgenic mice are generated to express human antigens that tolerize them to humanized antibodies, something that will add significantly to development costs.

Moreover, in search of a solution to increase the penetration of antibodies in the brain, it is likely that all of the parameters described earlier, such as target interaction, FcRn binding, molecular size, and surface charge, are likely to play a part in the trafficking of anti-receptor antibodies across the BBB. As mentioned above, there is no consensus on the role of FcRn in influencing the blood-to-brain transcytosis of IgG across the brain endothelial cells (BECs), despite several notable studies that support the modifications of biophysical properties, such as pI, to achieve improved brain uptake of therapeutic IgGs [7,84]. Special attention is also being given to lipophilicity and overall surface hydrophobicity, since there is a tendency for those parameters to play a significant role in the BBB transport of proteins [90,92,102]. Only through the systematic evaluation of all of these parameters will it become clear which, if any, is the most important to have an effect on the PK of the brain interstitial space [103]. In the past decade, innumerable preclinical studies have been reported on the use of real-time imaging with targeted drug delivery, and this strategy has now matured with promises to assess the distribution and uptake of protein drugs [104]. For example, it has been shown that molecular imaging technologies like PET and SPECT have made important contributions to enable brain imaging of recombinant antibodies that are engineered for BBB transport, particularly in determining drug pharmacokinetics of directly labeled antibodies [35,36,105]. Additional evidence for the sensitivity of antibody PET imaging is provided by a study where a recombinant bispecific antibody was radiolabeled with I-124 and then administered in two transgenic AD and wild-type mice at different ages [73]. This study demonstrates that antibody-based PET is able to visualize and quantify early formed Aβ assemblies (Figure 3) and may become a valuable tool for disease staging of AD patients and for monitoring the effects of Aβ-directed treatment. Additionally valuable in the setting of advanced CNS imaging is the assessment of brain uptake and changes in BBB integrity, which will help to accelerate drug development by assisting in understanding and defining the challenges to translating molecularly targeted agents to the brain [10]. In this aspect, the current trend in drug discovery is to consider classical absorption, distribution, metabolism, and excretion (ADME) studies in parallel with imaging studies, enabling differentiation between biophysical and binding properties and their delivery to the brain. Such classical rules have the advantage of being very simple, as well as being easy to interpret. Their drawback, however, is that they do not take into consideration uncertainties in measurements and calculations as well as the pharmacological effect and toxicity requirements. Meanwhile, the release of an antibody drug in the brain should be accurately monitored and controlled in situ or in real-time [106,107]. It is also important to keep in mind that although no single technology currently provides all the answers, integrating different modalities into other in vivo methodologies (e.g., QWBA, microautoradiography, PET, and SPECT) can enhance our quantitative understanding of spatial brain distribution [32,36]. Furthermore, the brain is a highly vascularized organ with a relatively high proportion of endothelial cells. In determining the concentration of a therapeutic protein in the brain parenchyma, it is critical to ensure that the methods used for assessing distribution are capable of distinguishing endothelial uptake from parenchymal uptake [31]. Thus, this approach indicates that it would be more appropriate to establish a high-quality preclinical assessment of ADME,

PK, and safety/toxicity studies with an emphasis on activity in the CNS, which will permit the parallel optimization of pharmacological response and druggability properties.

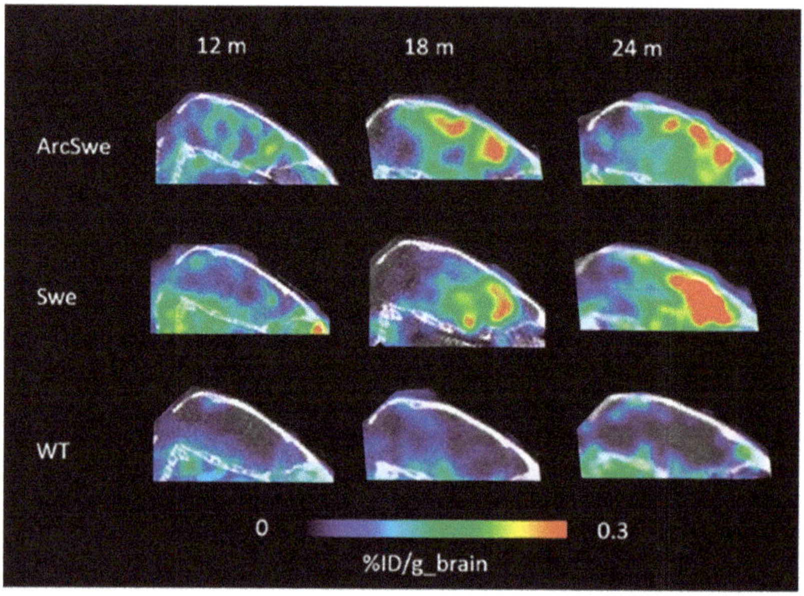

Figure 3. Sagittal PET images obtained at 3 days after administration of the bispecific antibody radiolabeled with I-124 in two transgenic mouse models of AD (ArcSwe and Swe) and wild-type (WT) mice at different ages (12, 18, and 24 months). Quantification of the radiolabeled antibody in brain tissue showed an increasing signal intensity with age (i.e., with increasing Aβ pathology) in the two transgenic AD animal models, while brains of WT mice were devoid of signal regardless of age. This figure is reproduced from Sehlin and Syvänen (2019) with permission of the copyright owner [73].

In addition to classical ADME studies, generation of in silico physiologically based pharmacokinetic (PBPK) models by incorporating PKPD data and safety profiles as a tool for the treatment of CNS diseases has attracted great interest from pharmaceutical scientists and are likely to be crucial to the development of novel antibody-based therapeutics [28,29,108–111]. Further, the high-throughput and low-cost nature of these models permit a more streamlined drug development process in which the identification of antibody structural optimization can be guided based on a parallel investigation of CNS uptake and safety, along with activity [112]. Hence, the development of in vivo and especially in silico models can be an instrumental tool for predicting the association between BBB penetration and the profile of expected human response for a specific antibody drug against a specific target. This approach will greatly help to simplify the practical difficulties and circumvent potential ethical controversies [106]. In essence, by simultaneously optimizing the antibody molecule in the light of their biophysical and molecular properties, BBB penetration, and activity, it should prove possible to identify a highly qualified clinical candidate and consequently enable faster development of therapeutic antibodies [70]. Although delivery of antibodies to the CNS shows great promise, a greater understanding of CNS physiology and pathophysiology is still needed. Accordingly, it would be vital to characterize further the physiological and vascular attributes such as perfusion, blood volume, and permeability to protein drugs in various CNS compartments [30,43]. Nevertheless, it is believed that the various methods historically used to assess BBB permeability or dysfunction in mouse models of human disease have led to many disparate findings. For example, early studies showed that the BBB is disrupted in Alzheimer's disease models, potentially increasing drug permeability [113]. However, more recent data have shown that the BBB remains intact in multiple preclinical models of Alzheimer's disease (AD) [38]. Thus, the current lack of in vivo validation of BBB permeability in neurodegenerative diseases and the lack of controlled studies hinder the understanding of antibody delivery through the BBB. Moreover, robust characterization of preclinical disease models is necessary for predicting drug delivery to target tissues and for interpreting correctly the pharmacodynamic responses to disease-modifying biotherapeutic candidates.

After a decade of intensive engineering of antibodies followed by preclinical testing, scientists are still seeking a variety of strategies for optimizing their use as powerful therapeutic agents, particularly for targeted delivery to the CNS for the treatment of neurological disorders. With recent advances in scaffold design, construction, and selection methodologies, there is now a rapid process for recombinant synthesis of specific antibodies differing in affinity and molecular properties against virtually any BBB target [49,114]. For example, in vivo studies showed an enhanced brain uptake of antibodies with novel BBB targets but doing so, while remaining in the range of manageable safety and efficacy, is still challenging [115]. In the case of antibody modifications, it remains to be seen whether modern genetic engineering may affect the pharmacokinetics, biodistribution, therapeutic index, or safety profiles due to immunogenicity [116]. As a consequence of all these minor modifications, immunogenicity concerns are still under investigation by drug regulatory agencies, since their potential for immunogenicity can alter ADME properties, thereby greatly confounding the interpretation of PK/PD assessments [116,117].

To date, great progress has been made with the brain shuttle approach, which has proved to be successful in improving the CNS exposure of some of the large molecules with poor brain permeability, such as bispecific TfR antibodies [4,108,109]. However, further developments are still needed for this approach to become a more robust technology. Until then, fine-tuning of the biophysical and binding properties for optimal brain exposure will remain a staple of CNS drug discovery and development [42]. More importantly, in order to increase further our knowledge regarding the effects of antibody modification on brain-targeted uptake and efficacy, additional clinical studies using relevant animal species and disease models need to be implemented [118,119]. Finally, MRI-guided FUS delivery to the CNS still has great promise and provides the opportunity to improve biotherapeutics' bioavailability locally and to improve their therapeutic profiles. In summary, targeted CNS biotherapeutics is an ever expanding and challenging but important field of study [120,121]. In fact, until now, there is only one human monoclonal antibody aducanumab (under the brand name Adulhelm^{TM}), that has been FDA-approved for the treatment of people with AD. The approval was granted this year based on data from clinical trials demonstrating that aducanumab targets aggregated forms of β-amyloid, a biomarker that is reasonably likely to predict clinical benefits. Thus, since more investigators across academia and industry have joined the race to increase the uptake of antibodies across the BBB, there is good reason for optimism for additional FDA-approved CNS biotherapeutics in the near future.

Author Contributions: All other authors (A.K., T.K., V.P., P.H., A.L.E. and L.A.K.) contributed substantially to the discussions, writing, and referencing of the paper. In addition, all authors contributed to editing and reviewing the manuscript during the submission process. All authors have read and agreed to the published version of the manuscript.

Funding: This research received no external funding.

Data Availability Statement: The data presented in this review are available and can be found in the cited references.

Acknowledgments: We thank our colleagues Kevin Brady at UCB (Slough, United Kingdom) and Sherri Dudal at Roche (Basel, Switzerland) for scientific exchange and discussions. Leslie Khawli conceived the paper and wrote the outline of the manuscript.

Conflicts of Interest: The authors declare no conflict of interest.

References

1. Tucker, I.G. Drug delivery to the brain via the blood-brain barrier: A review of the literature and some recent patent disclosures. *Ther. Deliv.* **2011**, *2*, 311–327. [CrossRef]
2. Alavijeh, M.S.; Chishty, M.; Qaiser, M.Z.; Palmer, A.M. Drug metabolism and pharmacokinetics, the blood-brain barrier, and central nervous system drug discovery. *NeuroRx* **2005**, *2*, 554–571. [CrossRef]
3. Grabrucker, A.M.; Ruozi, B.; Belletti, D.; Pederzoli, F.; Forni, F.; Vandelli, M.A.; Tosi, G. Nanoparticle transport across the blood brain barrier. *Tissue Barriers* **2016**, *4*, e1153568. [CrossRef]
4. Yu, Y.J.; Watts, R.J. Developing therapeutic antibodies for neurodegenerative disease. *Neurotherapeutics* **2013**, *10*, 459–472. [CrossRef]
5. Dimitrov, D.S. Engineered CH2 domains (nanoantibodies). *MAbs* **2009**, *1*, 26–28. [CrossRef] [PubMed]
6. Lajoie, J.M.; Shusta, E.V. Targeting receptor-mediated transport for delivery of biologics across the blood-brain barrier. *Annu. Rev. Pharmacol. Toxicol.* **2015**, *55*, 613–631. [CrossRef]
7. Goulatis, L.I.; Shusta, E.V. Protein engineering approaches for regulating blood-brain barrier transcytosis. *Curr. Opin. Struct. Biol.* **2017**, *45*, 109–115. [CrossRef] [PubMed]
8. Pardridge, W.M.; Boado, R.J. Reengineering biopharmaceuticals for targeted delivery across the blood-brain barrier. *Methods Enzymol.* **2012**, *503*, 269–292. [CrossRef]
9. Gao, H. Progress and perspectives on targeting nanoparticles for brain drug delivery. *Acta Pharm. Sin. B* **2016**, *6*, 268–286. [CrossRef] [PubMed]
10. Sweeney, M.D.; Sagare, A.P.; Zlokovic, B.V. Blood-brain barrier breakdown in Alzheimer disease and other neurodegenerative disorders. *Nat. Rev. Neurol.* **2018**, *14*, 133–150. [CrossRef] [PubMed]
11. Salameh, T.S.; Banks, W.A. Delivery of therapeutic peptides and proteins to the CNS. *Adv. Pharmacol.* **2014**, *71*, 277–299. [CrossRef]
12. Xiao, G.; Gan, L.S. Receptor-mediated endocytosis and brain delivery of therapeutic biologics. *Int. J. Cell Biol.* **2013**, *2013*, 703545. [CrossRef]
13. Oller-Salvia, B.; Sanchez-Navarro, M.; Giralt, E.; Teixido, M. Blood-brain barrier shuttle peptides: An emerging paradigm for brain delivery. *Chem. Soc. Rev.* **2016**, *45*, 4690–4707. [CrossRef] [PubMed]
14. Gabathuler, R. Approaches to transport therapeutic drugs across the blood-brain barrier to treat brain diseases. *Neurobiol. Dis.* **2010**, *37*, 48–57. [CrossRef]
15. Pulgar, V.M. Transcytosis to Cross the Blood Brain Barrier, New Advancements and Challenges. *Front. Neurosci.* **2018**, *12*, 1019. [CrossRef] [PubMed]
16. Strazielle, N.; Ghersi-Egea, J.F. Physiology of blood-brain interfaces in relation to brain disposition of small compounds and macromolecules. *Mol. Pharm.* **2013**, *10*, 1473–1491. [CrossRef] [PubMed]
17. Vieira, D.B.; Gamarra, L.F. Getting into the brain: Liposome-based strategies for effective drug delivery across the blood-brain barrier. *Int. J. Nanomed.* **2016**, *11*, 5381–5414. [CrossRef]
18. Papisov, M.I.; Belov, V.V.; Gannon, K.S. Physiology of the intrathecal bolus: The leptomeningeal route for macromolecule and particle delivery to CNS. *Mol. Pharm.* **2013**, *10*, 1522–1532. [CrossRef] [PubMed]
19. Bagchi, S.; Chhibber, T.; Lahooti, B.; Verma, A.; Borse, V.; Jayant, R.D. In-Vitro blood-brain barrier models for drug screening and permeation studies: An overview. *Drug Des. Devel. Ther.* **2019**, *13*, 3591–3605. [CrossRef] [PubMed]
20. Conner, K.P.; Devanaboyina, S.C.; Thomas, V.A.; Rock, D.A. The biodistribution of therapeutic proteins: Mechanism, implications for pharmacokinetics, and methods of evaluation. *Pharmacol. Ther.* **2020**, *212*, 107574. [CrossRef]
21. Herda, L.M.; Polo, E.; Kelly, P.M.; Rocks, L.; Hudecz, D.; Dawson, K.A. Designing the future of nanomedicine: Current barriers to targeted brain therapeutics. *Eur. J. Nanomed.* **2014**, *6*, 127–139. [CrossRef]
22. Cavaco, M.; Gaspar, D.; Arb Castanho, M.; Neves, V. Antibodies for the Treatment of Brain Metastases, a Dream or a Reality? *Pharmaceutics* **2020**, *12*, 62. [CrossRef]
23. Modarres, H.P.; Janmaleki, M.; Novin, M.; Saliba, J.; El-Hajj, F.; RezayatiCharan, M.; Seyfoori, A.; Sadabadi, H.; Vandal, M.; Nguyen, M.D.; et al. In Vitro models and systems for evaluating the dynamics of drug delivery to the healthy and diseased brain. *J. Control. Release* **2018**, *273*, 108–130. [CrossRef] [PubMed]
24. Hammarlund-Udenaes, M.; Paalzow, L.K.; de Lange, E.C. Drug equilibration across the blood-brain barrier—pharmacokinetic considerations based on the microdialysis method. *Pharm. Res.* **1997**, *14*, 128–134. [CrossRef]
25. Taccola, C.; Barneoud, P.; Cartot-Cotton, S.; Valente, D.; Schussler, N.; Saubamea, B.; Chasseigneaux, S.; Cochois, V.; Mignon, V.; Curis, E.; et al. Modifications of physical and functional integrity of the blood-brain barrier in an inducible mouse model of neurodegeneration. *Neuropharmacology* **2021**, 108588. [CrossRef] [PubMed]
26. Darvesh, A.S.; Carroll, R.T.; Geldenhuys, W.J.; Gudelsky, G.A.; Klein, J.; Meshul, C.K.; Van der Schyf, C.J. In Vivo brain microdialysis: Advances in neuropsychopharmacology and drug discovery. *Expert Opin. Drug Discov.* **2011**, *6*, 109–127. [CrossRef]
27. Chang, H.Y.; Morrow, K.; Bonacquisti, E.; Zhang, W.; Shah, D.K. Antibody pharmacokinetics in rat brain determined using microdialysis. *MAbs* **2018**, *10*, 843–853. [CrossRef]
28. Chang, H.Y.; Wu, S.; Li, Y.; Zhang, W.; Burrell, M.; Webster, C.I.; Shah, D.K. Brain pharmacokinetics of anti-transferrin receptor antibody affinity variants in rats determined using microdialysis. *MAbs* **2021**, *13*, 1874121. [CrossRef] [PubMed]

29. Chang, H.Y.; Wu, S.; Meno-Tetang, G.; Shah, D.K. A translational platform PBPK model for antibody disposition in the brain. *J. Pharmacokinet. Pharmacodyn.* **2019**, *46*, 319–338. [CrossRef]
30. Boswell, C.A.; Mundo, E.E.; Johnstone, B.; Ulufatu, S.; Schweiger, M.G.; Bumbaca, D.; Fielder, P.J.; Prabhu, S.; Khawli, L.A. Vascular physiology and protein disposition in a preclinical model of neurodegeneration. *Mol. Pharm.* **2013**, *10*, 1514–1521. [CrossRef] [PubMed]
31. Tibbitts, J.; Canter, D.; Graff, R.; Smith, A.; Khawli, L.A. Key factors influencing ADME properties of therapeutic proteins: A need for ADME characterization in drug discovery and development. *MAbs* **2016**, *8*, 229–245. [CrossRef]
32. Solon, E.G. Autoradiography techniques and quantification of drug distribution. *Cell Tissue Res.* **2015**, *360*, 87–107. [CrossRef] [PubMed]
33. Pardridge, W.M. CSF, blood-bra in barrier, and brain drug delivery. *Expert Opin. Drug Deliv.* **2016**, *13*, 963–975. [CrossRef]
34. Warnders, F.J.; Lub-de Hooge, M.N.; de Vries, E.G.E.; Kosterink, J.G.W. Influence of protein properties and protein modification on biodistribution and tumor uptake of anticancer antibodies, antibody derivatives, and non-Ig scaffolds. *Med. Res. Rev.* **2018**, *38*, 1837–1873. [CrossRef] [PubMed]
35. Sehlin, D.; Fang, X.T.; Cato, L.; Antoni, G.; Lannfelt, L.; Syvanen, S. Antibody-based PET imaging of amyloid beta in mouse models of Alzheimer's disease. *Nat. Commun.* **2016**, *7*, 10759. [CrossRef] [PubMed]
36. Lesniak, W.G.; Chu, C.; Jablonska, A.; Behnam Azad, B.; Zwaenepoel, O.; Zawadzki, M.; Lisok, A.; Pomper, M.G.; Walczak, P.; Gettemans, J.; et al. PET imaging of distinct brain uptake of a nanobody and similarly-sized PAMAM dendrimers after intra-arterial administration. *Eur. J. Nucl. Med. Mol. Imaging* **2019**, *46*, 1940–1951. [CrossRef]
37. Bien-Ly, N.; Yu, Y.J.; Bumbaca, D.; Elstrott, J.; Boswell, C.A.; Zhang, Y.; Luk, W.; Lu, Y.; Dennis, M.S.; Weimer, R.M.; et al. Transferrin receptor (TfR) trafficking determines brain uptake of TfR antibody affinity variants. *J. Exp. Med.* **2014**, *211*, 233–244. [CrossRef]
38. Bien-Ly, N.; Boswell, C.A.; Jeet, S.; Beach, T.G.; Hoyte, K.; Luk, W.; Shihadeh, V.; Ulufatu, S.; Foreman, O.; Lu, Y.; et al. Lack of Widespread BBB Disruption in Alzheimer's Disease Models: Focus on Therapeutic Antibodies. *Neuron* **2015**, *88*, 289–297. [CrossRef]
39. Bayir, E.; Sendemir, A. In Vitro Human Blood-Brain Barrier Model for Drug Permeability Testing. *Methods Mol. Biol.* **2021**. [CrossRef]
40. Banks, W.A. From blood-brain barrier to blood-brain interface: New opportunities for CNS drug delivery. *Nat. Rev. Drug Discov.* **2016**, *15*, 275–292. [CrossRef]
41. Murugan, K.; Choonara, Y.E.; Kumar, P.; Bijukumar, D.; du Toit, L.C.; Pillay, V. Parameters and characteristics governing cellular internalization and trans-barrier trafficking of nanostructures. *Int. J. Nanomed.* **2015**, *10*, 2191–2206. [CrossRef]
42. Rankovic, Z. CNS drug design: Balancing physicochemical properties for optimal brain exposure. *J. Med. Chem.* **2015**, *58*, 2584–2608. [CrossRef]
43. Boswell, C.A.; Tesar, D.B.; Mukhyala, K.; Theil, F.P.; Fielder, P.J.; Khawli, L.A. Effects of charge on antibody tissue distribution and pharmacokinetics. *Bioconjug. Chem.* **2010**, *21*, 2153–2163. [CrossRef]
44. Patel, M.M.; Goyal, B.R.; Bhadada, S.V.; Bhatt, J.S.; Amin, A.F. Getting into the brain: Approaches to enhance brain drug delivery. *CNS Drugs* **2009**, *23*, 35–58. [CrossRef] [PubMed]
45. Watts, R.J.; Dennis, M.S. Bispecific antibodies for delivery into the brain. *Curr. Opin. Chem. Biol.* **2013**, *17*, 393–399. [CrossRef] [PubMed]
46. Coloma, M.J.; Lee, H.J.; Kurihara, A.; Landaw, E.M.; Boado, R.J.; Morrison, S.L.; Pardridge, W.M. Transport across the primate blood-brain barrier of a genetically engineered chimeric monoclonal antibody to the human insulin receptor. *Pharm. Res.* **2000**, *17*, 266–274. [CrossRef]
47. Boado, R.J.; Hui, E.K.; Lu, J.Z.; Pardridge, W.M. Glycemic control and chronic dosing of rhesus monkeys with a fusion protein of iduronidase and a monoclonal antibody against the human insulin receptor. *Drug Metab. Dispos.* **2012**, *40*, 2021–2025. [CrossRef]
48. Karim, R.; Palazzo, C.; Evrard, B.; Piel, G. Nanocarriers for the treatment of glioblastoma multiforme: Current state-of-the-art. *J. Control. Release* **2016**, *227*, 23–37. [CrossRef]
49. Thom, G.; Hatcher, J.; Hearn, A.; Paterson, J.; Rodrigo, N.; Beljean, A.; Gurrell, I.; Webster, C. Isolation of blood-brain barrier-crossing antibodies from a phage display library by competitive elution and their ability to penetrate the central nervous system. *MAbs* **2018**, *10*, 304–314. [CrossRef] [PubMed]
50. Zhang, T.T.; Li, W.; Meng, G.; Wang, P.; Liao, W. Strategies for transporting nanoparticles across the blood-brain barrier. *Biomater. Sci.* **2016**, *4*, 219–229. [CrossRef]
51. Neuwelt, E.A.; Diehl, J.T.; Vu, L.H.; Hill, S.A.; Michael, A.J.; Frenkel, E.P. Monitoring of methotrexate delivery in patients with malignant brain tumors after osmotic blood-brain barrier disruption. *Ann. Intern. Med.* **1981**, *94*, 449–454. [CrossRef] [PubMed]
52. Toman, P.; Lien, C.F.; Ahmad, Z.; Dietrich, S.; Smith, J.R.; An, Q.; Molnar, E.; Pilkington, G.J.; Gorecki, D.C.; Tsibouklis, J.; et al. Nanoparticles of alkylglyceryl-dextran-graft-poly(lactic acid) for drug delivery to the brain: Preparation and in vitro investigation. *Acta Biomater.* **2015**, *23*, 250–262. [CrossRef] [PubMed]
53. Etame, A.B.; Diaz, R.J.; O'Reilly, M.A.; Smith, C.A.; Mainprize, T.G.; Hynynen, K.; Rutka, J.T. Enhanced delivery of gold nanoparticles with therapeutic potential into the brain using MRI-guided focused ultrasound. *Nanomedicine* **2012**, *8*, 1133–1142. [CrossRef] [PubMed]

54. Liu, H.L.; Hua, M.Y.; Yang, H.W.; Huang, C.Y.; Chu, P.C.; Wu, J.S.; Tseng, I.C.; Wang, J.J.; Yen, T.C.; Chen, P.Y.; et al. Magnetic resonance monitoring of focused ultrasound/magnetic nanoparticle targeting delivery of therapeutic agents to the brain. *Proc. Natl. Acad. Sci. USA* **2010**, *107*, 15205–15210. [CrossRef]
55. Aryal, M.; Vykhodtseva, N.; Zhang, Y.Z.; McDannold, N. Multiple sessions of liposomal doxorubicin delivery via focused ultrasound mediated blood-brain barrier disruption: A safety study. *J. Control. Release* **2015**, *204*, 60–69. [CrossRef] [PubMed]
56. Dennis, M.S.; Watts, R.J. Transferrin antibodies into the brain. *Neuropsychopharmacology* **2012**, *37*, 302–303. [CrossRef] [PubMed]
57. Niewoehner, J.; Bohrmann, B.; Collin, L.; Urich, E.; Sade, H.; Maier, P.; Rueger, P.; Stracke, J.O.; Lau, W.; Tissot, A.C.; et al. Increased brain penetration and potency of a therapeutic antibody using a monovalent molecular shuttle. *Neuron* **2014**, *81*, 49–60. [CrossRef] [PubMed]
58. Yu, Y.J.; Zhang, Y.; Kenrick, M.; Hoyte, K.; Luk, W.; Lu, Y.; Atwal, J.; Elliott, J.M.; Prabhu, S.; Watts, R.J.; et al. Boosting brain uptake of a therapeutic antibody by reducing its affinity for a transcytosis target. *Sci. Transl. Med.* **2011**, *3*, 84ra44. [CrossRef]
59. Kariolis, M.S.; Wells, R.C.; Getz, J.A.; Kwan, W.; Mahon, C.S.; Tong, R.; Kim, D.J.; Srivastava, A.; Bedard, C.; Henne, K.R.; et al. Brain delivery of therapeutic proteins using an Fc fragment blood-brain barrier transport vehicle in mice and monkeys. *Sci. Transl. Med.* **2020**, *12*. [CrossRef]
60. Atwal, J.K.; Chen, Y.; Chiu, C.; Mortensen, D.L.; Meilandt, W.J.; Liu, Y.; Heise, C.E.; Hoyte, K.; Luk, W.; Lu, Y.; et al. A therapeutic antibody targeting BACE1 inhibits amyloid-beta production in vivo. *Sci. Transl. Med.* **2011**, *3*, 84ra43. [CrossRef] [PubMed]
61. Haqqani, A.S.; Caram-Salas, N.; Ding, W.; Brunette, E.; Delaney, C.E.; Baumann, E.; Boileau, E.; Stanimirovic, D. Multiplexed evaluation of serum and CSF pharmacokinetics of brain-targeting single-domain antibodies using a NanoLC-SRM-ILIS method. *Mol. Pharm.* **2013**, *10*, 1542–1556. [CrossRef]
62. Tanha, J.; Muruganandam, A.; Stanimirovic, D. Phage display technology for identifying specific antigens on brain endothelial cells. *Methods Mol. Med.* **2003**, *89*, 435–449. [CrossRef]
63. Demeule, M.; Currie, J.C.; Bertrand, Y.; Che, C.; Nguyen, T.; Regina, A.; Gabathuler, R.; Castaigne, J.P.; Beliveau, R. Involvement of the low-density lipoprotein receptor-related protein in the transcytosis of the brain delivery vector angiopep-2. *J. Neurochem.* **2008**, *106*, 1534–1544. [CrossRef]
64. Huile, G.; Shuaiqi, P.; Zhi, Y.; Shijie, C.; Chen, C.; Xinguo, J.; Shun, S.; Zhiqing, P.; Yu, H. A cascade targeting strategy for brain neuroglial cells employing nanoparticles modified with angiopep-2 peptide and EGFP-EGF1 protein. *Biomaterials* **2011**, *32*, 8669–8675. [CrossRef]
65. Muruganandam, A.; Tanha, J.; Narang, S.; Stanimirovic, D. Selection of phage-displayed llama single-domain antibodies that transmigrate across human blood-brain barrier endothelium. *FASEB J.* **2002**, *16*, 240–242. [CrossRef] [PubMed]
66. Boado, R.J.; Zhang, Y.; Zhang, Y.; Wang, Y.; Pardridge, W.M. GDNF fusion protein for targeted-drug delivery across the human blood-brain barrier. *Biotechnol. Bioeng.* **2008**, *100*, 387–396. [CrossRef] [PubMed]
67. Herz, J.; Strickland, D.K. LRP: A multifunctional scavenger and signaling receptor. *J. Clin. Investig.* **2001**, *108*, 779–784. [CrossRef] [PubMed]
68. Paterson, J.; Webster, C.I. Exploiting transferrin receptor for delivering drugs across the blood-brain barrier. *Drug Discov. Today Technol.* **2016**, *20*, 49–52. [CrossRef] [PubMed]
69. Zvonova, E.A.; Tyurin, A.A.; Soloviev, A.A.; Goldenkova-Pavlova, I.V. Strategies for Modulation of Pharmacokinetics of Recombinant Therapeutic Proteins. *Biol. Bull. Rev.* **2018**, *8*, 124–141. [CrossRef]
70. Kuramochi, T.; Igawa, T.; Tsunoda, H.; Hattori, K. Humanization and simultaneous optimization of monoclonal antibody. *Methods Mol. Biol.* **2014**, *1060*, 123–137. [CrossRef]
71. Carter, P.J. Potent antibody therapeutics by design. *Nat. Rev. Immunol.* **2006**, *6*, 343–357. [CrossRef]
72. Khawli, L.A.; Biela, B.; Hu, P.; Epstein, A.L. Comparison of recombinant derivatives of chimeric TNT-3 antibody for the radioimaging of solid tumors. *Hybrid Hybridomics* **2003**, *22*, 1–9. [CrossRef]
73. Sehlin, D.; Syvanen, S.; Faculty, M. Engineered antibodies: New possibilities for brain PET? *Eur. J. Nucl. Med. Mol. Imaging* **2019**, *46*, 2848–2858. [CrossRef]
74. Yeung, Y.A.; Leabman, M.K.; Marvin, J.S.; Qiu, J.; Adams, C.W.; Lien, S.; Starovasnik, M.A.; Lowman, H.B. Engineering human IgG1 affinity to human neonatal Fc receptor: Impact of affinity improvement on pharmacokinetics in primates. *J. Immunol.* **2009**, *182*, 7663–7671. [CrossRef]
75. Roopenian, D.C.; Christianson, G.J.; Sproule, T.J.; Brown, A.C.; Akilesh, S.; Jung, N.; Petkova, S.; Avanessian, L.; Choi, E.Y.; Shaffer, D.J.; et al. The MHC class I-like IgG receptor controls perinatal IgG transport, IgG homeostasis, and fate of IgG-Fc-coupled drugs. *J. Immunol.* **2003**, *170*, 3528–3533. [CrossRef]
76. Deane, R.; Sagare, A.; Hamm, K.; Parisi, M.; LaRue, B.; Guo, H.; Wu, Z.; Holtzman, D.M.; Zlokovic, B.V. IgG-assisted age-dependent clearance of Alzheimer's amyloid beta peptide by the blood-brain barrier neonatal Fc receptor. *J. Neurosci.* **2005**, *25*, 11495–11503. [CrossRef]
77. Pardridge, W.M. Blood-Brain Barrier and Delivery of Protein and Gene Therapeutics to Brain. *Front Aging Neurosci.* **2019**, *11*, 373. [CrossRef]
78. Abuqayyas, L.; Balthasar, J.P. Investigation of the role of FcgammaR and FcRn in mAb distribution to the brain. *Mol. Pharm.* **2013**, *10*, 1505–1513. [CrossRef] [PubMed]
79. Garg, A.; Balthasar, J.P. Investigation of the influence of FcRn on the distribution of IgG to the brain. *AAPS J.* **2009**, *11*, 553–557. [CrossRef] [PubMed]

80. Chen, N.; Wang, W.; Fauty, S.; Fang, Y.; Hamuro, L.; Hussain, A.; Prueksaritanont, T. The effect of the neonatal Fc receptor on human IgG biodistribution in mice. *MAbs* **2014**, *6*, 502–508. [CrossRef] [PubMed]
81. Eigenmann, M.J.; Fronton, L.; Grimm, H.P.; Otteneder, M.B.; Krippendorff, B.F. Quantification of IgG monoclonal antibody clearance in tissues. *MAbs* **2017**, *9*, 1007–1015. [CrossRef] [PubMed]
82. Cooper, P.R.; Ciambrone, G.J.; Kliwinski, C.M.; Maze, E.; Johnson, L.; Li, Q.; Feng, Y.; Hornby, P.J. Efflux of monoclonal antibodies from rat brain by neonatal Fc receptor, FcRn. *Brain Res.* **2013**, *1534*, 13–21. [CrossRef]
83. Schlachetzki, F.; Zhu, C.; Pardridge, W.M. Expression of the neonatal Fc receptor (FcRn) at the blood-brain barrier. *J. Neurochem.* **2002**, *81*, 203–206. [CrossRef] [PubMed]
84. Ruano-Salguero, J.S.; Lee, K.H. Antibody transcytosis across brain endothelial-like cells occurs nonspecifically and independent of FcRn. *Sci. Rep.* **2020**, *10*, 3685. [CrossRef] [PubMed]
85. Friden, P.M.; Walus, L.R.; Musso, G.F.; Taylor, M.A.; Malfroy, B.; Starzyk, R.M. Anti-transferrin receptor antibody and antibody-drug conjugates cross the blood-brain barrier. *Proc. Natl. Acad. Sci. USA* **1991**, *88*, 4771–4775. [CrossRef] [PubMed]
86. Sade, H.; Baumgartner, C.; Hugenmatter, A.; Moessner, E.; Freskgard, P.O.; Niewoehner, J. A human blood-brain barrier transcytosis assay reveals antibody transcytosis influenced by pH-dependent receptor binding. *PLoS ONE* **2014**, *9*, e96340. [CrossRef]
87. Levin, V.A. Relationship of octanol/water partition coefficient and molecular weight to rat brain capillary permeability. *J. Med. Chem.* **1980**, *23*, 682–684. [CrossRef]
88. Pan, W.; Kastin, A.J. Changing the chemokine gradient: CINC1 crosses the blood-brain barrier. *J. Neuroimmunol.* **2001**, *115*, 64–70. [CrossRef]
89. Heyl, D.L.; Sefler, A.M.; He, J.X.; Sawyer, T.K.; Wustrow, D.J.; Akunne, H.C.; Davis, M.D.; Pugsley, T.A.; Heffner, T.G.; Corbin, A.E.; et al. Structure-activity and conformational studies of a series of modified C-terminal hexapeptide neurotensin analogues. *Int. J. Pept. Protein Res.* **1994**, *44*, 233–238. [CrossRef]
90. Gentry, C.L.; Egleton, R.D.; Gillespie, T.; Abbruscato, T.J.; Bechowski, H.B.; Hruby, V.J.; Davis, T.P. The effect of halogenation on blood-brain barrier permeability of a novel peptide drug. *Peptides* **1999**, *20*, 1229–1238. [CrossRef]
91. Sola, R.J.; Griebenow, K. Glycosylation of therapeutic proteins: An effective strategy to optimize efficacy. *BioDrugs* **2010**, *24*, 9–21. [CrossRef]
92. Poduslo, J.F.; Curran, G.L. Glycation increases the permeability of proteins across the blood-nerve and blood-brain barriers. *Brain Res. Mol. Brain Res.* **1994**, *23*, 157–162. [CrossRef]
93. Bickel, U.; Lee, V.M.Y.; Pardridge, W.M. Pharmacokinetic differences between111In- and125I-Labeled cationized monoclonal antibody against β-Amyloid in mouse and dog. *Drug Delivery* **2008**, *2*, 128–135. [CrossRef]
94. Triguero, D.; Buciak, J.B.; Yang, J.; Pardridge, W.M. Blood-brain barrier transport of cationized immunoglobulin G: Enhanced delivery compared to native protein. *Proc. Natl. Acad. Sci. USA* **1989**, *86*, 4761–4765. [CrossRef]
95. Kang, Y.S.; Pardridge, W.M. Brain delivery of biotin bound to a conjugate of neutral avidin and cationized human albumin. *Pharm. Res.* **1994**, *11*, 1257–1264. [CrossRef]
96. Pardridge, W.M.; Triguero, D.; Buciak, J.L. Beta-endorphin chimeric peptides: Transport through the blood-brain barrier in vivo and cleavage of disulfide linkage by brain. *Endocrinology* **1990**, *126*, 977–984. [CrossRef] [PubMed]
97. Nau, R.; Sorgel, F.; Eiffert, H. Penetration of drugs through the blood-cerebrospinal fluid/blood-brain barrier for treatment of central nervous system infections. *Clin Microbiol. Rev.* **2010**, *23*, 858–883. [CrossRef]
98. Vendel, E.; Rottschafer, V.; de Lange, E.C.M. The 3D Brain Unit Network Model to Study Spatial Brain Drug Exposure under Healthy and Pathological Conditions. *Pharm. Res.* **2020**, *37*, 137. [CrossRef] [PubMed]
99. Tanha, J.; Dubuc, G.; Hirama, T.; Narang, S.A.; MacKenzie, C.R. Selection by phage display of llama conventional V(H) fragments with heavy chain antibody V(H)H properties. *J. Immunol. Methods* **2002**, *263*, 97–109. [CrossRef]
100. Abulrob, A.; Sprong, H.; Van Bergen en Henegouwen, P.; Stanimirovic, D. The blood-brain barrier transmigrating single domain antibody: Mechanisms of transport and antigenic epitopes in human brain endothelial cells. *J. Neurochem.* **2005**, *95*, 1201–1214. [CrossRef] [PubMed]
101. Chacko, A.M.; Li, C.; Pryma, D.A.; Brem, S.; Coukos, G.; Muzykantov, V. Targeted delivery of antibody-based therapeutic and imaging agents to CNS tumors: Crossing the blood-brain barrier divide. *Expert Opin. Drug Deliv.* **2013**, *10*, 907–926. [CrossRef]
102. Bumbaca Yadav, D.; Sharma, V.K.; Boswell, C.A.; Hotzel, I.; Tesar, D.; Shang, Y.; Ying, Y.; Fischer, S.K.; Grogan, J.L.; Chiang, E.Y.; et al. Evaluating the Use of Antibody Variable Region (Fv) Charge as a Risk Assessment Tool for Predicting Typical Cynomolgus Monkey Pharmacokinetics. *J. Biol. Chem.* **2015**, *290*, 29732–29741. [CrossRef]
103. Naseri Kouzehgarani, G.; Feldsien, T.; Engelhard, H.H.; Mirakhur, K.K.; Phipps, C.; Nimmrich, V.; Clausznitzer, D.; Lefebvre, D.R. Harnessing cerebrospinal fluid circulation for drug delivery to brain tissues. *Adv. Drug Deliv. Rev.* **2021**, *173*, 20–59. [CrossRef]
104. Boado, R.J.; Hui, E.K.; Lu, J.Z.; Sumbria, R.K.; Pardridge, W.M. Blood-brain barrier molecular trojan horse enables imaging of brain uptake of radioiodinated recombinant protein in the rhesus monkey. *Bioconjug. Chem.* **2013**, *24*, 1741–1749. [CrossRef]
105. Hultqvist, G.; Syvanen, S.; Fang, X.T.; Lannfelt, L.; Sehlin, D. Bivalent Brain Shuttle Increases Antibody Uptake by Monovalent Binding to the Transferrin Receptor. *Theranostics* **2017**, *7*, 308–318. [CrossRef] [PubMed]
106. He, Q.; Liu, J.; Liang, J.; Liu, X.; Li, W.; Liu, Z.; Ding, Z.; Tuo, D. Towards Improvements for Penetrating the Blood-Brain Barrier-Recent Progress from a Material and Pharmaceutical Perspective. *Cells* **2018**, *7*, 24. [CrossRef] [PubMed]

107. Vallianatou, T.; Giaginis, C.; Tsantili-Kakoulidou, A. The impact of physicochemical and molecular properties in drug design: Navigation in the "drug-like" chemical space. *Adv. Exp. Med. Biol.* **2015**, *822*, 187–194. [CrossRef]
108. Gadkar, K.; Yadav, D.B.; Zuchero, J.Y.; Couch, J.A.; Kanodia, J.; Kenrick, M.K.; Atwal, J.K.; Dennis, M.S.; Prabhu, S.; Watts, R.J.; et al. Mathematical PKPD and safety model of bispecific TfR/BACE1 antibodies for the optimization of antibody uptake in brain. *Eur. J. Pharm. Biopharm.* **2016**, *101*, 53–61. [CrossRef] [PubMed]
109. Kanodia, J.S.; Gadkar, K.; Bumbaca, D.; Zhang, Y.; Tong, R.K.; Luk, W.; Hoyte, K.; Lu, Y.; Wildsmith, K.R.; Couch, J.A.; et al. Prospective Design of Anti-Transferrin Receptor Bispecific Antibodies for Optimal Delivery into the Human Brain. *CPT Pharmacomet. Syst. Pharmacol.* **2016**, *5*, 283–291. [CrossRef]
110. Pearlstein, R.A.; McKay, D.J.J.; Hornak, V.; Dickson, C.; Golosov, A.; Harrison, T.; Velez-Vega, C.; Duca, J. Building New Bridges between In Vitro and In Vivo in Early Drug Discovery: Where Molecular Modeling Meets Systems Biology. *Curr. Top Med. Chem.* **2017**, *17*, 2642–2662. [CrossRef]
111. Morales, J.F.; Montoto, S.S.; Fagiolino, P.; Ruiz, M.E. Current State and Future Perspectives in QSAR Models to Predict Blood-Brain Barrier Penetration in Central Nervous System Drug R&D. *Mini. Rev. Med. Chem.* **2017**, *17*, 247–257. [CrossRef]
112. Wang, Y.; Xing, J.; Xu, Y.; Zhou, N.; Peng, J.; Xiong, Z.; Liu, X.; Luo, X.; Luo, C.; Chen, K.; et al. In silico ADME/T modelling for rational drug design. *Q Rev. Biophys.* **2015**, *48*, 488–515. [CrossRef]
113. Blair, L.J.; Frauen, H.D.; Zhang, B.; Nordhues, B.A.; Bijan, S.; Lin, Y.C.; Zamudio, F.; Hernandez, L.D.; Sabbagh, J.J.; Selenica, M.L.; et al. Tau depletion prevents progressive blood-brain barrier damage in a mouse model of tauopathy. *Acta Neuropathol. Commun.* **2015**, *3*, 8. [CrossRef] [PubMed]
114. Lalatsa, A.; Leite, D.M. Single-Domain Antibodies for Brain Targeting. *Biopharm. Int.* **2014**, *27*, 20–26.
115. Zuchero, Y.J.; Chen, X.; Bien-Ly, N.; Bumbaca, D.; Tong, R.K.; Gao, X.; Zhang, S.; Hoyte, K.; Luk, W.; Huntley, M.A.; et al. Discovery of Novel Blood-Brain Barrier Targets to Enhance Brain Uptake of Therapeutic Antibodies. *Neuron* **2016**, *89*, 70–82. [CrossRef]
116. Lu, Y.; Khawli, L.A.; Purushothama, S.; Theil, F.P.; Partridge, M.A. Recent Advances in Assessing Immunogenicity of Therapeutic Proteins: Impact on Biotherapeutic Development. *J. Immunol. Res.* **2016**, *2016*, 8141269. [CrossRef] [PubMed]
117. Smith, A.; Manoli, H.; Jaw, S.; Frutoz, K.; Epstein, A.L.; Khawli, L.A.; Theil, F.P. Unraveling the Effect of Immunogenicity on the PK/PD, Efficacy, and Safety of Therapeutic Proteins. *J. Immunol. Res.* **2016**, *2016*, 2342187. [CrossRef]
118. Khawli, L.A.; Prabhu, S. Drug delivery across the blood-brain barrier. *Mol. Pharm.* **2013**, *10*, 1471–1472. [CrossRef]
119. Deo, A.K.; Theil, F.P.; Nicolas, J.M. Confounding parameters in preclinical assessment of blood-brain barrier permeation: An overview with emphasis on species differences and effect of disease states. *Mol. Pharm.* **2013**, *10*, 1581–1595. [CrossRef] [PubMed]
120. Lu, C.T.; Zhao, Y.Z.; Wong, H.L.; Cai, J.; Peng, L.; Tian, X.Q. Current approaches to enhance CNS delivery of drugs across the brain barriers. *Int. J. Nanomed.* **2014**, *9*, 2241–2257. [CrossRef]
121. Terstappen, G.C.; Meyer, A.H.; Bell, R.D.; Zhang, W. Strategies for delivering therapeutics across the blood-brain barrier. *Nat. Rev. Drug Discov.* **2021**, *20*, 362–383. [CrossRef] [PubMed]

International Journal of *Molecular Sciences*

MDPI

Review

Antibody-Based Therapeutics for Atherosclerosis and Cardiovascular Diseases

Eunhye Ji [1] and Sahmin Lee [1,2,*]

[1] Division of Cardiology, Heart Institute, Asan Medical Center, Seoul 05505, Korea; jieunhye7@gmail.com
[2] Department of Medical Science, Asan Medical Institute of Convergence Science and Technology, University of Ulsan College of Medicine, Seoul 05505, Korea
* Correspondence: sahmin.lee@amc.seoul.kr

Abstract: Cardiovascular disease is the leading cause of death worldwide, and its prevalence is increasing due to the aging of societies. Atherosclerosis, a type of chronic inflammatory disease that occurs in arteries, is considered to be the main cause of cardiovascular diseases such as ischemic heart disease or stroke. In addition, the inflammatory response caused by atherosclerosis confers a significant effect on chronic inflammatory diseases such as psoriasis and rheumatic arthritis. Here, we review the mechanism of action of the main causes of atherosclerosis such as plasma LDL level and inflammation; furthermore, we review the recent findings on the preclinical and clinical effects of antibodies that reduce the LDL level and those that neutralize the cytokines involved in inflammation. The apolipoprotein B autoantibody and anti-PCSK9 antibody reduced the level of LDL and plaques in animal studies, but failed to significantly reduce carotid inflammation plaques in clinical trials. The monoclonal antibodies against PCSK9 (alirocumab, evolocumab), which are used as a treatment for hyperlipidemia, lowered cholesterol levels and the incidence of cardiovascular diseases. Antibodies that neutralize inflammatory cytokines (TNF-α, IL-1β, IL-6, IL-17, and IL-12/23) have shown promising but contradictory results and thus warrant further research.

Keywords: atherosclerosis; inflammation; antibody therapy

Citation: Ji, E.; Lee, S. Antibody-Based Therapeutics for Atherosclerosis and Cardiovascular Diseases. *Int. J. Mol. Sci.* **2021**, *22*, 5770. https://doi.org/10.3390/ijms22115770

Academic Editors: Yong-Seok Heo and Gaetano Santulli

Received: 31 March 2021
Accepted: 26 May 2021
Published: 28 May 2021

1. Introduction

Cardiovascular disease is the leading cause of death in populations worldwide, and the prevalence of aging-related chronic diseases is increasing every year. According to a survey by the World Health Organization (WHO), 17.9 million people died due to cardiovascular disease in 2016, accounting for 31% of total deaths worldwide [1]. Of the cardiovascular disease-related deaths, 85% are caused by heart attacks and strokes, and the most significant cause of the two diseases is the blockage of blood vessels. Atherosclerotic lipid-laden plaques are the major etiology factors for blood vessel blockage, and as these plaques are stacked inside the sub-endothelial space (i.e., the intima), the walls of the vessel become narrow and physically interfere with the blood flow [2,3]. Since atherosclerosis is asymptomatic until the occurrence of remarkable phenomena, early detection is difficult. As such, the prognosis is poor in most cases, which directly links to the high mortality rates [2].

Yet, the currently available modes of treatment for atherosclerosis are limited to statin, ACE inhibitor, and β-blocker, among which statin is the most studied and used as first-line therapy [4]. Statin, which is used as a treatment for hyperlipidemia, functions by lowering the LDL levels; importantly, a meta-analysis of several randomized controlled studies on statin reported that statin reduced both the mortality from all causes and the incidence rates of atherosclerotic cardiovascular diseases [5]. This suggests that lipid is a critical factor in atherosclerosis.

Atherosclerosis has been considered to be caused by increases in cholesterol. The complexity of atherosclerosis and the involvement of various risk factors call for further research, but it is well-known that increases in cholesterol mark the beginning of atherosclerosis [6–9]. Increase in the concentration of LDL-C (low-density lipoprotein cholesterol) above the physiological need leads to the accumulation of LDL in the intima of the arteries and the development of atherosclerosis [10]. The lipid infiltrated into the intima becomes oxidized LDL (oxLDL) through oxidative modification and is engulfed by macrophages derived from monocytes to generate foam cells [11]. The form cells are held in the intima and their migration is inhibited, and thereby build up the lipid-rich center (necrotic core) of atherosclerotic plaques by being combined with cholesterol and apoptotic, necrotic cells (Figure 1) [12,13].

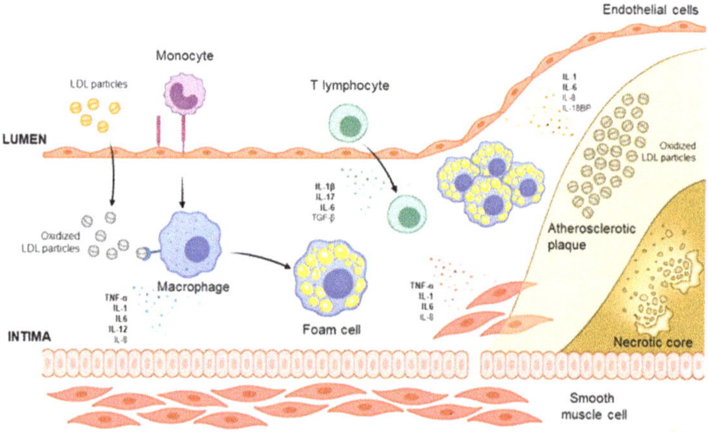

Figure 1. Mechanism of atherosclerosis formation.The development of atherosclerosis begins when low-density lipoprotein (LDL) particles infiltrate the intima layer and accumulate. Within the intima, LDLs form oxidized LDL (oxLDL) through myeloperoxidase and lipoxygenase, bind to the scavenger receptor of macrophage-derived foam cells, and activate the foam cells. Activated foam cells induce inflammation by secreting cytokines through several downstream signals. Concurrently, smooth muscle cells in the media layer migrate to the intima and are transdifferentiated into macrophage-like cells, and under the influence of the cytokines secreted from foam cells, secrete cytokines such as IL-6 to promote inflammation. In the intima, oxLDL increases the expression of adhesion molecules at the endothelial cell surface, leading to the recruitment of monocytes and other immune cells, and promote synergy with the aforementioned phenomena to induce the formation of atherosclerotic plaques.

Another key mechanism that drives the development of atherosclerosis is immune/inflammation [14]. Endothelial cells at the site of the accumulation of the modified lipoprotein express VCAM-1 (vascular cell adhesion protein 1), which functions as an adhesion molecule to recruit circulating monocytes and other immune cells [15]. All cells that contribute to the development of atherosclerosis—macrophages differentiated from monocytes, recruited leukocytes, and smooth muscle cells that migrated from the media to the intima—produce and secrete various cytokines, such as tumor necrosis factor (TNF)-α, interleukin (IL)-1β, and IL-6 to promote plaque growth [16]. Through the effects of several pro-inflammatory cytokines, atherosclerosis develops and the plaques are destabilized. Accordingly, a number of antibodies have been developed to specifically target and neutralize the pro-inflammatory cytokines that are involved in the development of atherosclerotic plaques (Figure 2).

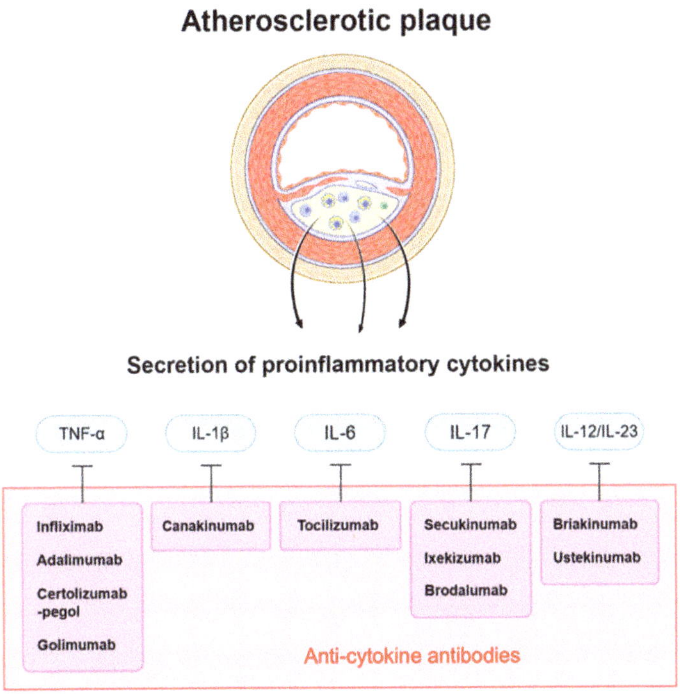

Figure 2. Antibodies targeting cytokines and cytokines acting on atherosclerotic plaque. Atherosclerotic plaque consists of lipid, apoptotic cells, immune cells, smooth muscle cells, and endothelial cells. These cells induce inflammation by secreting specific cytokines. Among them, IL-1β, TNF-α, IL-17, IL-6, and IL-12/23 are under investigation as therapeutic targets for atherosclerosis, and a number of antibodies have been developed to target each cytokine.

Along with the aforementioned pathogenesis studies on atherosclerosis, many pharmacological and clinical studies have been carried out [17]. This review will focus on the studies of antibody-based treatments targeting LDL and pro-inflammatory cytokines (Table 1). Therapeutic antibodies are stable molecules to be used as targeting reagents. They have an ability to bind to target proteins with high specificity and affinity. Despite of several limitations including unclear mode of action, inefficient tissue penetration and impaired immune reactions, current technological advances in antibody engineering have enabled the successful translation of antibody drugs to the clinic [18,19]. Currently, more than 79 antibody drugs are approved by the United States Food and Drug Administration (US FDA), and more than 570 antibody therapies around the world are under study [20]. Development of antibody drugs against pro-atherosclerotic factors also will play a major role in the treatment of cardiovascular diseases and inflammation.

Table 1. Summary of antibody based clinical trials.

Therapeutic/Study Name	Antibody Name	Target	Patients	Result
GLACIER	MLDL1278A	oxLDL (MDA-modified human ApoB-100)	CVD patients	Non significantly reduce carotid plaque
FOURIER	Evolocumab	PCSK9	patients with clinically evident CVD(prior MI, stroke or PAD)	LDL-C level and primary outcomes (MI, stroke, cardiovascular death, coronary revascularization, unstable angina) reduction
ODYSSEY	Alirocumab	PCSK9	patients diagnosed with ACS	LDL-C level and primary outcomes (non-fatal MI, ischemic stroke, unstable angina) reduction
SPIRE	Bococizumab	PCSK9	CV or high risk patients	LDL-C level and primary ennpoint reduction in LDL-C >100 mg/dL group
ATTACH	Infliximab	TNF-α	Heart failure	Deteriorated heart failure
STROBE (follow up study)	Infliximab	TNF-α	Psoriasis	Significantly reduce the cardiovascular risk
Di Minno et al. [21]	Adalimumab, Infliximab	TNF-A	Psoriatic arthritis	Decreased atherosclerosis of carotid artery
CANTOS	Canakinumab	IL-1B	CAD after MI + hsCRP	Decreased hsCRP level and incidence of the primary endpoint (nonfatal myocardial infarction, stroke, cardiovascular death)
ASSIL-MI	Tocilizumab	IL-6	ACS	Increased myocardial salvage
Mease et al. [22]	Secukinumab	IL-17	Psoriatic arthritis	Non significant increased MACE
Uncover	Ixekizumab	IL-17	Moderate to severe psoriasis	Reduced Psoriasis Area and Severity Index (PASI) score
Langley et al. [23]	Briakinumab	IL-12/23	Psoriasis	Increased MACE
Uniti	Ustekinumab	IL-12/23	Moderate to severe Crohn's disease	Significantly higher rate of response

2. LDL- or oxLDL-Lowering Therapies

2.1. Apolipoprotein B Autoantibody

Previous studies reported that high concentrations of autoantibodies that recognize various epitopes of oxidized LDL are found in atherosclerotic plaques [24,25]. In addition, animal studies using IgG antibodies specific to the epitope of oxidized LDL showed the atheroprotective effects such as decreases in atherosclerotic plaque inflammation and plaque area [26,27]. The immunization of apoE-deficient mice with MDA-p45, an MDA-modified apo B-100 peptide, increased the levels of MDA-p45 IgG and decreased atherosclerotic plaques. Experiments using anti-p45 IgG consistently demonstrated the inhibition of the development of atherosclerotic plaques, and showed the potential benefit of anti-p45 therapy [26,28]. MLDL1278a, which targets oxLDL (MDA-modified human ApoB-100), confers an anti-inflammatory effect by regulating Syk, p38 MAPK phosphorylation, and NF-κB. In subsequent experiments in obese Rhesus macaques, MLDL1278a was shown to significantly reduce pro-inflammatory cytokines and enhance the function of immune cells [29]. However, clinical results showed that the levels of MDA-modified peptide p45 and p210 autoantibody were inversely proportional to the severity of arterial disease; moreover, the GLACIER (Goal of Oxidized LDL and Activated Macrophage Inhibition by Exposure to a Recombinant Antibody) study, which was a multicenter, randomized, double-blind trial, showed that anti-oxLDL antibody did not significantly reduce carotid plaque inflammation in stable patients with cardiovascular disease [30–32]. In response to this trial, it was suggested that the plaque inflammation level of the patients included in the clinical trial was not high enough to be effective for the antibody therapy; however, there was no explanation for the contradiction in the results [31]. Despite some uncertainty, multiple experiments and clinical studies have demonstrated the atheroprotective effects of autoantibodies targeting oxLDL, which suggest its potential for use as an atherosclerosis antibody therapy [33].

2.2. PCSK9 Inhibitor

High concentration of LDL-C in the plasma is a crucial factor for atherosclerosis [34,35]. Therefore, reducing LDL-C is a key mechanism for the alleviation of the disease, and the molecular mechanism for LDL-C reduction involves PCSK9. Circulating LDL in the plasma is internalized by binding with LDL receptors on the cell surface. The internalized LDL particles are then moved to the lysosome and degraded, and the LDL receptor is recycled and expressed on the cell surface [36]. However, in the presence of PCSK9, the LDL receptor binds to PCSK9 and forms a PCSK9-LDL receptor-LDL complex. This complex is internalized into the cell and transferred to the lysosome, resulting in the degradation of both LDL and LDL receptors [37,38]. Consequentially, LDL receptors cannot be reused, and the abundance of LDL receptors on the cell surface is reduced, thereby leading to increases in the plasma level of LDL particles that serve as the trigger of atherosclerosis [37,39,40].

Accordingly, a previous study suggested that the serum level of PCSK9 may be useful as a predictive factor for early atherosclerosis, considering that the expression of PCSK9 was high in the plasma of patients with carotid IMT [41]. The E670G mutation in PCSK9 leads to an increase in enzyme activity, increases the intima-media thickness (D374Y), and decreases the level of hepatic LDL and the development of atherosclerotic plaque in pigs [42,43]. In contrast, a study using loss-of-function mutation for PCSK9 demonstrated that it was associated with the maintenance of low cholesterol levels and subsequent reduction in atherosclerotic disease [44,45]. Based on these results, PSCK9 was highlighted as the therapeutic target of atherosclerosis, and several studies have been conducted to test the potential for functional inhibition of PCSK9 using antibody mechanisms. The monoclonal antibodies that could interfere with the interaction of LDLR and PCSK9 were obtained [46,47] and it was found that these monoclonal antibodies increase the cellular LDL receptor and lower the level of LDL-C, so the clinical studies of the antibody as a PCSK9 inhibitor were promoted [48–50].

Two of the most well-known human monoclonal antibodies targeting PCSK9 are alirocumab (Praluent) and evolocumab (Repatha), both of which were approved in the U.S. and European Union [51]. The FOURIER (Further Cardiovascular Outcomes Research with PCSK9 Inhibition in Subjects with Elevated Risk) trial, which was conducted to verify the clinical effect of evolocumab, enrolled 27,564 high-risk patients with a history of myocardial infarction, non-hemorrhagic stroke, or symptomatic peripheral artery disease, all of whom continued to take statin while being administered with evolocumab or placebo [52,53]. The study patients were followed-up for 2.2 years and the incidence of cardiovascular abnormalities was evaluated by dividing into the primary and secondary outcomes according to gradual decreases in the LDL levels [54]. After 48 weeks, the LDL-C levels in the evolocumab group decreased by 59% compared with that in the placebo group; moreover, the incidence of the primary outcomes of MI, stroke, cardiovascular death, coronary revascularization, and unstable angina was lower in the evolocumab group (9.8%) than in the placebo group (11.3%) [34,44,52,53].

The ODYSSEY (Evaluation of Cardiovascular Outcomes After an Acute Coronary Syndrome During Treatment With Alirocumab) trial is a representative clinical trial on the safety and efficacy of alirocumab, another human monoclonal antibody targeting PCSK9. From 1315 sites, the ODYSSEY trial enrolled 18,924 patients diagnosed with acute coronary syndrome (ACS) within 12 months prior to study inclusion [55]. After 2.8 years, the LDL-c level in the alirocumab group was 54.7% lower than that in the placebo group, and the incidence of the primary outcome of non-fatal MI, fatal or non-fatal ischemic stroke, and unstable angina requiring hospitalization was lower in the alirocumab group (9.5%) than in the placebo group (11.1%) [52,56].

Unlike the evolocumab and alirocumab, the bococizumab, another antibody against PCSK9, is a humanized mouse antibody. Two large scale trials were conducted in parallel, Studies of PCSK9 Inhibition and the Reduction of Vascular Events (SPIRE) −1 and −2′, and the trials randomized 27,438 cardiovascular disease or high risk patients. The participants received 150 mg of bococizumab or placebo subcutaneously every 2 weeks. After 14 weeks, LDL-C level of bococizumab group showing 59% reduction compared with placebo. And primary endpoints were 21% lower in high-risk patients with LDL-C >100 mg/dL, but no significant results were obtained in lower-risk patients. More studies are being conducted based on these clinical results [52,57–59].

These clinical trials demonstrated that monoclonal antibodies against PCSK9 could dramatically lower the LDL-C level and reduce the risk of atherosclerotic cardiovascular disease. Based on these results, the 2018 ACC/AHA Multisociety guidelines recommended the use of PCSK9 inhibitors in patients with a very high risk of atherosclerotic cardiovascular disease [60,61]. In addition to the antibodies mentioned above, many studies have investigated the efficacies of LDL-lowering drugs such as PCSK9 siRNA, and bempedoic acid [53,62].

3. Cytokine-Targeting Therapy

3.1. Anti-TNF-α

TNF-α is an essential cytokine involved in adaptive immunity during the process of atherosclerosis [63]. The mRNA of TNF-α is synthesized from smooth muscle cells and macrophages present in the atherosclerotic plaques [64]. Importantly, TNF-α was steadily increased in patients after MI who were being monitored for recurrent MACE (major adverse cardiovascular events). As inflammation was shown to play a critical role in cardiovascular disease, the pro-inflammatory cytokine TNF-α was highlighted as a potent therapeutic target for cardiovascular disease [65].

In an animal experiment investigating the pathological effect of TNF-α on atherosclerosis, it was found that when the TNF-α gene was deficient, the expression levels of adhesion molecules and chemokines were altered and led to the inhibition of the development of atherosclerosis [66]. However, experiments with mice with genetic deletion of the TNF-α receptor showed contrasting results. Since TNF-α is a pro-inflammatory cytokine, it was expected that the deficiency of TNF-α would protect against atherosclerosis; however, the size of aortic atherosclerosis lesion in TNF-α-null mice was 2.3 times larger than that in wild-type mice [67].

Anti-TNF-α therapy using monoclonal antibodies that specifically bind to and neutralizes TNF-α has been studied for a long time and has led to significant advances in the treatment of rheumatoid arthritis [68]. In pilot clinical trials determining the effectiveness of anti-TNF-α monoclonal antibody on psoriatic arthritis, carotid atherosclerotic plaques were found in 15.8% of patients who received TNF-α blockers, in contrast to 40.4% of those who received traditional DMARD consisting of sulfasalazine, methotrexate, cyclosporine, and leflunomide [21]. A clinical trial using the anti-TNF-α antibody infliximab also showed that the use of TNF blocker resulted in lower events of cardiovascular disease in patients with rheumatic diseases compared with no treatment [69]. In another clinical trial that examined the 5-year cardiovascular events in patients with psoriasis, which was associated with cardiovascular disease, anti-TNF-α antibody therapy was shown to significantly reduce the cardiovascular risk compared with other treatments [70].

Aside from infliximab, other antibodies such as adalimumab, golimumab, and certolizumab pegol also target TNF-α. Adalimumab and golimumab are human monoclonal antibodies, and certolizumab pegol is a PEGylated fragment of an anti-TNF-α antibody [71]. Adalimumab therapy in psoriasis patients for 2 years significantly reduced hsCRP, E-selectin, and IL-22, and had a positive effect on reducing systemic inflammation [72]. A phase 3 clinical trial showed that compared with those who received placebo, patients with moderate-to-severe psoriasis who received certolizumab pegol were more likely to show reductions in PASI score 75 (Psoriasis Area and Severity Index score >75%) [73]. Golimumab has been approved as a monotherapy for the treatment of inflammatory arthritis such as rheumatoid arthritis and psoriatic arthritis; [74] the stability and effectiveness of golimumab were verified in several phase 3 studies, and the effect was not inferior when indirectly compared with other anti-TNF-α therapies [75].

Despite the body of experimental and clinical evidence, there are limitations in the role of anti-TNF-α therapy as its clinical benefit has not been demonstrated in heart failure. The randomized, double-blind Anti-TNF Therapy Against Congestive Heart failure study was conducted in patients with moderate-to-severe heart failure, in whom infliximab therapy for 6 weeks did not result in symptom improvement and the risk of heart failure aggravation was increased when infliximab was administered at a high dose (10 mg/kg) [76]. The mechanism of the negative outcome of high-dose anti-TNF-α therapy has not been identified. Moreover, the results in lupus, obesity, metabolic syndrome, and type 2 diabetes are inconsistent, and further studies are needed for anti-TNF-α therapy to be used in a variety of diseases [77].

3.2. *Anti-IL-1β*

IL-1 signaling leads to the expression of secondary inflammatory cytokines such as IL-6; therefore, IL-1 is a critical factor in the process of atherosclerosis [78]. The IL1 gene is translated into two forms, IL-1α and IL-1β, of which the β form plays a more important role in inflammation [79]. IL-1β exists in the inactive form, pro-IL-1β, and is cleaved by caspase 1 enzyme to be converted into the biologically active form, IL-1β [80]. The expression of IL-1β is increased through mediators such as cholesterol crystals and TNF-α [81]. IL-1β has not been studied as a biomarker for cardiovascular disease because unlike hsCRP and IL-6, it is difficult to directly measure its levels in the plasma; nevertheless, many studies have been conducted to examine its role as a therapeutic target in atherosclerosis [79].

In a murine experiment, mice with double-knockout of ApoE and IL-1β had significantly smaller sizes of atherosclerotic lesions in the aortic sinus and the ratio of atherosclerotic areas of the aorta compared with single ApoE-knockout mice [82]. On the contrary, a gain-of-function animal study on the effects of IL-1β on atherosclerosis in pigs showed that artificial expression of IL-1β on one side of the coronary artery led to increases in the coronary stenosis and aggravation of vascular diseases [83]. This result is likely due to the increase in pro-inflammatory cytokines caused by the activation of immune cells and the increase in the expression of adhesion molecules in endothelial cells [84,85]. The results of these animal experiments served as the basis for clinical trials on anti-IL-1β therapy.

Canakinumab, a human monoclonal antibody for IL-1β, has been approved for use in a variety of rheumatic inflammatory diseases including cryopyrin-associated periodic syndrome, systemic juvenile idiopathic arthritis, and adult-onset Still's disease [86]. In addition, studies have shown that canakinumab significantly reduces inflammation, regardless of LDL-C or HDH-C, which suggests that canakinumab can be used as a therapeutic agent that inhibits the inflammatory response of atherosclerosis [87].

The Canakinumab Anti-Inflammatory Thrombosis Outcome Study (CANTOS) was carried out by enrolling 17,200 patients with coronary artery disease after MI whose high-sensitivity C-reactive protein (hsCRP) level steadily increased and remained at high cardiovascular risk despite secondary prevention medical therapy such as statin [88]. The patients were administered either placebo or canakinumab (50, 150, or 300 mg) for three months, and examination at 48-months showed that the hsCRP levels in the canakinumab 50 mg group, 150 mg group, and 300 mg group were 26%, 37%, and 41% of that of the placebo group [89]. At an intermediate follow-up of 44 months, the incidence of the primary endpoints was lower in the canakinumab-treated groups (50 mg: 4.11/100, 100 mg: 3.86/100, 300 mg: 3.9/100) compared with that of the placebo group (4.5/100) [89]. In conclusion, CANTOS showed that canakinumab can reduce the risk of cardiovascular disease by lowering inflammation without altering the lipids [77,90]

3.3. Anti-IL-6

IL-6, which is induced by pro-inflammatory cytokines such as IL-1 and TNF cytokines, acts as a central hub for atherosclerosis inflammatory signaling. IL-6 is produced in various cells such as smooth muscle cells, endothelial cells, and immune cells, and is a soluble cytokine that can move away from the source of inflammation and reach a target tissue by blood circulation [91]. In a study investigating the association of calcified coronary atherosclerosis and IL-6 in patients with type 2 diabetes, the level of IL-6 identified a significant association with the coronary arterial calcium score independent of other cardiovascular risk factors [92]. This study demonstrated the potential use of IL-6 as a risk factor for coronary atherosclerosis and as a therapeutic target for atherosclerosis.

One study examined the effects of IL-6 on the development of early atherosclerosis in non-obese diabetic male mice and ApoE-deficient mice that were fed a high-fat or normal chow diet for 15 weeks while receiving recombinant IL-6 or saline once a week. Regardless of the genetic alteration and diet, all mice treated with recombinant IL-6 showed significant increases in the levels of the pro-inflammatory cytokines IL-1β, TNF-α, and fibrinogen; more importantly, the area of fatty streak lesion were 1.9- to 5.1- fold larger compared with that in saline-treated mice [93]. However, IL-6 has a two-sided role in the development of atherosclerosis. In mice with double-knockout of ApoE and IL-6, serum cholesterol concentration and atherosclerotic lesion area were significantly higher compared with ApoE single-knockout mice [94]. Another study using young IL-6 and ApoE double-knockout mice showed no significant differences in the development of fatty streaks in comparison with mice of other genotypes (IL-$6^{+/+}$ApoE$^{-/-}$, IL-$6^{+/-}$ApoE$^{-/-}$) [95]. IL-6 is generally recognized as a pro-inflammatory cytokine, but it also plays a role in lowering pro-inflammatory activity by releasing soluble TNF receptors; therefore, the balance of IL-6 activity is critical in the pathogenesis of atherosclerosis [16].

IL-6 is also expressed in human atherosclerotic plaque, and an investigation of the correlation between IL-6 and risk factors of cardiovascular disease in healthy individuals showed that high IL-6 levels were associated with the risk of atherosclerosis-associated MI [96]. In addition, the variant (rs7529229) of the IL-6 receptor, which increases the level of circulating IL-6 and lowers the concentration of C-reactive protein and fibrinogen, reduced the risk of coronary heart disease events [97]. As a result of several studies commonly showing the relationship between IL-6 and atherosclerosis, IL-6 became a therapeutic target for atherosclerosis [68].

Tocilizumab, a humanized monoclonal antibody for the IL-6 receptor, interferes with the binding between IL-6 and IL-6 receptors and has been approved as a treatment in RA [63]. Tocilizumab raises the level of LDL-cholesterol, triglycerides, and HDL-cholesterol to deteriorate the lipid profile; [98] however, several studies have also reported positive results. In cohort studies using claims data from Medicare, IMS PharMetrics, and MarketScan, tocilizumab was not associated with an increased risk of cardiovascular while being associated with protective effects against MACE outbreaks [99]. Similar studies have been published in Italy [100] and Japan as well [101]. Overall, tocilizumab increases the plasma levels of LDL-C and triglyceride, but reduces the incidence of MACE. The ongoing Assessing the Effect of Anti-IL-6 Treatment in Myocardial Infraction (ASSIL-MI) phase II trial will evaluate whether tocilizumab can reduce myocardial damage in patients with ACS [102].

3.4. Anti-IL-17

IL-17 is divided into 6 members from A to F, of which A and F are the most critical members. IL-17 is produced from immune cells, such as CD4+ T helper cells, Tc17 cells, natural killer cells, and natural killer T cells [103]. IL-17a plays a role in the protection against bacterial or fungal infection, and it was found that the sensitivity to infection increases in cases with defects in IL-17A or malfunctions in the IL-17 receptor [104]. In addition, IL-17 has shown therapeutic benefits in chronic inflammatory disorders such as psoriasis, rheumatoid arthritis, and inflammatory bowel disease, a type of Crohn's disease [105,106].

The mechanism of IL-17 for atherosclerosis remains under debate. Several studies have shown that IL-17A increases the formation of atherosclerotic plaques [107–109], but not others [110,111]. The ambivalence of the role of IL-17A may be due to differences in the surrounding environment such as the location of the plaque and the level of other cytokines and chemokines [112]. Other studies reported the protective effect of IL-17A by reducing endothelial expression of VCAM-1 used for monocyte adhesion and stabilizing atherosclerotic plaque [111,113,114]. In addition, in a cohort study of more than 1000 patients with acute MI, low IL-17 levels were associated with the relapse of major adverse cardiovascular events within one year after cardiovascular risk factor treatment [115].

Secukinumab is the first human monoclonal antibody among antibody drugs targeting IL-17 that has been approved for clinical use, and has shown positive effects in psoriasis, psoriatic arthritis, and ankylosing spondylitis [22,116–119]. Secukinumab has shown significantly better effects than Ethanercept, a receptor that targets TNF-α [116,120], and adalimumab, an antibody that targets TNF-α to offset its functionality [121]. In addition, long-term use of secukinumab was associated with only low-risk side effects such as cold and diarrhea [103]. Another monoclonal antibody targeting IL-17A is lxekizumab, which was recently approved for use in plaque psoriasis. In a clinical trial conducted on patients with plaque psoriasis, the plaque was completely cured in 34% to 37% of all patients [122]. Brodalumab acts on the A chain of the IL-17 receptor and blocks the binding of IL-17 and the receptor, thereby interfering with the downstream signaling pathway. Compared to secukinumab, brodalumab showed a better effect on psoriasis [123]. However, IL-17 neutralization studies conducted on patients with rheumatoid arthritis did not report consistent results [124,125]. Therefore, it is necessary to further study the mechanism of functional changes in IL-17 in various situations and environments and to discover therapeutic candidates to offset the function of IL-17.

3.5. Anti-IL-12/23

IL-23 and IL-12 are cytokines constituting the same IL-12 family and act as heterodimers, each of which shares IL-12p40 and forms a dimer with IL-23p19 and IL-12p35. These two cytokines are produced by immune cells such as macrophages and bind to respective receptors to activate the JAK-STAT signaling and regulate inflammation [126,127]. High levels of serum IL-12 were detected in animal experiments using atherosclerosis-induced ApoE knockout mice [128]. Treatment with recombinant murine IL-12 in ApoE knockout mice and LDLR-deficient mice significantly increased the aortic atherosclerotic plaque areas [129]. Conversely, when the function of IL-12 was neutralized using vaccination in LDL receptor-knockout mice, atherogenesis was reduced by 68.5% [130,131]. The levels of IL-12 family cytokines are also significantly higher in patients with atherosclerosis associated with cardiovascular disease [132,133].

Since IL-12 and IL-23 share the IL-12p40 subunit, briakinumab and ustekinumab targeting IL-12p40 are able to neutralize both IL-12 and IL-23. Briakinumab is a human monoclonal antibody, and its efficacy was tested in a small-sized preclinical study involving patients with moderate-to-severe Crohn's disease who received either placebo or briakinumab (1 or 3 mg/kg) for 7 weeks [134]. In the initial treatment results, the 3 mg/kg injection group showed a significantly higher response rate compared with the 1 mg/kg injection and the placebo group, but the statistical significance of the difference disappeared during the 18-week follow-up period [134]. In addition, several meta-analyses compared antibody-based inflammatory agents with briakinumab and showed that MACE was more common in the briakinumab-treated groups [23].

Another monoclonal antibody targeting the human IL-12p40 is ustekinumab, which has been recently approved for use in Crohn's disease, following its approval for psoriasis and psoriatic arthritis [126]. Ustekinumab was found to be effective in a phase 2a study conducted in patients with moderate-to-severe Crohn's disease, and a randomized, double-blind phase 2b study showed an increased response rate in patients with moderate-to-severe Crohn's disease in whom anti-TNF therapy was not effective [135]. The subsequent phase 3 trial was designed more precisely and showed that the 6-week induction trial had significantly higher responses rates in the ustekinumab group than in the placebo group, and some of the patients who received ustekinumab in the induction trial were enrolled in the main maintenance study [136]. The main study measured the rate of remission of the disease at week 44, and the rate of remission was higher in the ustekinumab group than in the placebo group (placebo: 35.9%, ustekinumab every 8 weeks: 53.1%, ustekinumab: 48.8%). These results demonstrated the effectiveness of ustekinumab in alleviating the symptoms of patients with moderate-to-severe Crohn's disease [136]. A small-scale pilot study examined the atherosclerosis parameters in patients with psoriasis treated with ustekinumab, and reported that while there was a noticeable relief of skin lesions after 6 months of treatment, there was no notable change in the pulse wave velocity and intima-media thickness [137].

4. Discussion

This review summarized the mechanisms of action of antibody-based treatments targeting LDL and cytokines, which are the major causes of cardiovascular disease and atherosclerosis, and their results in recent clinical trials. The results of antibody therapy are ambivalent, with some cases showing significant alleviation of symptoms and others experiencing adverse events such as the aggravation of cardiovascular diseases. Antibodies targeting IL-17a and IL-12/23 also acted as pathogens in some cases, and briakinumab was withdrawn from the market due to increases in MACE. Therefore, it is important to monitor the side effects of new antibody therapies in terms of cardiovascular disease. Delineating the exact mechanism of action of the target molecules would be very helpful in overcoming the side effects or applying the appropriate treatment according to the situation and environment of each patient. In addition to the antibodies mentioned in the text, development and clinical trials of antibodies that inhibit a variety of molecules continue, such as ANGPTL family, CD47, CD31 [138–141]. Through these efforts, more targets will be found in the future, and mediators such as specific antibodies will be developed and eventually lead to the conquering of many diseases.

Funding: This research was supported by Basic Science Research Program through the National Research Foundation of Korea (NRF) funded by the Ministry of Education (2019R1I1A2A01060702). It was also supported by a grant of the Korea Health Technology R&D Project through the Korea Health Industry Development Institute (KHIDI), funded by the Ministry of Health & Welfare, Republic of Korea (HR20C0026) and by grants (2020IP-086, 2021IP-0038) from the Asan Institute for Life Sciences, Asan Medical Center, Seoul, Korea.

Institutional Review Board Statement: Not applicable.

Informed Consent Statement: Not applicable.

Conflicts of Interest: The authors declare no conflict of interest.

References

1. Otreba, M.; Kosmider, L.; Rzepecka-Stojko, A. Polyphenols' Cardioprotective Potential: Review of Rat Fibroblasts as Well as Rat and Human Cardiomyocyte Cell Lines Research. *Molecules* **2021**, *26*, 774. [CrossRef] [PubMed]
2. Chen, J.; Zhang, X.; Millican, R.; Sherwood, J.; Martin, S.; Jo, H.; Yoon, Y.S.; Brott, B.C.; Jun, H.W. Recent advances in nanomaterials for therapy and diagnosis for atherosclerosis. *Adv. Drug Deliv. Rev.* **2021**, *170*, 142–199. [CrossRef] [PubMed]
3. Palasubramaniam, J.; Wang, X.W.; Peter, K. Myocardial Infarction-From Atherosclerosis to Thrombosis Uncovering New Diagnostic and Therapeutic Approaches. *Arter. Throm. Vas.* **2019**, *39*, E176–E185. [CrossRef]
4. Adhyaru, B.B.; Jacobson, T.A. Safety and efficacy of statin therapy. *Nat. Rev. Cardiol.* **2018**, *15*, 757–769. [CrossRef] [PubMed]
5. Cholesterol Treatment Trialists Collaborators; Mihaylova, B.; Emberson, J.; Blackwell, L.; Keech, A.; Simes, J.; Barnes, E.H.; Voysey, M.; Gray, A.; Collins, R.; et al. The effects of lowering LDL cholesterol with statin therapy in people at low risk of vascular disease: Meta-analysis of individual data from 27 randomised trials. *Lancet* **2012**, *380*, 581–590. [CrossRef]
6. Wu, M.-Y.; Li, C.-J.; Hou, M.-F.; Chu, P.-Y. New Insights into the Role of Inflammation in the Pathogenesis of Atherosclerosis. *Int. J. Mol. Sci.* **2017**, *18*, 2034. [CrossRef]

7. Shah, P.K.; Lecis, D. Inflammation in atherosclerotic cardiovascular disease. *F1000Research* **2019**, *8*, 1402. [CrossRef]
8. Libby, P.; Buring, J.E.; Badimon, L.; Hansson, G.K.; Deanfield, J.; Bittencourt, M.S.; Tokgözoğlu, L.; Lewis, E.F. Atherosclerosis. *Nat. Rev. Dis. Primers* **2019**, *5*, 56. [CrossRef]
9. Valanti, E.-K.; Dalakoura-Karagkouni, K.; Siasos, G.; Kardassis, D.; Eliopoulos, A.G.; Sanoudou, D. Advances in biological therapies for dyslipidemias and atherosclerosis. *Metabolism* **2021**, *116*, 154461. [CrossRef]
10. Gistera, A.; Hansson, G.K. The immunology of atherosclerosis. *Nat. Rev. Nephrol.* **2017**, *13*, 368–380. [CrossRef]
11. Goldstein, J.L.; Ho, Y.K.; Basu, S.K.; Brown, M.S. Binding site on macrophages that mediates uptake and degradation of acetylated low density lipoprotein, producing massive cholesterol deposition. *Proc. Natl. Acad. Sci. USA* **1979**, *76*, 333–337. [CrossRef]
12. Park, Y.M.; Febbraio, M.; Silverstein, R.L. CD36 modulates migration of mouse and human macrophages in response to oxidized LDL and may contribute to macrophage trapping in the arterial intima. *J. Clin. Investig.* **2009**, *119*, 136–145. [CrossRef]
13. Robbins, C.S.; Hilgendorf, I.; Weber, G.F.; Theurl, I.; Iwamoto, Y.; Figueiredo, J.-L.; Gorbatov, R.; Sukhova, G.K.; Gerhardt, L.M.S.; Smyth, D.; et al. Local proliferation dominates lesional macrophage accumulation in atherosclerosis. *Nat. Med.* **2013**, *19*, 1166–1172. [CrossRef]
14. Libby, P. Targeting Inflammatory Pathways in Cardiovascular Disease: The Inflammasome, Interleukin-1, Interleukin-6 and Beyond. *Cells* **2021**, *10*, 951. [CrossRef] [PubMed]
15. Cybulsky, M.I.; Gimbrone, M.A., Jr. Endothelial expression of a mononuclear leukocyte adhesion molecule during atherogenesis. *Science* **1991**, *251*, 788–791. [CrossRef] [PubMed]
16. Ait-Oufella, H.; Taleb, S.; Mallat, Z.; Tedgui, A. Recent advances on the role of cytokines in atherosclerosis. *Arter. Thromb. Vasc. Biol.* **2011**, *31*, 969–979. [CrossRef] [PubMed]
17. Niu, N.; Xu, S.; Xu, Y.; Little, P.J.; Jin, Z.G. Targeting Mechanosensitive Transcription Factors in Atherosclerosis. *Trends Pharm. Sci.* **2019**, *40*, 253–266. [CrossRef]
18. Tiller, K.E.; Tessier, P.M. Advances in Antibody Design. *Annu. Rev. Biomed. Eng.* **2015**, *17*, 191–216. [CrossRef]
19. Chames, P.; Van Regenmortel, M.; Weiss, E.; Baty, D. Therapeutic antibodies: Successes, limitations and hopes for the future. *Br. J. Pharmacol.* **2009**, *157*, 220–233. [CrossRef]
20. Lu, R.-M.; Hwang, Y.-C.; Liu, I.J.; Lee, C.-C.; Tsai, H.-Z.; Li, H.-J.; Wu, H.-C. Development of therapeutic antibodies for the treatment of diseases. *J. Biomed. Sci.* **2020**, *27*, 1–30. [CrossRef]
21. Di Minno, M.N.D.; Iervolino, S.; Peluso, R.; Scarpa, R.; Di Minno, G. Carotid Intima-Media Thickness in Psoriatic Arthritis. *Arterioscler. Thromb. Vasc. Biol.* **2011**, *31*, 705–712. [CrossRef]
22. Mease, P.J.; McInnes, I.B.; Kirkham, B.; Kavanaugh, A.; Rahman, P.; Van Der Heijde, D.; Landewé, R.; Nash, P.; Pricop, L.; Yuan, J.; et al. Secukinumab Inhibition of Interleukin-17A in Patients with Psoriatic Arthritis. *N. Engl. J. Med.* **2015**, *373*, 1329–1339. [CrossRef] [PubMed]
23. Langley, R.G.; Papp, K.; Gottlieb, A.B.; Krueger, G.G.; Gordon, K.B.; Williams, D.; Valdes, J.; Setze, C.; Strober, B. Safety results from a pooled analysis of randomized, controlled phase II and III clinical trials and interim data from an open-label extension trial of the interleukin-12/23 monoclonal antibody, briakinumab, in moderate to severe psoriasis. *J. Eur. Acad. Derm. Venereol.* **2012**. [CrossRef] [PubMed]
24. Fredrikson, G.N.; Hedblad, B.; Berglund, G.; Alm, R.; Ares, M.; Cercek, B.; Chyu, K.Y.; Shah, P.K.; Nilsson, J. Identification of immune responses against aldehyde-modified peptide sequences in apoB associated with cardiovascular disease. *Arter. Thromb. Vasc. Biol.* **2003**, *23*, 872–878. [CrossRef] [PubMed]
25. Gonçalves, I.; Nitulescu, M.; Ares, M.P.S.; Fredrikson, G.N.; Jansson, B.; Li, Z.-C.; Nilsson, J. Identification of the target for therapeutic recombinant anti-apoB-100 peptide antibodies in human atherosclerotic lesions. *Atherosclerosis* **2009**, *205*, 96–100. [CrossRef] [PubMed]
26. Schiopu, A.; Bengtsson, J.; Soderberg, I.; Janciauskiene, S.; Lindgren, S.; Ares, M.P.; Shah, P.K.; Carlsson, R.; Nilsson, J.; Fredrikson, G.N. Recombinant human antibodies against aldehyde-modified apolipoprotein B-100 peptide sequences inhibit atherosclerosis. *Circulation* **2004**, *110*, 2047–2052. [CrossRef]
27. Schiopu, A.; Frendéus, B.; Jansson, B.; Söderberg, I.; Ljungcrantz, I.; Araya, Z.; Shah, P.K.; Carlsson, R.; Nilsson, J.; Fredrikson, G.N. Recombinant Antibodies to an Oxidized Low-Density Lipoprotein Epitope Induce Rapid Regression of Atherosclerosis in Apobec-1−/−/Low-Density Lipoprotein Receptor−/−Mice. *J. Am. Coll. Cardiol.* **2007**, *50*, 2313–2318. [CrossRef] [PubMed]
28. Fredrikson, G.N.; Andersson, L.; Soderberg, I.; Dimayuga, P.; Chyu, K.Y.; Shah, P.K.; Nilsson, J. Atheroprotective immunization with MDA-modified apo B-100 peptide sequences is associated with activation of Th2 specific antibody expression. *Autoimmunity* **2005**, *38*, 171–179. [CrossRef]
29. Li, S.; Kievit, P.; Robertson, A.-K.; Kolumam, G.; Li, X.; Von Wachenfeldt, K.; Valfridsson, C.; Bullens, S.; Messaoudi, I.; Bader, L.; et al. Targeting oxidized LDL improves insulin sensitivity and immune cell function in obese Rhesus macaques. *Mol. Metab.* **2013**, *2*, 256–269. [CrossRef]
30. Björkbacka, H.; Alm, R.; Persson, M.; Hedblad, B.; Nilsson, J.; Fredrikson, G.N. Low Levels of Apolipoprotein B-100 Autoantibodies Are Associated With Increased Risk of Coronary Events. *Arterioscler. Thromb. Vasc. Biol.* **2016**, *36*, 765–771. [CrossRef]
31. Asciutto, G.; Wigren, M.; Fredrikson, G.N.; Mattisson, I.Y.; Grönberg, C.; Alm, R.; Björkbacka, H.; Dias, N.V.; Edsfeldt, A.; Gonçalves, I.; et al. Apolipoprotein B-100 Antibody Interaction With Atherosclerotic Plaque Inflammation and Repair Processes. *Stroke* **2016**, *47*, 1140–1143. [CrossRef]

32. Lehrer-Graiwer, J.; Singh, P.; Abdelbaky, A.; Vucic, E.; Korsgren, M.; Baruch, A.; Fredrickson, J.; Van Bruggen, N.; Tang, M.T.; Frendeus, B.; et al. FDG-PET Imaging for Oxidized LDL in Stable Atherosclerotic Disease: A Phase II Study of Safety, Tolerability, and Anti-Inflammatory Activity. *JACC Cardiovasc. Imaging* **2015**, *8*, 493–494. [CrossRef] [PubMed]
33. Dunér, P.; Mattisson, I.Y.; Fogelstrand, P.; Glise, L.; Ruiz, S.; Farina, C.; Borén, J.; Nilsson, J.; Bengtsson, E. Antibodies against apoB100 peptide 210 inhibit atherosclerosis in apoE-/- mice. *Sci. Rep.* **2021**, *11*, 9022. [CrossRef]
34. Lin, X.-L.; Xiao, L.-L.; Tang, Z.-H.; Jiang, Z.-S.; Liu, M.-H. Role of PCSK9 in lipid metabolism and atherosclerosis. *Biomed. Pharmacother.* **2018**, *104*, 36–44. [CrossRef]
35. Tang, Y.; Li, S.-L.; Hu, J.-H.; Sun, K.-J.; Liu, L.-L.; Xu, D.-Y. Research progress on alternative non-classical mechanisms of PCSK9 in atherosclerosis in patients with and without diabetes. *Cardiovasc. Diabetol.* **2020**, *19*, 33. [CrossRef]
36. Morelli, M.B.; Wang, X.; Santulli, G. Functional role of gut microbiota and PCSK9 in the pathogenesis of diabetes mellitus and cardiovascular disease. *Atherosclerosis* **2019**, *289*, 176–178. [CrossRef]
37. Horton, J.D.; Cohen, J.C.; Hobbs, H.H. PCSK9: A convertase that coordinates LDL catabolism. *J. Lipid Res.* **2009**, *50*, S172–S177. [CrossRef] [PubMed]
38. Kasichayanula, S.; Grover, A.; Emery, M.G.; Gibbs, M.A.; Somaratne, R.; Wasserman, S.M.; Gibbs, J.P. Clinical Pharmacokinetics and Pharmacodynamics of Evolocumab, a PCSK9 Inhibitor. *Clin. Pharmacokinet.* **2018**, *57*, 769–779. [CrossRef] [PubMed]
39. Catapano, A.L.; Pirillo, A.; Norata, G.D. New Pharmacological Approaches to Target PCSK9. *Curr. Atheroscler. Rep.* **2020**, *22*, 24. [CrossRef]
40. Kosenko, T.; Golder, M.; Leblond, G.; Weng, W.; Lagace, T.A. Low density lipoprotein binds to proprotein convertase subtilisin/kexin type-9 (PCSK9) in human plasma and inhibits PCSK9-mediated low density lipoprotein receptor degradation. *J. Biol. Chem.* **2013**, *288*, 8279–8288. [CrossRef] [PubMed]
41. Lee, C.J.; Lee, Y.-H.; Park, S.W.; Kim, K.J.; Park, S.; Youn, J.-C.; Lee, S.-H.; Kang, S.-M.; Jang, Y. Association of serum proprotein convertase subtilisin/kexin type 9 with carotid intima media thickness in hypertensive subjects. *Metabolism* **2013**, *62*, 845–850. [CrossRef]
42. Chen, S.N.; Ballantyne, C.M.; Gotto, A.M., Jr.; Tan, Y.; Willerson, J.T.; Marian, A.J. A common PCSK9 haplotype, encompassing the E670G coding single nucleotide polymorphism, is a novel genetic marker for plasma low-density lipoprotein cholesterol levels and severity of coronary atherosclerosis. *J. Am. Coll. Cardiol.* **2005**, *45*, 1611–1619. [CrossRef] [PubMed]
43. Norata, G.D.; Garlaschelli, K.; Grigore, L.; Raselli, S.; Tramontana, S.; Meneghetti, F.; Artali, R.; Noto, D.; Cefalù, A.B.; Buccianti, G.; et al. Effects of PCSK9 variants on common carotid artery intima media thickness and relation to ApoE alleles. *Atherosclerosis* **2010**, *208*, 177–182. [CrossRef]
44. Shapiro, M.D.; Tavori, H.; Fazio, S. PCSK9. *Circ. Res.* **2018**, *122*, 1420–1438. [CrossRef] [PubMed]
45. Brandts, J.; Dharmayat, K.I.; Vallejo-Vaz, A.J.; Azar Sharabiani, M.T.; Jones, R.; Kastelein, J.J.P.; Raal, F.J.; Ray, K.K. A meta-analysis of medications directed against PCSK9 in familial hypercholesterolemia. *Atherosclerosis* **2021**, *325*, 46–56. [CrossRef] [PubMed]
46. Duff, C.J.; Scott, M.J.; Kirby, I.T.; Hutchinson, S.E.; Martin, S.L.; Hooper, N.M. Antibody-mediated disruption of the interaction between PCSK9 and the low-density lipoprotein receptor. *Biochem. J.* **2009**, *419*, 577–584. [CrossRef] [PubMed]
47. Chan, J.C.Y.; Piper, D.E.; Cao, Q.; Liu, D.; King, C.; Wang, W.; Tang, J.; Liu, Q.; Higbee, J.; Xia, Z.; et al. A proprotein convertase subtilisin/kexin type 9 neutralizing antibody reduces serum cholesterol in mice and nonhuman primates. *Proc. Natl. Acad. Sci. USA* **2009**, *106*, 9820–9825. [CrossRef]
48. Maxwell, K.N.; Breslow, J.L. Antibodies to PCSK9. *Circ. Res.* **2012**, *111*, 274–277. [CrossRef]
49. Stein, E.A.; Mellis, S.; Yancopoulos, G.D.; Stahl, N.; Logan, D.; Smith, W.B.; Lisbon, E.; Gutierrez, M.; Webb, C.; Wu, R.; et al. Effect of a Monoclonal Antibody to PCSK9 on LDL Cholesterol. *N. Engl. J. Med.* **2012**, *366*, 1108–1118. [CrossRef]
50. Catapano, A.L.; Papadopoulos, N. The safety of therapeutic monoclonal antibodies: Implications for cardiovascular disease and targeting the PCSK9 pathway. *Atherosclerosis* **2013**, *228*, 18–28. [CrossRef]
51. Solanki, A.; Bhatt, L.K.; Johnston, T.P. Evolving targets for the treatment of atherosclerosis. *Pharmacol. Ther.* **2018**, *187*, 1–12. [CrossRef]
52. Gallego-Colon, E.; Daum, A.; Yosefy, C. Statins and PCSK9 inhibitors: A new lipid-lowering therapy. *Eur. J. Pharmacol.* **2020**, *878*, 173114. [CrossRef] [PubMed]
53. Jia, X.; Lorenz, P.; Ballantyne, C.M. Poststatin Lipid Therapeutics: A Review. *Methodist Debakey Cardiovasc. J.* **2019**, *15*, 32–38. [CrossRef] [PubMed]
54. Sabatine, M.S.; Giugliano, R.P.; Keech, A.C.; Honarpour, N.; Wiviott, S.D.; Murphy, S.A.; Kuder, J.F.; Wang, H.; Liu, T.; Wasserman, S.M.; et al. Evolocumab and Clinical Outcomes in Patients with Cardiovascular Disease. *N. Engl. J. Med.* **2017**, *376*, 1713–1722. [CrossRef]
55. Schwartz, G.G.; Steg, P.G.; Szarek, M.; Bhatt, D.L.; Bittner, V.A.; Diaz, R.; Edelberg, J.M.; Goodman, S.G.; Hanotin, C.; Harrington, R.A.; et al. Alirocumab and Cardiovascular Outcomes after Acute Coronary Syndrome. *N. Engl. J. Med.* **2018**, *379*, 2097–2107. [CrossRef]
56. Whayne, T.F. PCSK9 inhibitors in the current management of atherosclerosis. *Arch. Cardiol. México* **2017**, *87*, 43–48. [CrossRef]
57. Adamstein, N.H.; Macfadyen, J.G.; Rose, L.M.; Glynn, R.J.; Dey, A.K.; Libby, P.; Tabas, I.A.; Mehta, N.N.; Ridker, P.M. The neutrophil–lymphocyte ratio and incident atherosclerotic events: Analyses from five contemporary randomized trials. *Eur. Heart J.* **2021**, *42*, 896–903. [CrossRef]

58. Ridker, P.M.; Revkin, J.; Amarenco, P.; Brunell, R.; Curto, M.; Civeira, F.; Flather, M.; Glynn, R.J.; Gregoire, J.; Jukema, J.W.; et al. Cardiovascular Efficacy and Safety of Bococizumab in High-Risk Patients. *N. Engl. J. Med.* **2017**, *376*, 1527–1539. [CrossRef]
59. Wiciński, M.; Żak, J.; Malinowski, B.; Popek, G.; Grześk, G. PCSK9 signaling pathways and their potential importance in clinical practice. *EPMA J.* **2017**, *8*, 391–402. [CrossRef] [PubMed]
60. Jia, X.; Al Rifai, M.; Birnbaum, Y.; Smith, S.C.; Virani, S.S. The 2018 Cholesterol Management Guidelines: Topics in Secondary ASCVD Prevention Clinicians Need to Know. *Curr. Atheroscler. Rep.* **2019**, *21*, 20. [CrossRef] [PubMed]
61. Wong, N.D.; Shapiro, M.D. Interpreting the Findings From the Recent PCSK9 Monoclonal Antibody Cardiovascular Outcomes Trials. *Front. Cardiovasc. Med.* **2019**, *6*, 14. [CrossRef] [PubMed]
62. Ruscica, M.; Tokgözoğlu, L.; Corsini, A.; Sirtori, C.R. PCSK9 inhibition and inflammation: A narrative review. *Atherosclerosis* **2019**, *288*, 146–155. [CrossRef]
63. Khambhati, J.; Engels, M.; Allard-Ratick, M.; Sandesara, P.B.; Quyyumi, A.A.; Sperling, L. Immunotherapy for the prevention of atherosclerotic cardiovascular disease: Promise and possibilities. *Atherosclerosis* **2018**, *276*, 1–9. [CrossRef] [PubMed]
64. Rayment, N.; Moss, E.; Faulkner, L.; Brickell, P.; Davies, M.; Woolf, N.; Katz, D. Synthesis of TNFα and TGFβ mRNA in the different micro-environments within atheromatous plaques. *Cardiovasc. Res.* **1996**, *32*, 1123–1130. [CrossRef]
65. Ridker, P.M.; Rifai, N.; Pfeffer, M.; Sacks, F.; Lepage, S.; Braunwald, E. Elevation of Tumor Necrosis Factor-α and Increased Risk of Recurrent Coronary Events After Myocardial Infarction. *Circulation* **2000**, *101*, 2149–2153. [CrossRef] [PubMed]
66. Ohta, H.; Wada, H.; Niwa, T.; Kirii, H.; Iwamoto, N.; Fujii, H.; Saito, K.; Sekikawa, K.; Seishima, M. Disruption of tumor necrosis factor-α gene diminishes the development of atherosclerosis in ApoE-deficient mice. *Atherosclerosis* **2005**, *180*, 11–17. [CrossRef] [PubMed]
67. Schreyer, S.A.; Peschon, J.J.; Leboeuf, R.C. Accelerated Atherosclerosis in Mice Lacking Tumor Necrosis Factor Receptor p55. *J. Biol. Chem.* **1996**, *271*, 26174–26178. [CrossRef] [PubMed]
68. Ait-Oufella, H.; Libby, P.; Tedgui, A. Anticytokine Immune Therapy and Atherothrombotic Cardiovascular Risk. *Arterioscler. Thromb. Vasc. Biol.* **2019**, *39*, 1510–1519. [CrossRef]
69. Jacobsson, L.T.; Turesson, C.; Gulfe, A.; Kapetanovic, M.C.; Petersson, I.F.; Saxne, T.; Geborek, P. Treatment with tumor necrosis factor blockers is associated with a lower incidence of first cardiovascular events in patients with rheumatoid arthritis. *J. Rheumatol.* **2005**, *32*, 1213–1218.
70. Ahlehoff, O.; Skov, L.; Gislason, G.; Gniadecki, R.; Iversen, L.; Bryld, L.E.; Lasthein, S.; Lindhardsen, J.; Kristensen, S.L.; Torp-Pedersen, C.; et al. Cardiovascular outcomes and systemic anti-inflammatory drugs in patients with severe psoriasis: 5-year follow-up of a Danish nationwide cohort. *J. Eur. Acad. Dermatol. Venereol.* **2015**, *29*, 1128–1134. [CrossRef]
71. Lebwohl, M.; Blauvelt, A.; Paul, C.; Sofen, H.; Węgłowska, J.; Piguet, V.; Burge, D.; Rolleri, R.; Drew, J.; Peterson, L.; et al. Certolizumab pegol for the treatment of chronic plaque psoriasis: Results through 48 weeks of a phase 3, multicenter, randomized, double-blind, etanercept- and placebo-controlled study (CIMPACT). *J. Am. Acad. Dermatol.* **2018**, *79*, 266–276.e265. [CrossRef]
72. Gkalpakiotis, S.; Arenbergerova, M.; Gkalpakioti, P.; Potockova, J.; Arenberger, P.; Kraml, P. Long-term impact of adalimumab therapy on biomarkers of systemic inflammation in psoriasis: Results of a 2 year study. *Dermatol. Ther.* **2020**, *33*. [CrossRef]
73. Lee, A.; Scott, L.J. Certolizumab Pegol: A Review in Moderate to Severe Plaque Psoriasis. *BioDrugs* **2020**, *34*, 235–244. [CrossRef]
74. Frampton, J.E. Golimumab: A Review in Inflammatory Arthritis. *BioDrugs* **2017**, *31*, 263–274. [CrossRef]
75. Pelechas, E.; Voulgari, P.; Drosos, A. Golimumab for Rheumatoid Arthritis. *J. Clin. Med.* **2019**, *8*, 387. [CrossRef]
76. Chung, E.S.; Packer, M.; Lo, K.H.; Fasanmade, A.A.; Willerson, J.T. Randomized, Double-Blind, Placebo-Controlled, Pilot Trial of Infliximab, a Chimeric Monoclonal Antibody to Tumor Necrosis Factor-α, in Patients With Moderate-to-Severe Heart Failure. *Circulation* **2003**, *107*, 3133–3140. [CrossRef] [PubMed]
77. Ait-Oufella, H.; Libby, P.; Tedgui, A. Antibody-based immunotherapy targeting cytokines and atherothrombotic cardiovascular diseases. *Arch. Cardiovasc. Dis.* **2020**, *113*, 5–8. [CrossRef] [PubMed]
78. Lukens, J.R.; Gross, J.M.; Kanneganti, T.-D. IL-1 family cytokines trigger sterile inflammatory disease. *Front. Immunol.* **2012**, *3*, 315. [CrossRef] [PubMed]
79. Moriya, J. Critical roles of inflammation in atherosclerosis. *J. Cardiol.* **2019**, *73*, 22–27. [CrossRef]
80. Singer, I.I.; Scott, S.; Chin, J.; Bayne, E.K.; Limjuco, G.; Weidner, J.; Miller, D.K.; Chapman, K.; Kostura, M.J. The interleukin-1 beta-converting enzyme (ICE) is localized on the external cell surface membranes and in the cytoplasmic ground substance of human monocytes by immuno-electron microscopy. *J. Exp. Med.* **1995**, *182*, 1447–1459. [CrossRef]
81. Libby, P. Interleukin-1 Beta as a Target for Atherosclerosis Therapy. *J. Am. Coll. Cardiol.* **2017**, *70*, 2278–2289. [CrossRef] [PubMed]
82. Kirii, H.; Niwa, T.; Yamada, Y.; Wada, H.; Saito, K.; Iwakura, Y.; Asano, M.; Moriwaki, H.; Seishima, M. Lack of Interleukin-1β Decreases the Severity of Atherosclerosis in ApoE-Deficient Mice. *Arterioscler. Thromb. Vasc. Biol.* **2003**, *23*, 656–660. [CrossRef] [PubMed]
83. Shimokawa, H.; Ito, A.; Fukumoto, Y.; Kadokami, T.; Nakaike, R.; Sakata, M.; Takayanagi, T.; Egashira, K.; Takeshita, A. Chronic treatment with interleukin-1 beta induces coronary intimal lesions and vasospastic responses in pigs in vivo. The role of platelet-derived growth factor. *J. Clin. Investig.* **1996**, *97*, 769–776. [CrossRef]
84. Dinarello, C.A. Interleukin-1 in the pathogenesis and treatment of inflammatory diseases. *Blood* **2011**, *117*, 3720–3732. [CrossRef] [PubMed]
85. Dinarello, C.A.; Simon, A.; Van Der Meer, J.W.M. Treating inflammation by blocking interleukin-1 in a broad spectrum of diseases. *Nat. Rev. Drug Discov.* **2012**, *11*, 633–652. [CrossRef]

86. Kedor, C.; Listing, J.; Zernicke, J.; Weiß, A.; Behrens, F.; Blank, N.; Henes, J.C.; Kekow, J.; Rubbert-Roth, A.; Schulze-Koops, H.; et al. Canakinumab for Treatment of Adult-Onset Still's Disease to Achieve Reduction of Arthritic Manifestation (CONSIDER): Phase II, randomised, double-blind, placebo-controlled, multicentre, investigator-initiated trial. *Ann. Rheum. Dis.* **2020**, *79*, 1090–1097. [CrossRef]
87. Ridker, P.M.; Howard, C.P.; Walter, V.; Everett, B.; Libby, P.; Hensen, J.; Thuren, T. Effects of Interleukin-1β Inhibition With Canakinumab on Hemoglobin A1c, Lipids, C-Reactive Protein, Interleukin-6, and Fibrinogen. *Circulation* **2012**, *126*, 2739–2748. [CrossRef] [PubMed]
88. Ridker, P.M.; Thuren, T.; Zalewski, A.; Libby, P. Interleukin-1β inhibition and the prevention of recurrent cardiovascular events: Rationale and Design of the Canakinumab Anti-inflammatory Thrombosis Outcomes Study (CANTOS). *Am. Heart J.* **2011**, *162*, 597–605. [CrossRef]
89. Ridker, P.M.; Everett, B.M.; Thuren, T.; Macfadyen, J.G.; Chang, W.H.; Ballantyne, C.; Fonseca, F.; Nicolau, J.; Koenig, W.; Anker, S.D.; et al. Antiinflammatory Therapy with Canakinumab for Atherosclerotic Disease. *N. Engl. J. Med.* **2017**, *377*, 1119–1131. [CrossRef]
90. Everett, B.M.; Macfadyen, J.G.; Thuren, T.; Libby, P.; Glynn, R.J.; Ridker, P.M. Inhibition of Interleukin-1β and Reduction in Atherothrombotic Cardiovascular Events in the CANTOS Trial. *J. Am. Coll. Cardiol.* **2020**, *76*, 1660–1670. [CrossRef]
91. Libby, P.; Rocha, V.Z. All roads lead to IL-6: A central hub of cardiometabolic signaling. *Int. J. Cardiol.* **2018**, *259*, 213–215. [CrossRef] [PubMed]
92. Saremi, A.; Anderson, R.J.; Luo, P.; Moritz, T.E.; Schwenke, D.C.; Allison, M.; Reaven, P.D. Association between IL-6 and the extent of coronary atherosclerosis in the veterans affairs diabetes trial (VADT). *Atherosclerosis* **2009**, *203*, 610–614. [CrossRef] [PubMed]
93. Huber, S.A.; Sakkinen, P.; Conze, D.; Hardin, N.; Tracy, R. Interleukin-6 Exacerbates Early Atherosclerosis in Mice. *Arterioscler. Thromb. Vasc. Biol.* **1999**, *19*, 2364–2367. [CrossRef] [PubMed]
94. Schieffer, B.; Selle, T.; Hilfiker, A.; Hilfiker-Kleiner, D.; Grote, K.; Tietge, U.J.F.; Trautwein, C.; Luchtefeld, M.; Schmittkamp, C.; Heeneman, S.; et al. Impact of Interleukin-6 on Plaque Development and Morphology in Experimental Atherosclerosis. *Circulation* **2004**, *110*, 3493–3500. [CrossRef]
95. Elhage, R. Involvement of interleukin-6 in atherosclerosis but not in the prevention of fatty streak formation by 17β-estradiol in apolipoprotein E-deficient mice. *Atherosclerosis* **2001**, *156*, 315–320. [CrossRef]
96. Ridker, P.M.; Rifai, N.; Stampfer, M.J.; Hennekens, C.H. Plasma Concentration of Interleukin-6 and the Risk of Future Myocardial Infarction Among Apparently Healthy Men. *Circulation* **2000**, *101*, 1767–1772. [CrossRef]
97. The interleukin-6 receptor as a target for prevention of coronary heart disease: A mendelian randomisation analysis. *Lancet* **2012**, *379*, 1214–1224. [CrossRef]
98. Gabay, C.; Riek, M.; Hetland, M.L.; Hauge, E.-M.; Pavelka, K.; Tomšič, M.; Canhao, H.; Chatzidionysiou, K.; Lukina, G.; Nordström, D.C.; et al. Effectiveness of tocilizumab with and without synthetic disease-modifying antirheumatic drugs in rheumatoid arthritis: Results from a European collaborative study. *Ann. Rheum. Dis.* **2016**, *75*, 1336–1342. [CrossRef]
99. Kim, S.C.; Solomon, D.H.; Rogers, J.R.; Gale, S.; Klearman, M.; Sarsour, K.; Schneeweiss, S. Cardiovascular Safety of Tocilizumab Versus Tumor Necrosis Factor Inhibitors in Patients With Rheumatoid Arthritis: A Multi-Database Cohort Study. *Arthritis Rheumatol.* **2017**, *69*, 1154–1164. [CrossRef]
100. Generali, E.; Carrara, G.; Selmi, C.; Verstappen, S.M.M.; Zambon, A.; Bortoluzzi, A.; Silvagni, E.; Scire, C.A. Comparison of the risks of hospitalisation for cardiovascular events in patients with rheumatoid arthritis treated with tocilizumab and etanercept. *Clin. Exp. Rheumatol.* **2018**, *36*, 310–313.
101. Yamamoto, K.; Goto, H.; Hirao, K.; Nakajima, A.; Origasa, H.; Tanaka, K.; Tomobe, M.; Totsuka, K. Longterm Safety of Tocilizumab: Results from 3 Years of Followup Postmarketing Surveillance of 5573 Patients with Rheumatoid Arthritis in Japan. *J. Rheumatol.* **2015**, *42*, 1368–1375. [CrossRef] [PubMed]
102. Anstensrud, A.K.; Woxholt, S.; Sharma, K.; Broch, K.; Bendz, B.; Aakhus, S.; Ueland, T.; Amundsen, B.H.; Damås, J.K.; Hopp, E.; et al. Rationale for the ASSAIL-MI-trial: A randomised controlled trial designed to assess the effect of tocilizumab on myocardial salvage in patients with acute ST-elevation myocardial infarction (STEMI). *Open Heart* **2019**, *6*, e001108. [CrossRef] [PubMed]
103. Kurschus, F.C.; Moos, S. IL-17 for therapy. *J. Dermatol. Sci.* **2017**, *87*, 221–227. [CrossRef] [PubMed]
104. Ye, P.; Rodriguez, F.H.; Kanaly, S.; Stocking, K.L.; Schurr, J.; Schwarzenberger, P.; Oliver, P.; Huang, W.; Zhang, P.; Zhang, J.; et al. Requirement of Interleukin 17 Receptor Signaling for Lung Cxc Chemokine and Granulocyte Colony-Stimulating Factor Expression, Neutrophil Recruitment, and Host Defense. *J. Exp. Med.* **2001**, *194*, 519–528. [CrossRef]
105. O'Connor, W., Jr.; Kamanaka, M.; Booth, C.J.; Town, T.; Nakae, S.; Iwakura, Y.; Kolls, J.K.; Flavell, R.A. A protective function for interleukin 17A in T cell–mediated intestinal inflammation. *Nat. Immunol.* **2009**, *10*, 603–609. [CrossRef]
106. Hawkes, J.E.; Yan, B.Y.; Chan, T.C.; Krueger, J.G. Discovery of the IL-23/IL-17 Signaling Pathway and the Treatment of Psoriasis. *J. Immunol.* **2018**, *201*, 1605–1613. [CrossRef]
107. Erbel, C.; Chen, L.; Bea, F.; Wangler, S.; Celik, S.; Lasitschka, F.; Wang, Y.; Böckler, D.; Katus, H.A.; Dengler, T.J. Inhibition of IL-17A Attenuates Atherosclerotic Lesion Development in ApoE-Deficient Mice. *J. Immunol.* **2009**, *183*, 8167–8175. [CrossRef] [PubMed]
108. Smith, E.; Prasad, K.-M.R.; Butcher, M.; Dobrian, A.; Kolls, J.K.; Ley, K.; Galkina, E. Blockade of Interleukin-17A Results in Reduced Atherosclerosis in Apolipoprotein E–Deficient Mice. *Circulation* **2010**, *121*, 1746–1755. [CrossRef]

109. Butcher, M.J.; Gjurich, B.N.; Phillips, T.; Galkina, E.V. The IL-17A/IL-17RA Axis Plays a Proatherogenic Role via the Regulation of Aortic Myeloid Cell Recruitment. *Circ. Res.* **2012**, *110*, 675–687. [CrossRef]
110. Madhur, M.S.; Funt, S.A.; Li, L.; Vinh, A.; Chen, W.; Lob, H.E.; Iwakura, Y.; Blinder, Y.; Rahman, A.; Quyyumi, A.A.; et al. Role of Interleukin 17 in Inflammation, Atherosclerosis, and Vascular Function in Apolipoprotein E–Deficient Mice. *Arterioscler. Thromb. Vasc. Biol.* **2011**, *31*, 1565–1572. [CrossRef]
111. Danzaki, K.; Matsui, Y.; Ikesue, M.; Ohta, D.; Ito, K.; Kanayama, M.; Kurotaki, D.; Morimoto, J.; Iwakura, Y.; Yagita, H.; et al. Interleukin-17A Deficiency Accelerates Unstable Atherosclerotic Plaque Formation in Apolipoprotein E-Deficient Mice. *Arterioscler. Thromb. Vasc. Biol.* **2012**, *32*, 273–280. [CrossRef]
112. Ge, S.; Hertel, B.; Koltsova, E.K.; Sörensen-Zender, I.; Kielstein, J.T.; Ley, K.; Haller, H.; Von Vietinghoff, S. Increased Atherosclerotic Lesion Formation and Vascular Leukocyte Accumulation in Renal Impairment Are Mediated by Interleukin-17A. *Circ. Res.* **2013**, *113*, 965–974. [CrossRef] [PubMed]
113. Taleb, S.; Romain, M.; Ramkhelawon, B.; Uyttenhove, C.; Pasterkamp, G.; Herbin, O.; Esposito, B.; Perez, N.; Yasukawa, H.; Van Snick, J.; et al. Loss of SOCS3 expression in T cells reveals a regulatory role for interleukin-17 in atherosclerosis. *J. Exp. Med.* **2009**, *206*, 2067–2077. [CrossRef] [PubMed]
114. Gisterå, A.; Robertson, A.-K.L.; Andersson, J.; Ketelhuth, D.F.J.; Ovchinnikova, O.; Nilsson, S.K.; Lundberg, A.M.; Li, M.O.; Flavell, R.A.; Hansson, G.K. Transforming Growth Factor–β Signaling in T Cells Promotes Stabilization of Atherosclerotic Plaques Through an Interleukin-17–Dependent Pathway. *Sci. Transl. Med.* **2013**, *5*, 196ra100–196ra191. [CrossRef]
115. Simon, T.; Taleb, S.; Danchin, N.; Laurans, L.; Rousseau, B.; Cattan, S.; Montely, J.-M.; Dubourg, O.; Tedgui, A.; Kotti, S.; et al. Circulating levels of interleukin-17 and cardiovascular outcomes in patients with acute myocardial infarction. *Eur. Heart J.* **2013**, *34*, 570–577. [CrossRef]
116. Langley, R.G.; Elewski, B.E.; Lebwohl, M.; Reich, K.; Griffiths, C.E.M.; Papp, K.; Puig, L.; Nakagawa, H.; Spelman, L.; Sigurgeirsson, B.; et al. Secukinumab in Plaque Psoriasis—Results of Two Phase 3 Trials. *N. Engl. J. Med.* **2014**, *371*, 326–338. [CrossRef]
117. McInnes, I.B.; Sieper, J.; Braun, J.; Emery, P.; Van Der Heijde, D.; Isaacs, J.D.; Dahmen, G.; Wollenhaupt, J.; Schulze-Koops, H.; Kogan, J.; et al. Efficacy and safety of secukinumab, a fully human anti-interleukin-17A monoclonal antibody, in patients with moderate-to-severe psoriatic arthritis: A 24-week, randomised, double-blind, placebo-controlled, phase II proof-of-concept trial. *Ann. Rheum. Dis.* **2014**, *73*, 349–356. [CrossRef]
118. Gisondi, P.; Dalle Vedove, C.; Girolomoni, G. Efficacy and Safety of Secukinumab in Chronic Plaque Psoriasis and Psoriatic Arthritis Therapy. *Dermatol. Ther.* **2014**, *4*, 1–9. [CrossRef] [PubMed]
119. Baeten, D.; Baraliakos, X.; Braun, J.; Sieper, J.; Emery, P.; Van Der Heijde, D.; McInnes, I.; Van Laar, J.M.; Landewé, R.; Wordsworth, P.; et al. Anti-interleukin-17A monoclonal antibody secukinumab in treatment of ankylosing spondylitis: A randomised, double-blind, placebo-controlled trial. *Lancet* **2013**, *382*, 1705–1713. [CrossRef]
120. Burkett, P.R.; Kuchroo, V.K. IL-17 Blockade in Psoriasis. *Cell* **2016**, *167*, 1669. [CrossRef]
121. Nash, P.; McInnes, I.B.; Mease, P.; Thom, H.; Cure, S.; Palaka, E.; Gandhi, K.; Mpofu, S.; Jugl, S. Secukinumab for the Treatment of Psoriatic Arthritis: Comparative Effectiveness Results Versus Adalimumab up to 48 Weeks Using a Matching-Adjusted Indirect Comparison. *Ann. Rheum. Dis.* **2016**, *75*, 353–354. [CrossRef]
122. Gordon, K.B.; Blauvelt, A.; Papp, K.A.; Langley, R.G.; Luger, T.; Ohtsuki, M.; Reich, K.; Amato, D.; Ball, S.G.; Braun, D.K.; et al. Phase 3 Trials of Ixekizumab in Moderate-to-Severe Plaque Psoriasis. *N. Engl. J. Med.* **2016**, *375*, 345–356. [CrossRef] [PubMed]
123. Papp, K.A.; Leonardi, C.; Menter, A.; Ortonne, J.-P.; Krueger, J.G.; Kricorian, G.; Aras, G.; Li, J.; Russell, C.B.; Thompson, E.H.Z.; et al. Brodalumab, an Anti–Interleukin-17–Receptor Antibody for Psoriasis. *N. Engl. J. Med.* **2012**, *366*, 1181–1189. [CrossRef] [PubMed]
124. Kunwar, S.; Dahal, K.; Sharma, S. Anti-IL-17 therapy in treatment of rheumatoid arthritis: A systematic literature review and meta-analysis of randomized controlled trials. *Rheumatol. Int.* **2016**, *36*, 1065–1075. [CrossRef] [PubMed]
125. Kugyelka, R.; Kohl, Z.; Olasz, K.; Mikecz, K.; Rauch, T.A.; Glant, T.T.; Boldizsar, F. Enigma of IL-17 and Th17 Cells in Rheumatoid Arthritis and in Autoimmune Animal Models of Arthritis. *Mediat. Inflamm.* **2016**, *2016*, 6145810. [CrossRef]
126. Moschen, A.R.; Tilg, H.; Raine, T. IL-12, IL-23 and IL-17 in IBD: Immunobiology and therapeutic targeting. *Nat. Rev. Gastroenterol. Hepatol.* **2019**, *16*, 185–196. [CrossRef] [PubMed]
127. Ye, J.; Wang, Y.; Wang, Z.; Liu, L.; Yang, Z.; Wang, M.; Xu, Y.; Ye, D.; Zhang, J.; Zhou, Q.; et al. The Expression of IL-12 Family Members in Patients with Hypertension and Its Association with the Occurrence of Carotid Atherosclerosis. *Mediat. Inflamm.* **2020**, *2020*, 2369279. [CrossRef]
128. Jääskeläinen, A.E.; Seppälä, S.; Kakko, T.; Jaakkola, U.; Kallio, J. Systemic treatment with neuropeptide Y receptor Y1-antagonist enhances atherosclerosis and stimulates IL-12 expression in ApoE deficient mice. *Neuropeptides* **2013**, *47*, 67–73. [CrossRef]
129. Lee, T.-S.; Yen, H.-C.; Pan, C.-C.; Chau, L.-Y. The Role of Interleukin 12 in the Development of Atherosclerosis in ApoE-Deficient Mice. *Arterioscler. Thromb. Vasc. Biol.* **1999**, *19*, 734–742. [CrossRef] [PubMed]
130. Davenport, P.; Tipping, P.G. The Role of Interleukin-4 and Interleukin-12 in the Progression of Atherosclerosis in Apolipoprotein E-Deficient Mice. *Am. J. Pathol.* **2003**, *163*, 1117–1125. [CrossRef]
131. Hauer, A.D.; Uyttenhove, C.; De Vos, P.; Stroobant, V.; Renauld, J.C.; Van Berkel, T.J.C.; Van Snick, J.; Kuiper, J. Blockade of Interleukin-12 Function by Protein Vaccination Attenuates Atherosclerosis. *Circulation* **2005**, *112*, 1054–1062. [CrossRef] [PubMed]

132. Sun, J.; Yu, H.; Liu, H.; Pu, D.; Gao, J.; Jin, X.; Liu, X.; Yan, A. Correlation of pre-operative circulating inflammatory cytokines with restenosis and rapid angiographic stenotic progression risk in coronary artery disease patients underwent percutaneous coronary intervention with drug-eluting stents. *J. Clin. Lab. Anal.* **2020**, *34*. [CrossRef] [PubMed]
133. Ye, J.; Wang, Y.; Wang, Z.; Liu, L.; Yang, Z.; Wang, M.; Xu, Y.; Ye, D.; Zhang, J.; Lin, Y.; et al. Roles and Mechanisms of Interleukin-12 Family Members in Cardiovascular Diseases: Opportunities and Challenges. *Front. Pharmacol.* **2020**, *11*. [CrossRef] [PubMed]
134. Mannon, P.J.; Fuss, I.J.; Mayer, L.; Elson, C.O.; Sandborn, W.J.; Present, D.; Dolin, B.; Goodman, N.; Groden, C.; Hornung, R.L.; et al. Anti–Interleukin-12 Antibody for Active Crohn's Disease. *N. Engl. J. Med.* **2004**, *351*, 2069–2079. [CrossRef]
135. Sandborn, W.J.; Gasink, C.; Gao, L.L.; Blank, M.A.; Johanns, J.; Guzzo, C.; Sands, B.E.; Hanauer, S.B.; Targan, S.; Rutgeerts, P.; et al. Ustekinumab induction and maintenance therapy in refractory Crohn's disease. *N. Engl. J. Med.* **2012**, *367*, 1519–1528. [CrossRef] [PubMed]
136. Feagan, B.G.; Sandborn, W.J.; Gasink, C.; Jacobstein, D.; Lang, Y.; Friedman, J.R.; Blank, M.A.; Johanns, J.; Gao, L.-L.; Miao, Y.; et al. Ustekinumab as Induction and Maintenance Therapy for Crohn's Disease. *N. Engl. J. Med.* **2016**, *375*, 1946–1960. [CrossRef]
137. Marovt, M.; Marko, P.B.; Pirnat, M.; Ekart, R. Effect of biologics targeting interleukin-23/-17 axis on subclinical atherosclerosis: Results of a pilot study. *Clin. Exp. Dermatol.* **2020**, *45*, 560–564. [CrossRef]
138. Morelli, M.B.; Chavez, C.; Santulli, G. Angiopoietin-like proteins as therapeutic targets for cardiovascular disease: Focus on lipid disorders. *Expert Opin. Ther. Targets* **2020**, *24*, 79–88. [CrossRef]
139. Geladari, E.; Tsamadia, P.; Vallianou, N.G. ANGPTL3 Inhibitors- Their Role in Cardiovascular Disease Through Regulation of Lipid Metabolism. *Circ. J.* **2019**, *83*, 267–273. [CrossRef]
140. Jarr, K.-U.; Nakamoto, R.; Doan, B.H.; Kojima, Y.; Weissman, I.L.; Advani, R.H.; Iagaru, A.; Leeper, N.J. Effect of CD47 Blockade on Vascular Inflammation. *N. Engl. J. Med.* **2021**, *384*, 382–383. [CrossRef]
141. Caligiuri, G. CD31 as a Therapeutic Target in Atherosclerosis. *Circ. Res.* **2020**, *126*, 1178–1189. [CrossRef] [PubMed]

International Journal of
Molecular Sciences

MDPI

Review

Bioassay Development for Bispecific Antibodies—Challenges and Opportunities

Ames C. Register [1], Somayeh S. Tarighat [2] and Ho Young Lee [2,*]

[1] Biological Technologies, Department of Analytical Development and Quality Control, Genentech—A Member of the Roche Group, 1 DNA Way, South San Francisco, CA 94080, USA; register.ames@gene.com
[2] Cell Therapy Analytical Development, Department of Cell Therapy Engineering and Development, Genentech—A Member of the Roche Group, South San Francisco, CA 94080, USA; tarighat.somayeh@gene.com
* Correspondence: lee.ho-young@gene.com

Abstract: Antibody therapeutics are expanding with promising clinical outcomes, and diverse formats of antibodies are further developed and available for patients of the most challenging disease areas. Bispecific antibodies (BsAbs) have several significant advantages over monospecific antibodies by engaging two antigen targets. Due to the complicated mechanism of action, diverse structural variations, and dual-target binding, developing bioassays and other types of assays to characterize BsAbs is challenging. Developing bioassays for BsAbs requires a good understanding of the mechanism of action of the molecule, principles and applications of different bioanalytical methods, and phase-appropriate considerations per regulatory guidelines. Here, we review recent advances and case studies to provide strategies and insights for bioassay development for different types of bispecific molecules.

Keywords: bispecific antibodies; bioassays; mechanisms of action; binding assays; potency assays

Citation: Register, A.C.; Tarighat, S.S.; Lee, H.Y. Bioassay Development for Bispecific Antibodies—Challenges and Opportunities. *Int. J. Mol. Sci.* **2021**, *22*, 5350. https://doi.org/10.3390/ijms22105350

Academic Editor: Yong-Seok Heo

Received: 1 April 2021
Accepted: 15 May 2021
Published: 19 May 2021

1. Introduction

The concept of the bispecific antibody (BsAb) has been around for more than 50 years, but within the last 20 years, activity and interest in the field of study has skyrocketed [1,2]. Publications describing hundreds of BsAbs can be found in the scientific literature, and more than 100 BsAb clinical candidates are currently under development [3,4]. A handful of BsAbs have obtained health authority approval for use and are currently marketed as therapeutics in a number of disease areas (e.g., blinatumomab, emicizumab) around the world, highlighting the therapeutic potential of engaging two targets within a single molecule [4]. This is attributed to advanced biotechnologies, enhanced manufacturing knowledge of therapeutic antibody products, and strong scientific rationale for the development of biologics with the ability to engage more than one target [5,6].

BsAbs are typically designed to possess the epitope specificity and manufacturability of a conventional monoclonal antibody (mAb) but are engineered to bind two distinct targets instead of one. The actual structure of a BsAb can vary widely, and depends on a number of factors including the intended mechanism of action (MoA) of the BsAb and desired pharmacokinetic/pharmacodynamic (PK/PD) properties [7,8]. Development and commercialization of BsAbs, to engage multiple targets using only one therapeutic, has gained significant attention recently, shifting industry focus and investments on this effective therapeutic strategy.

In this review, we discuss challenges and opportunities associated with developing bioassays for BsAbs with a particular focus on recent advances in bioanalytical approaches, as supported by multiple case studies.

1.1. Diverse Formats of BsAb

There are more than 100 distinct BsAb formats described and reviewed in the literature, but they generally fall into two categories: IgG-like and fragment-based (see Figure 1 and Wang et al. [9]).

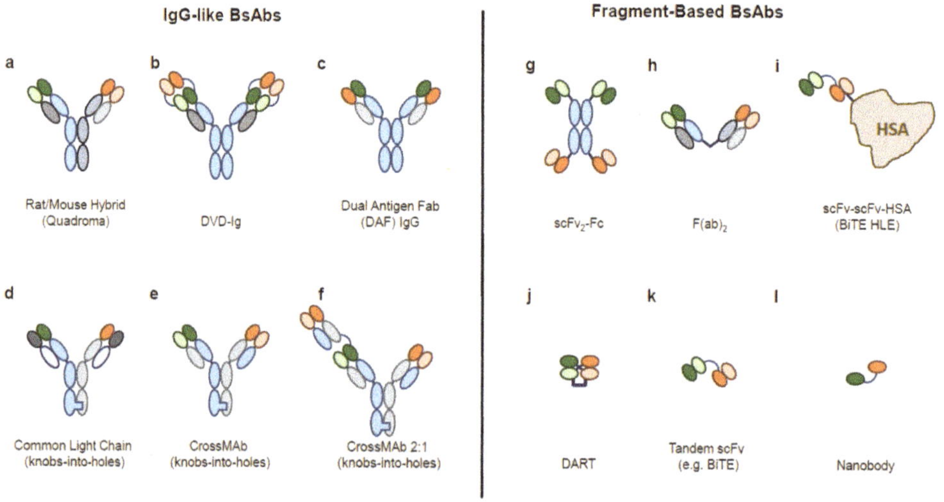

Figure 1. Examples of BsAb formats and structural diversity: (**a–f**) IgG-like BsAbs and (**g–l**) fragment-based BsAbs.

DVD-Ig: dual variable domain immunoglobulin; scFv: single-chain variable fragment; Fab: antigen-binding fragment; HSA: human serum albumin; BiTE: bispecific T-cell engager; HLE: half-life extended; DART: dual-affinity re-targeting antibody.

The IgG-like BsAbs approximate the structure of a traditional mAb and typically contain an Fc domain and two antigen binding domains. However, many designs incorporate multiple copies of one or more antigen binding domains, allowing for avidity binding of one or more targets (Figure 1a–f; [10]). For example, an IgG-like anti-human epidermal growth factor receptor 2 (aHer2)/aCD3 bispecific molecule was engineered to include two low-affinity Her2 binding domains, thereby increasing the selectivity of the BsAb for cells overexpressing Her2 and increasing selective killing of tumor cells over Her2-expressing bystander cells [11]. IgG-like BsAbs tend to have longer serum half-lives due to the presence of an Fc domain that can interact with neonatal Fc Receptor (FcRn), and they can be easily engineered to either maximize or minimize interactions with FcgammaRs, allowing for flexibility in regards to effector function activity such as antibody-dependent cellular cytolysis (ADCC), antibody-dependent cellular phagocytosis (ADCP), and complement-dependent cytotoxicity (CDC) as desired [12]. IgG-like BsAbs can be challenging to manufacture, as many platforms require in-vitro or in-vivo assembly of two distinct half antibody pairs, resulting in product-related impurities stemming from chain mispairing events that can be difficult to separate from the desired product [9]. However, a number of technologies have been developed to overcome these challenges and maximize BsAb formation including knobs-into-holes, Cross mAb, and common light chain, among others [13–16].

In contrast, fragment-based BsAbs are typically much simpler to manufacture, as they are smaller and less structurally complex. Many fragment-based BsAbs are made by combining scFv fragments of different specificities (see Figure 1g–l), and they often self assemble from a single polypeptide chain (no opportunity for chain mispairing) [17]. Their small size can lead to better tissue penetration, and it has been postulated that their small size and conformational flexibility enable a more potent receptor activation, for example when bridging two cell types, compared to their larger counterparts [7,10]. However, they tend to have very short serum half lives due to the lack of an Fc domain. For example, while efficacious, blinatumomab treatment requires continuous infusion due to its extremely short serum half life (~2h; [18]). Several fragment-based structures have been developed to increase serum half, including appending scFv fragments to Fc domains or Human Serum Albumin (HSA) [10,19]. As with IgG-like BsAbs, there is a wide range of structural variability and avidity of binding available with this class of BsAb molecules.

1.2. *Mechanisms of Action of BsAb*

Due largely to the high level of interest in BsAbs as potential therapeutics and because of their structural diversity in design, both the scientific literature and clinical development pipeline contain numerous examples of BsAbs whose MoAs span a wide range [3]. For the purpose of this review, we will sort the BsAbs into four general classes: cell-bridging BsAbs, receptor/ligand blockers or activators, cofactor mimetics, and "homing" BsAbs (Figure 2; [3,20]).

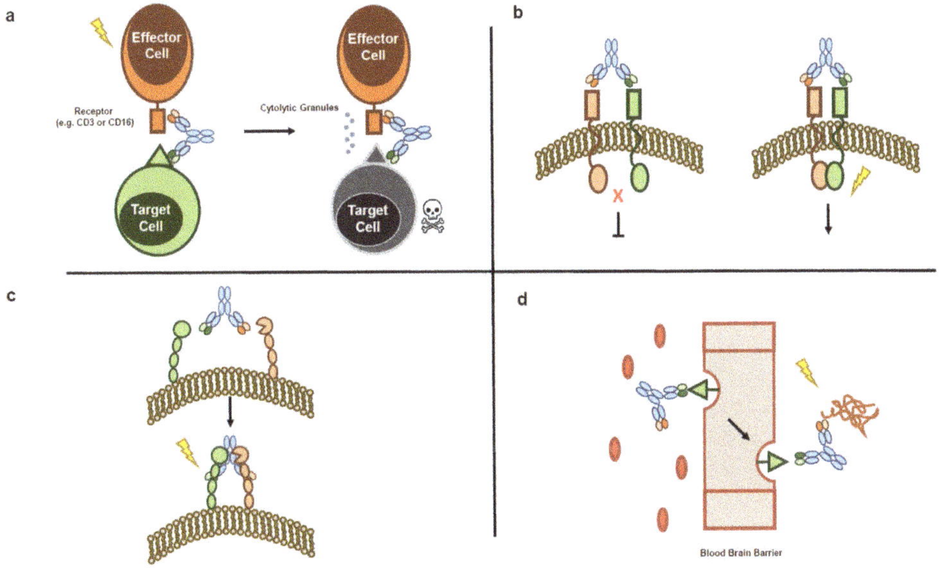

Figure 2. Mechanisms of actions of BsAb: (**a**) Schematic diagram of cell-bridging BsAb MoA (e.g., TDB or NK-recruiting BsAb); (**b**) Schematic diagram of receptor activating/inhibiting MoA (e.g., receptor dimerization inhibitor or activator); (**c**) Schematic diagram of cofactor mimicking MoA (e.g., emicizumab); and (**d**) Schematic diagram of "homing" BsAb MoA (e.g., blood brain barrier crosser).

1.2.1. MoA Type 1—Cell-bridging BsAbs

Cell-bridging BsAbs bind two distinct cell surface receptors—one on the surface of an effector cell and one on the surface of a target/tumor cell—resulting in activation of downstream signaling networks and killing of the target cell. One of the most prevalent examples of this MoA currently under clinical development is the T-cell dependent BsAbs (TDBs; [1]). These molecules most often target CD3e within the T-cell receptor (TCR) of cytolytic T cells and a tumor-specific antigen on the surface of target cells [8,21–34]. However, there are examples of BsAbs that activate T cells by engaging other epitopes, such as CD5 or co-stimulatory receptors such as CD28 [35,36]. Bridging of the target cell and the T cell by the BsAb leads to the formation of an immunological synapse, inducing T-cell activation and resulting in the release of perforin and granzymes that lyse the target cell [37]. Thus, TDBs harness a patient's own immune system to kill tumor cells independent of TCR epitope specificity by circumventing activation through the major histocompatability complex [2]. TDB immunotherapy is similar in concept to CAR-T therapy, in which a patient's T cells are extracted and engineered with a chimeric antigen receptor (CAR) designed to recognize and kill tumor cells [38]. However, while TDBs are often more complex and difficult to produce than a standard mAb biologic, they are currently cheaper and less logistically challenging to manufacture than CAR-T therapies, which must be prepared individually for each patient [39]. Additionally, TDBs can have more favorable safety profiles compared to CAR-T therapies, with fewer and less severe adverse events such as systemic cytokine release syndrome—the most common adverse event associated with immune-modulating therapies [27,40,41]. In addition to TDBs, there are several examples of BsAbs that recruit and activate NK cells by simultaneously binding CD16 (FcgammaRIII) and a tumor-specific receptor [42–45], as well as a BsAb that recruits and activates macrophages by targeting CD89 [46].

1.2.2. MoA Type 2—Receptor/Ligand-Blocking or -Activating BsAbs

By virtue of their ability to target more than one receptor, BsAbs can be developed to target and activate a receptor in a specific cellular context (e.g., a therapeutically-relevant complex). This allows for a level of selectivity that cannot be achieved with conventional mAbs alone or in combination. For example, the anti-Fibroblast Growth Factor Receptor (aFGFRI)/anti-β-Klotho (aKLB) BsAb activates the FGFRI/KLB receptor complex, leading to weight loss and a reduction in obesity-linked disorders in preclinical models [47]. By selectively targeting FGFRI/KLB, the molecule activates FGFRI when complexed with KLB, thereby avoiding widespread FGFRI activation—FGFRI receptor is expressed in a wide range of tissues—and reducing the unintended side effects associated with mAb FGFRI agonists.

In addition to acting as receptor agonists, BsAbs can also be effective receptor antagonists. Resistance to various Her2-targeting mAbs (e.g., trastuzumab) has led to the development of novel therapeutics for blocking Her2-associated signaling, including several BsAbs [48]. While many of these molecules are TDBs (MoA discussed above), there are also examples of BsAbs that bind to Her2 and Her3, preventing ligand-activated Her3 from heterodimerizing with Her2, and dampening PI3K signaling in Her2-overexpressing cancers [48]. There is also an example of an antibody-drug conjugate (ADC) BsAb that targets two distinct, non-overlapping epitopes on Her2, leading to more efficient internalization, lysosomal degradation, and release of cytotoxic payload [49]. Beyond treatments for Her2-overexpressing cancers, there are many examples of BsAbs that target combinations of receptors and/or cognate ligands, as well as cytokines [50–59]. These BsAbs sometimes serve the same purpose as that of a combination treatment of mAb therapeutics, but there are instances in which a BsAb provides a particular advantage. For example, an aCTLA4/PD1 BsAb was developed to preferentially inhibit CTLA-4 on PD1+ cells, leading to fewer adverse events associated with immune activation than have been observed when treating patients with combinations of the conventional mAb aCTLA-4 and aPD1/L checkpoint inhibitors [60]. Monovalent targeting of CTLA-4 significantly reduces the ability of the BsAb to inhibit CTLA-4, but monovalent binding has a much lower impact on the ability of the molecule to inhibit PD1 compared to a conventional bivalent aPD1 mAb. As a result, the BsAb is able to saturate CTLA-4 receptors on PD1+ cells, without widespread inhibition of CTLA-4 leading to fewer adverse events. Bispecific targeting of CTLA-4 and PD1 with this BsAb also leads to internalization and degradation of PD1—an effect that is not observed with combinations of aCTLA-4 and aPD1 mAbs.

1.2.3. MoA Type 3—Cofactor Mimicking BsAbs

Emicizumab (marketed name Hemlibra®®) is a BsAb that was developed to treat hemophilia A. The BsAb binds to coagulation Factors X and IX and is therefore able to play the role of Factor XIII—the coagulation factor missing in many hemophilia A patients [61,62].

1.2.4. MoA Type 4—"Homing" BsAbs

For the purposes of this review, "homing" BsAbs are molecules in which one arm serves to deliver the molecule to a specific, often hard-to-reach location. There are multiple examples with a diverse range of therapeutic targets. Several BsAbs have been developed that are able to cross the blood-brain barrier by targeting the transferase receptor [63–65]. Once across the barrier, the non-transferase receptor arm can target the therapeutic target of interest (typically amyloid beta-protein and other Alzheimer's Disease targets). Additionally, there is an example of a tandem scFv BsAb that targets activated platelets and sca-1, helping to bring stem cells to the location of injury; it is being explored for the treatment of myocardial infarction [66]. An aCD63/aHER2-ADC has been developed, in which binding to CD64 targets the molecule to the lysosome while the aHer2 portion provides tumor specificity, leading to a more efficient release of the conjugated drug [67]. There is also an example of a BsAb with one epitope designed to gain entry into the late endosome, where it is able to neutralize Ebola virus [68].

1.3. *Challenges and Opportunities of BsAb Bioassay Development*

Concurrent to the development of these complex biological products with multiple modalities is the need to develop bioassays that are not only accurate and reproducible, but also adequately reflective of the proposed mechanism(s) of action. Well-developed bioassays are critical to the characterization and control of biological products, as well as to the interpretation of clinical study results. BsAb bioassay development presents a unique set of challenges for assay design, such as the ability to fulfill the desired performance of the assay (i.e., to capture the dual activities and potential synergistic effects of the molecule) preferably using a single assay format, and to detect multifaceted structural changes [69]. Depending on the molecule's MoA, several bioassays might be necessary for characterization in addition to a main potency assay in the control system. For example, cell-killing, cytokine secretion, receptor internalization [70], effector function (ADCC, ADCP), and surface marker expression assays might need to be developed for the characterization of bispecific molecules for later stages of product development in addition to the one most MoA-relevant bioassay selected and validated for release, stability, and comparability testing for product licensure. A number of technologies were developed to overcome these challenges to characterize BsAb, and selected case studies are described in the Section 3.

2. Strategies and Considerations for BsAb Bioassay Development

2.1. *Phase-Appropriate Approach*

A phased approach to the development and implementation of bioassays for biotherapeutics is widely accepted by industry and regulatory agencies, and the similar principles apply to bispecific therapeutics. It is often advantageous and preferred to start with a binding method for the early phases of product development. Most commonly implemented binding assays include enzyme-linked immunosorbent assays (ELISAs) or surface-plasmon resonance (SPR) technologies. More complex and MoA-reflective cell-based bioassays are developed by later phases, and they are validated before marketing application submission. However, it is recommended that a relevant MoA-based bioassay is developed earlier, not only to gain a greater process and product understanding but also to gain a better understanding of the method's performance prior to pivotal clinical trials. Cell-based bioassays should be qualified and monitored over the span of the clinical development to have a true understanding of the critical steps and components of the assay in most cases. The selection of the bioassay should be driven by the product's therapeutic MoA. In cases where the MoA is simply binding to a target, a surrogate method, such as a protein binding or competitive binding assay, may be sufficient to determine potency. Developing robust and quality-control (QC)-suitable cell-based bioassays is more challenging than developing non-cell based binding assays [71,72]. There are case studies of implementing surrogate, non-cell-based bioassays in the commercial control system if the surrogate assay has demonstrated a good correlation in a bridging study using degraded product and other samples with the MoA-reflective cell-based assay.

2.2. Mechanism of Action

Design strategies for bioassays are driven by the drug's intended physiological MoA. Unlike other analytical techniques, bioassays are almost always unique for each therapeutic. A well-designed bioassay will accurately capture the biological activity of a drug candidate. As shown in Figure 2, common MoAs of bispecific therapeutics include direct binding to soluble targets (e.g., ligands, cytokines and enzymes), or to cell-surface receptors in either an inhibitory or agonistic manner.

Each MoA will require a different approach when considering the bioassay design. In the case of BsAbs and related recombinant proteins, secondary, tertiary, or synergistic MoAs may be discovered during development. This biological complexity further contributes to the challenge of developing MoA-reflective assays to capture the candidate molecule's putative therapeutic biological activity [50,73–76]. In some cases where multiple MoAs exist in a single molecule, a combination assay that measures all MoAs in a single assay may be suitable for product release and stability testing, with secondary characterization assays developed to measure the individual activities of each MoA if applicable. Otherwise, multiple bioassays would be necessary to fully characterize the molecule's activity. It is not required to have all bioassays for release, instead only the assay with the most MoA-relevant and stability indicating bioassay can be selected as the release potency assay while the other assays are used for characterization.

2.3. Overall BsAb Characterization Strategy

Efficacy and safety assessments of BsAbs rely on the successful development of a pharmacologically and clinically relevant bioanalytical strategy that most importantly can reflect the biological activities of these dual-targeting antibodies and can differentiate higher order structure, potency, and efficacy.

It is most vital to develop characterization and bioanalytical approaches to study important quality attributes [77] including overall stability, fragmentation/aggregation/ immunogenicity, antigen specificity, affinity, on and off rates, avidity (for molecules with two targets on the same cell), and MoA/biological activity.

While BsAbs require bioassays to measure two binding events, the choice of the appropriate bioassay will also depend on the assay format, assay platform, critical reagents, and, importantly, the BsAb target profile. Following the successful development of the pharmacologically relevant BsAb format, the analytical strategy is outlined to first characterize the independent or simultaneous binding affinities and the preferential binding of BsAb to their dual-antigen targets. Widely used bi-functional quantitative assay formats to enable target-specific capture and detection of binding properties include flow cytometry and ligand-binding immunoassay setups. A range of other assay platforms (ELISA, SPR, ADCC, competitive flow cytometry, etc.), whose selection relies on BsAb format, MoA, and target profile, are used to address bioanalytical questions for BsAbs. These assays are listed in Table 1 and further discussed in Section 3.

Meaningful bioanalytical approaches are also needed for immunogenicity and PK/PD assessments to determine the safety and efficacy of BsAbs [78,79]. Immunogenicity is defined as the unwanted immune response of the host against the therapeutic BsAb. In addition to altering the PK of a target through changing its clearance, immunogenicity is responsible for infusion-related reactions and in some cases, reduced treatment efficacy [80]. Immunogenicity is clinically assessed by the detection of anti-drug antibodies, consisting of IgM, IgG, IgE, and/or IgA isotypes [81]. The bioassays employed to assess immunogenicity include binding immunoassays such as ELISA to detect all isotypes capable of binding the therapeutic BsAbs, and neutralization assays (in-vitro cell-based assays or competitive ligand-binding assays) directed at the biologically active site, to inhibit the functional activity of BsAb. Major histocompatibility complex-II (MHC-II)-Associated Peptide Proteomics

(MAPPs) assay can screen and quantitate naturally processed and presented MHC-II peptides on the surface of antigen-presenting cells, which are then further characterized for immunogenicity using in-vitro assays. T-cell epitope-mapping prediction tools are also used to identify the CD4 T cell epitope within the amino acid sequence of the therapeutic antibody and determine the strength of peptide binding to HLA molecules [82,83]. PK for biologics is often at least partially determined by FcRn-mediated recycling. In-vitro assays designed to measure binding of a therapeutic antibody to FcRn via its Fc domain, including SPR-based FcRn binding assays and FcRn-affinity chromatography, have been shown to be indicative of FcRn-mediated clearance and are frequently used to assess potential impacts to PK [84,85].

Table 1. List of bioassays for bispecific molecules.

Bioassay	Method Principle	Examples
Bridging ELISA	To assess the ability of each arm of the BsAbs to bind two antigens simultaneously. The assay follows a sequential capture method, where antibody is allowed to bind the first coated antigen, followed by a wash step and addition of a biotinylated version of the second antigen. The bound biotinylated antigen can be detected using HRP-labeled streptavidin and luminescent substrate.	tetra-VH IgG bispecific tetravalent [86]
Sandwich ELISA	To assess binding specificity, including dual-specificity detection, of BsAbs. The assay format consists of antigen incubation with an immobilized capture antibody in the plate, followed by wash step to remove non-bound components. The antibody-antigen complex is then detected using a labeled antibody.	IgE receptor signaling blocking BsAb, FcεRI/FcγRIIb cross-link [87]
Bridging SPR	To measure the binding affinities of antibodies to their respective antigens. The assay follows Biacore™ SPR-based format, where two sequential binding events to a ligand immobilized on a chip and surface regeneration is used to measure a bridging signal and, as a result, the simultaneous binding of the assay to both antigens.	Ang-2/VEGF BsAb [88]
Dual-Binding SPR	A solution binding SPR-based assay for individual assessment of both targets in solution without the need for immobilization and regeneration of the target.	anti-VEGFA-121/Ang2 BsAb [89]
Direct Cell Killing	To evaluate cell killing potential by co-culturing the target and effector cells in the presence or absence of BsAb. Assay readout can be accomplished through luciferase reporter system or by flow cytometry-based methods to measure percent apoptotic cells or percent cytolysis of pre-labeled target cells by proliferation dye dilution analysis. Additional assays include labeling target cells with ^{51}Cr or measuring the presence of extracellular LDH, where the release of the label or LDH by lysed target cells is used as surrogate for cell-killing activity [90,91].	CD47 blocking BsAb specifically targeted to GPC3 expressing target cells [92]) PD-L1 blocking BsAb specifically directed to CSPG4-expressing target cells [93] CD3-bispecific (anti-HER2/CD3) TDB [94]
T Cell Activation	To assess BsAb effects on T-cell activation and proliferation potential. Assay readout mainly includes luciferase bioluminescence reporter signal using Jurkat T cells engineered with an NFAT-response-element driving luciferase expression. Depending on the MoA of the molecule, T-cell activation can be triggered either only by T cells expressing relevant receptors or in the presence of antigen-presenting target cells. In addition, activation and proliferation of T cells can be evaluated using an in-vitro mixed lymphocyte reaction followed by flow cytometry (proliferation dye dilution analysis or measurement of T-cell activation markers) and ELISA (for IFN-g and granzyme B secretion measurements).	CD3e-targeting TDB [95] PD-L1 blocking BsAb specifically directed to CSPG4-expressing target cells [93] CD3-bispecific (anti-HER2/CD3) TDB [94]

BsAbs: bispecific antibodies; ELISA: enzyme-linked immunosorbent assay; HRP: horseradish peroxidase; IFN-g: interferon gamma; LDH: lactate dehydrogenase; MoA: mechanism of action; NFAT: nuclear factor of activated T cells; SPR: surface-plasmon resonance; VH: variable heavy domain; Ang-2: angiopoietin-2; VEGF: vascular endothelial growth factor; PD-L1: programmed death-ligand 1; CSPG: chondroitin sulfate proteoglycan.

3. Bioassays for Bispecific Antibodies and Case Studies

3.1. Bioassays for Biotherapeutics

For biotherapeutics, a selective, physiologically relevant bioassay is essential to report on the product's potency and stability, by providing an assessment of the molecule's biological activity. Bioassays, in principle, can range from recognition of a particular antigen in a simple binding method, through systems as complex as blocking an inhibitory ligand that restores a co-stimulatory effect in a cell-based method. Selection of an appropriate method has its challenges rooted not only in the need to mimic the MoA, but also because bioassays can be costly to develop, perform, transfer, and maintain. Despite efforts to implement measures to ensure method control, cell-based bioassays can be inherently variable and often lack the precision and robustness of biophysical methods simply because they use living organisms, tissues, or cells.

While the general principles of bioassay design and strategy (e.g., measuring antigen target binding and biological activities) apply to bispecific antibodies, developing bioassays for bispecific antibodies requires unique considerations as bispecific antibodies bind two different targets with distinct mechanisms of action from monospecific biotherapeutics. A diverse range of bioanalytical assays have been developed and employed to study BsAbs, including methods designed to assess binding, potency, biological function, and purity. Figure 3 depicts a few of the methods involved in the various types of BsAb bioassays, which are further discussed in the following sections, and case studies are summarized in Table 2.

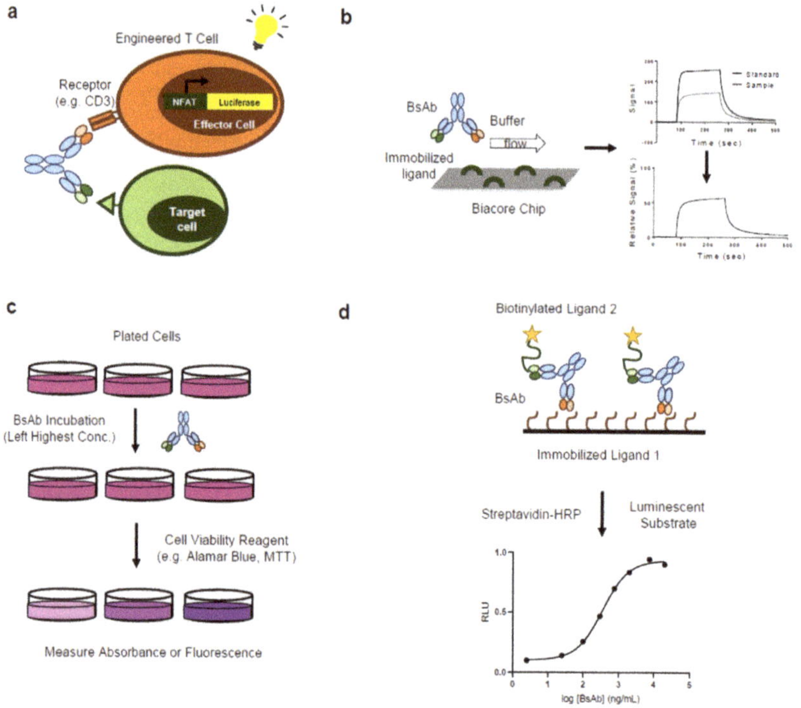

Figure 3. Representative bioassays for BsAb: (**a**) Reporter gene T-cell activation assay; (**b**) Single-arm binding SPR assay; (**c**) Cell proliferation assay; (**d**) Bridging ELISA. MTT:3-(4,5-dimethylthiazol-2-yl)-2,5-diphenyl-2H-tetrazolium bromide.

Table 2. BsAb categories and potential bioassays applicable: Summary of case studies.

	Type 1 Cell Bridging	Type 2 Receptor Blocking or Activating (Cis/Trans)	Type 3 Cofactor Mimicking	Type 4 Spatial Targeting ("Homing" BsAbs)
Binding	ELISA (binding to single target) [96], SPR (binding to single target) [96]	ELISA (binding to either target), SPR (affinity for either target) [50], bridging ELISA (dual target recognition) [50], bridging SPR [92], ELISA (ligand blocking) [74], SPR (stoichiometry of binding) [74]	SPR (characterize affinity for FIX, FIXa, FX, FXa) [61,62], ELISA (confirm specificity for FIX and FX) [62]	BLI (measure affinity of each arm, and support 1:1 binding) [68], Competition ELISA [63]
Bioactivity (Major MoA)	Reporter gene effector cell activation assay [96], direct cell killing assay [21,22,42]	Cell Proliferation [50,69,76], Apoptosis [73], cytokine neutralization [56]	Enzymatic assays (FXa activity) [61]	Viral Inactivation [68], TR-FRET AB assay [63]
Functional (other supporting MoA as characterization)	Cell depletion by flow cytometery [21,96], Cytokine release [42], cell surface marker expression (per MoA) [22,42,45,96]	Tyrosine phosphorylation [74], inhibition of antibody production/secretion [50], Calcium flux assay [50]	Thrombin generation assay [61,62]	Fluorescence microscopy to assess subcellular localization [63,65,68], transcytosis assay [65]
Effector Function	ADCC [97], ADCP [97]	CDC assay [75], ADCC/ADCP bioassay [92], binding to FcgRs [92]	NA	NA
Impurity Bioassay	T-cell activating impurities [95]	NA	NA	NA

BLI: biolayer interferometry; TR-FRET: time-resolved fluorescence resonance energy transfer.

3.2. BsAb Bioassay: Binding Assays

ELISA and SPR are commonly used for in-vitro characterization of antigen binding for BsAbs. ELISAs are advantageous in that they are sensitive, typically fast to develop compared to cell-based assays, relatively inexpensive, and can be performed in complex matrices (e.g., cell lysates) [98,99]. Bridging ELISAs and competitive binding ELISAs can also provide information on the ability of the BsAbs to bind both antigens simultaneously, and they can therefore potentially be used as MoA-reflective potency assays, at least during initial development phases. The case studies presented below provide examples of competitive and bridging ELISAs used to confirm the simultaneous binding of two different targets for a tetravalent IgG-like BsAb. Despite their advantages, ELISA assays have drawbacks, one of which is that they are end-point assays and do not provide information on binding kinetics such as on and off rates [100]. In contrast, SPR measures continuous binding in a flow cell without the need for chemical labels, and the entire binding event can be analyzed in real time (association and dissociation). This allows for the determination of both kinetic and thermodynamic parameters through various data analyses [101]. SPR assays can also be designed to measure binding to two targets simultaneously, and are also potential candidates for MoA-reflective potency by binding assays. The case studies presented below provide two examples of assay formats for the purpose of measuring concurrent antigen binding by SPR.

Drawbacks for both ELISA and SPR are that it can be difficult to measure the impact of either target density (avidity effects) on BsAb binding, which can be important factors for a BsAb's activity in an in-vivo context. SPR allows for control of target density by depositing different amounts of capture ligand on the sensor chip. Binding of the therapeutic antibody can then be characterized under the different conditions to investigate the effects of receptor density on binding affinity/avidity [102]. However, the fact that BsAbs bind two targets, with varying levels of avidity depending on structure/format, can make this type of experiment challenging to design and interpret using label-free mass-based detection by SPR [103]. Additionally, there are open questions with respect to the in-vivo relevance of binding events [e.g., how relevant is binding to an immobilized ligand on a chip, or is solution-based association of a truncated ligand (such as a peptide or extracellular domain) reflective of binding to a cell surface receptor?] [104]. Investigators have used SPR to measure binding of aCD20 mAbs to membrane bound CD20, and developed sophisticated software that makes it possible to extract and analyze individual binding events from heterogeneous mixtures. There have also been reports of affixing multiple ligands on a sensor surface in a solution-like context using DNA-directed immobilization using SPR, which would be useful for characterizing BsAbs. New biosensor technologies that allow for discrete detection of both binding events and precise control over surface density, as well as advances in SPR data analysis and experimental design, may provide avenues for more thoroughly investigating complex binding events under increasingly biologically relevant conditions in the future [105–109].

- Case Study: ELISA to detect simultaneous target binding by a tetravalent BsAb [86]: The authors developed a tetravalent BsAb composed of two different variable heavy (VH) domains on an IgG framework (tetra-VH IgG). The structure was meant to be an alternative to dual-action Fab (DAF) molecules, which are often difficult to generate via mutagenesis and additionally may not be able to bind both targets simultaneously, due to overlapping binding surfaces. Three bispecific tetra-VH IgGs were created (CD40/OX40, 4-1BB/CD40, OX40/4-1BB). In order to confirm that the BsAbs were able to bind both targets simultaneously, a competition ELISA assay was developed. The BsAb was immobilized on a plate and incubated with non-biotinylated ligand (for example OX40), followed by biotinylated ligand (for example OX40 or CD40). For each BsAb, binding of the biotinylated ligand was only inhibited by binding of the biotinylated ligand of the same specificity, while the ligand of the other specificity retained binding, suggesting that the BsAb is able to bind both targets simultaneously. To confirm that each arm of the BsAb (VH_{OX40}-$VH_{4\text{-}1BB}$ Fab) can simultaneously bind each target, a bridging ELISA assay was used. An assay plate was coated with OX40 and allowed to bind to the VH_{OX40}-VH_{41BB} Fab before being incubated with varying concentrations of biotinylated 4-1BB or biotinylated OX40. Dose-dependent binding of 4-1BB was observed, while no binding of OX40 was observed, supporting the conclusion that each arm of the BsAb is able to simultaneously bind both targets.
- Case Study: SPR to measure kinetics and binding affinity of Ang-2/VEGF BsAb [88,89]: The authors evaluated a humanized bivalent-BsAb generated for the neutralization of angiopoietin-2 (Ang-2) and vascular endothelial growth factor A (VEGF-A) [88]. Using SPR technology to characterize the kinetics and affinity of binding, the authors developed an assay to cover two binding events simultaneously, which can be reported as one response. Assay setup utilized a Biacore™ instrument and commonly used CM5 chips, and followed a scheme of sequential additions of the CrossMab and then Ang-2 to immobilized VEGF. The second binding event (Ang-2 binding to the VEGF-bound CrossMab) included surface regeneration. As a result, Ang-2-binding response is dependent on the amount of VEGF-bound CrossMab molecules and therefore reflects the actual bridging signal. In this assay, SPR-detected bridging signal reflects the active concentration of Ang-2- and VEGF-binding molecules, where the loss of overall binding can be attributed to either the VEGF or the Ang-2 binding contribution, and therefore, covers both antigen interactions. A modified SPR-based dual-binding assay was developed by Meschendoerfer et al. [89] to address the pitfalls associated with the bridging assay—specifically the change of antigen activity upon immobilization. The main objective was to allow for the individual assessment of both targets in solution while avoiding the need for immobilization and regeneration of the target. They determined the individual VEGFA-121 and Ang2 activities of an anti-VEGFA-121/Ang2 BsAb where an anti-human-Fab capture system (for the Ang2 antigen) was used to measure different antibody concentrations with the same Biosensor (regeneration cycles included). The findings suggested that comparable binding signals can be read from individual injections, when compared to an approach with sequential antigen injection. Using this assay, they showed that simultaneous binding can be calculated

based on both individual readouts: two binding events can be measured, and the third parameter can be accurately calculated based on these measurements.

Cell Surface Ligand Binding Assays

Binding properties of investigational BsAbs to their targets can also be assessed by flow cytometry, which can be used to measure binding specificity and selectivity of BsAbs in a cellular context—information that is not captured in a traditional SPR or ELISA-based binding assay. Flow cytometry, is a fluidics and optics-based method that evaluates fluorescently-labeled cell suspensions in a single cell flow to capture receptor- or antigen-binding events in intact cells. However, flow cytometric analysis of antibody binding is an indirect measurement of kinetic values and it should be used in combination with SPR analysis to provide truly comprehensive, label-free, and accurate kinetic data for the antibodies being studied.

In addition to flow-cytometry assays, cell-based reporter assays have been developed to measure gene expression in response to disruption of an inhibitory binding interaction, such as PD-L1/PD-1 [93]. As a result, these assays provide a functional measure of BsAb binding as opposed to, for example, directly measuring binding affinity by SPR. In the case studies discussed below, variations of flow cytometric analysis are used to demonstrate the preferential binding, receptor blocking, and avidity of binding to dual-antigen-expressing target cells. In addition, application of a reporter assay to assess BsAb-mediated blockade of receptor-ligand interaction between the antigen-expressing tumor cells and effector cells is reviewed.

- Case Study: Flow cytometry-based binding and blocking assays for GPC3/CD47 BsAb [92]: To develop a potential immune-modulating therapeutic to treat hepatocellular carcinoma (HCC), the authors designed a novel BsAb directed against the HCC-associated antigen Glypican-3 (GPC3) and CD47, an inhibitory innate immune checkpoint that inhibits ADCP by binding to SIRPa on myeloid cells. Due to the fact that CD47 is widely expressed on both healthy and cancerous cells, treatment with anti-CD47 mAbs is associated with toxicity. Therefore, the authors sought to direct the ADCP-enhancing activity of targeting CD47 to GPC3+ tumor cells using a bispecific approach. Several flow cytometry-based binding assays were used to demonstrate selective targeting of GPC3+ cells. For example, wild-type Raji cells (GPC3-) were labeled with a fluorescent dye and mixed in a 1:1 ratio with unlabeled Raji cells engineered to express GPC3 (Raji-GPC3^{H}) prior to incubation with GPC3/CD47 BsAb or anti-CD47 mAb. Following incubation with a FITC-labeled secondary antibody, labeled and unlabeled cells were separated by flow cytometry and the binding of the BsAb to each cell population was assessed. The results showed higher levels of BsAb binding to Raji-GPC3^{H} cells compared to the wild-type cells. In contrast, no difference in binding was observed for an anti-CD47 mAb. The authors further tested the ability of the BsAb to block the interaction between CD47 and SIRPa in each cell type using a competitive flow cytometry assay. Wild-type and Raji-GPC3^{H} cells were incubated with biotinylated SIRPa-mF in the presence of anti-CD47 mAb or GPC3/CD47 BsAb, followed by the addition of FITC-labeled streptavidin. The results showed that the BsAb prevented SIRPa binding more effectively in the Raji-GPC3^{H} cells, while the anti-CD47 mAb showed similar blocking activity in both cell types. The results of the flow cytometry-based binding assays demonstrate preferential binding and blocking activities of the GPC3/CD47 BsAb in GPC3+/CD47+ compared to GPC3-/CD47+ cells in vitro. These results suggest that the bispecific targeting of GPC3+ and CD47 may preferentially induce killing of GPC3+ tumor cells by ADCP.
- Case Study: Flow cytometry-based assay to characterize binding activity of PD-L1xCSPG4 BsAb [93]: To improve antibody-therapy efficacy in patients with advanced melanoma, the authors developed a BsAb, PD-L1xCSPG4, to selectively reactivate T cells by directing PD-1/PD-L1 disrupting activity to chondroitin sulfate proteoglycan 4 (CSPG4)-expressing tumor cells. A flow cytometry-based assay was employed to eval-

uate the binding activities of the investigational BsAb. Wild-type ectopically hPD-L1-expressing CHO cells (CHO.PD-L1) were incubated with test antibodies, labeled with a fluorescent secondary antibody, and analyzed by flow cytometry. Dose-dependent binding specific to CHO.PD-L1 cells was observed for the BsAb. These binding activities were replicated in several representative cancer cells endogenously expressing both CSPG4 or PD-L1. In addition, a flow cytometry-based competitive binding assay was used to assess the overall binding strength (avidity) of PD-L1xCSPG4 BsAb to CSPG4+/PD-L1+ cancer cells. BsAb binding was strongly inhibited in the presence of competing parental anti-CSPG4 mAb and only weakly inhibited in the presence of competing PD-L1-blocking mAb. These experiments demonstrate that PD-L1xCSPG4 binds to both PD-L1 and CSPG4 and that the strength of the interaction between the BsAb and CSPG4+/PD-L1+ cancer cells is primarily dominated by binding to CSGA4. To further show that the enhanced binding of the BsAb to CSPG4+/PD-L1+ cells is driven by avidity, cells were pre-incubated with a fluorescent anti-PD-L1 mAb, before being exposed to the test BsAb and a control BsAb, capable of binding PD-L1 but not CSPG4. The EC_{50} of PD-L1xCSPG4 for displacing the probe was substantially lower compared to the control BsAb. Performing the experiment in the presence of an anti-GSPG4 mAb increased the EC_{50} of the PD-L1xCSPG4 BsAb to a level similar to the control BsAb. Together these flow cytometry-based binding assays demonstrated that the PDL1xCSPG4 BsAb has enhanced selectivity for CSPG4+/PD-L1+ cancer cells driven by avidity binding.

- Case Study: Cell-based reporter assay to measure cell surface binding of PDL1xCSPG4 BsAb [93]: The authors further evaluated the role of CSPG4 in mediating the PD-L1-blocking capacity of the PDL1xCSPG4 BsAb using a PD-1/PD-L1 blockade reporter bioassay. The assay relies on co-culturing of Jurkat.PD-1-NFAT-luc reporter T cells (Jurkat cells engineered to express luciferase under the control of a NFAT response element and PD-1) and CHO.PDL1/CD3 cells (CHO cells engineered to express PD-L1 and a membrane-linked agonistic anti-CD3 antibody). Upon successful interaction of PD-1 and PD-L1 between the two cell types, TCR signaling and downstream NFAT-mediated luciferase activity in the Jurkat cells is inhibited. In contrast, interrupting the PD-1/PD-L1 interaction leads to NFAT-mediated luciferase activity. Addition of the PDL1xCSPG4 BsAb to the co-culture disrupted the PD-1/PD-L1 interaction between the two cell types in a dose-dependent manner, as measured by luminescence detection. Next, they tested the role of CSPG4 mAb in PD-1/PD-L1 blocking capacity of PDL1xCSPG4 BsAb by replacing the CHO.PD-L1/CD3 cells with a CSPG4+/PD-L1+ cancer cell line (the CD3 stimulation of T cells was achieved by pre-treating the cells with BIS1; an EpCAM-directed CD3-agonistic bsAb). Stimulated reporter T cells were co-cultured with the double-positive cells in the presence of PDL1xCSPG4 BsAb or controls, with and without anti-CSPG4 mAb. The ability of the PDL1xCSPG4 BsAb to block PD-1/PD-L1 interaction was reduced in the presence of anti-CSPG4 mAb. These findings suggest that the BsAb's PD-1/PD-L1-disrupting activity will be enhanced against CSPG4+/PD-L1+ cells compared to CSPG4-/PD-L1+ cells.

3.3. *BsAb Bioassay: Potency Assays*

In particular, the strategy of using a potency assay for BsAbs is challenging due to its complicated MoA with two target bindings, and it should be tailored to be MoA-reflective while meeting QC and regulatory expectations to be robust and sensitive methods to detect any structural changes in stability. One interesting question with respect to the BsAb potency assay is if two assays are needed for each target binding or if one potency assay would suffice. Depending on its MoA, either one or two potency assays would be suitable, but it is preferred to have one potency assay to measure synergistic biological effects of two target bindings or a dual read-out of the binding assays in a single assay.

A single assay that can fully capture the bioactivity of the therapeutic molecule is advantageous from both a cost/labor perspective and from a control perspective—synergistic effects resulting from dual antigen binding may be missed if data from multiple assays measuring discrete events are used. However, in order to show the assay is suitably MoA-reflective, the key events in the MoA must be relatively well understood, and characterization assays designed to measure each event (e.g., binding to either antigen, receptor activation, etc.) are needed. The two case studies below describe the development and justification of single QC potency assays to measure changes in bioactivity for (1) a TDB and (2) a DAF that inhibits ligand binding to two distinct cell surface receptors.

- Case Study: Reporter gene T cell activation assay to measure potency of CD3e-binding TDB [96]: The authors developed a reporter gene potency assay that measures T-cell activation in the presence of a CD3e-binding TDB, using Jurkat T-cells engineered to express luciferase under the control of a T-cell activation-sensitive transcriptional response element. The assay was shown to be quantitative and stability indicating. Additionally, it is robust and relatively fast/easy to perform compared to a traditional cell-based cell killing assay, such as a Cr51 release or dye release assay, making it more amenable to a QC testing environment. The MoA of the TDB is complex as it consists of multiple factors—concurrent antigen binding, T-cell activation, and target-cell depletion. In order to show that T-cell activation in an engineered context is a suitable surrogate measure of the TDB's overall bioactivity, the authors generated a characterization data package consisting of data from individual antigen binding assays (cell-based ELISA to measure binding to the target receptor, SPR to measure binding to CD3) and a flow cytometry-based cell killing assay that used human peripheral blood mononuclear cells as a source of cytolytic T-cells. By using the data generated from the characterization assays, the authors were able to show that changes in potency detected by the reporter gene assay agreed well with changes in affinity for either antigen and cell killing activity. The characterization results support the assertion that the reporter gene assay is sufficiently MoA-reflective to serve as a single potency assay on the control system without the need for additional assays. The authors' overall strategy can be applied to justify potency for other TDBs with similar MoAs.
- Case Study: Cell-based potency assay to measure biological activity of HER3/EGFR DAF BsAb [69]: In order to measure the activity of a DAF molecule designed to simultaneously inhibit HER3 and EGFR, the authors developed a cell-based potency assay that measures cell proliferation using a cell-permeable redox dye, in which the fluorescence signal is proportional to the number of viable cells. This method was selected based on the molecule's proposed MoA, which is characterized by blocking ligand binding to each receptor, prevention of receptor dimerization (hetero- and homo-), and inhibition of cell proliferation. A cell line that naturally expresses both receptors and their cognate ligands was selected in order to enable monitoring of the effects of inhibiting both receptors. As in the case study described above, the author's generated a characterization data package using the potency assay and individual ELISA binding assays for HER3 and EGFR to show that the single potency assay is reflective of the DAF's overall bioactivity. The fact that the potency assay was demonstrated to be sensitive to changes in affinity for either target and sensitive to inhibition of both receptors, with inhibition of both HER3 and EGFR by the DAF producing the most potent anti-proliferative activity, provides a strong justification that the potency assay sufficiently captures the molecule's MoA. This, combined with the potency assay's quantitative ability and stability indicating properties, provides a persuasive argument that it is suitable as a single control system assay for monitoring the impact of product quality on bioactivity.

3.4. BsAb Bioassay: Effector Function Assays

Some BsAbs target cell surface proteins or receptors with the intent of enhancing effector function. One arm often targets a tumor-associated antigen while the other targets an immune system-evading surface protein (such as CD47 or CD55/59), increasing susceptibility of the tumor cell to lysis by complement or NK cells, or phagocytosis by macrophages.

Other BsAbs have a primary MoA that does not involve effector function (e.g., TDB, or receptor blocker) but have an effector-competent Fc domain and can also exert cell killing activity through effector function. Depending on the MoA and other molecule-specific factors, effector function can be associated with unfavorable safety events, and so, effector-silenced Fc domains are preferred [110,111]. In other cases effector function enhances a molecule's activity [54,57].

- Case Study: ADCC reporter assay and competitive ADCP assay to measure enhanced Fc-mediated effector function of GPC3/CD47 BsAb [92]: As mediated by the Fc domain function of therapeutic antibodies, ADCC and ADCP assays are among the appropriate ones to assess the enhanced Fc-mediated effector functions of investigational BsAbs. The authors employed a cell-based reporter system to evaluate the ability of BsAb in inducing ADCC against dual-antigen-expressing Raji-GPC3^{H} cells. In this assay format, engineered Jurkat T lymphocyte cells were used as effector cells. Target cells, including wild-type Raji and Raji-GPC3^{H} cells, were incubated with each mAb and BsAb test antibodies and effector cells. A luminescent substrate was used to measure the luciferase activity at the end of co-incubation that corresponds to the extent of the effector activities. This bioassay revealed that GPC3/CD47 BsAb could induce ADCC against dual-antigen-expressing Raji-GPC3^{H} cells in a dose-dependent manner and to a greater extent compared to the wild-type Raji cells. The ability of BsAb to induce ADCP in vitro was also evaluated upon co-incubation of Raji-GPC3^{H} cells with macrophages. In this assay setup, the effector cells [mouse hSIRPa expressing bone marrow-derived macrophages (BMDMs) harvested from humanized mouse bone marrow] were Alexa Fluor647-labeled and incubated with target cells (Raji or Raji-GPC3^{H} cells) stained with a fluorescent proliferation dye and each antibody. Effector:target cell mixture was then evaluated for ADCP where the phagocytosis of fluorescent-labeled target cells by labeled BMDMs was recorded using a confocal microscope (unphagocytosed cells were washed away prior to microscopy). In this bioassay format, using fluorescence microscopy and quantification of phagocytosis, the authors showed a preferential phagocytosis of dual-antigen-expressing Raji-GPC3^{H} cells specifically in the presence of GPC3/CD47 BsAb.
- Case Study: Use of a CDC assay to assess activity of a complement-regulator neutralizing BsAbs directed against CD20 and CD55/CD59 [75]: The authors designed BsAbs to increase complement-mediated killing of CD20-expressing B cells. By simultaneous targeting CD20 and CD55/CD59, the BsAbs are able to neutralize the C-regulating proteins on B cells, leading to more efficient killing by CDC. Various CD20-expressing cells were treated with the BsAbs, followed by incubation with human sera (source of complement). Following an incubation period, cells were assessed for viability using MTT (a dye that is reduced to form a purple dye in the presence of metabolically active cells). Cell killing was enhanced by treatment with the BsAbs compared to treatment with an effector-competent aCD20 mAb. Additionally, cell killing levels remained consistent in the presence of CD20-bystander cells expressing CD55 and CD59, suggesting that the BsAbs are selectively killing CD20+ B cells. Flow cytometry-based binding assays were used to confirm binding to cells expressing CD20, CD55, and CD59.

3.5. BsAb Bioassay: Impurities Assays

Impurities assays for BsAbs are often physicochemical assays such as size-exclusion chromatography (to measure aggregates and fragments), imaging capillary isoelectric focusing/ion exchange chromatography (to measure charge variants), and mass spectrometry (to sensitively identify and/or quantify post-translational modifications and other trace variants) [112], which are commonly used to characterize impurities for conventional mAbs. However, the unique structure of BsAbs can produce unique product variants with impacts to safety and/or bioactivity that are not fully addressed by physicochemical assays. The nature/activity of such impurities is rooted in the structure of the molecule, its production process, and MoA. In order to illustrate this point a case study describing the development of a bioassay to measure T-cell activating impurities for a TDB is described below.

- Case Study: Luciferase reporter T cell activation assay to measure functional effects of impurities on CD3e-targeting TDB [95]: A CD3e-targeting TDB produced by knobs-into-holes technology and assembled in vitro contains a number of product-related impurities with the potential to activate T-cells in the absence of target cells. For example, aggregates and aCD3 homodimer, which result from the mispairing of aCD3 half antibody fragments during production, are characterized by multivalent binding to CD3 and can crosslink the TCR resulting in activation. These impurities are a safety concern because T-cell activation is linked to adverse events such as cytokine release syndrome. While aggregates and aCD3 HD can be measured using analytical methods, a bioassay is needed to assess their biological impact, such as target-independent T-cell activation. To address this need, the authors developed a reporter gene assay that measures T-cell activation in the absence of target cells using Jurkat T-cells engineered to express luciferase when activated. T-cell activation of product-related impurities present in the TDB formulation was quantified relative to T-cell activation by aCD3 HD standard. Using this assay, the authors were able to characterize the T-cell activating activities of aggregates and other product-related impurities, in order to get an idea of their potential impacts to safety and inform on the overall control strategy. Additionally, because the assay is a "catchall" assay that measures the combined T-cell activating activity of product-related impurities that may be present in a given sample, the method is able to provide reassurance that combinations of impurities are not leading to unexpected T-cell activation. Such combination effects would not be identified using physicochemical methods alone.

4. Conclusions

BsAbs represent a highly promising and emerging therapeutic area. Due to structural and biological differences from monospecific Abs, development of a bioassay strategy for the BsAb poses unique challenges and considerations. We reviewed currently available bioanalytical technological platforms, bioassays, and relevant case studies for BsAbs to provide insight into designing a BsAb release and characterization strategy. Understanding and developing good bioassays are critical for the overall control strategy of BsAbs to measure biological activities, and they will continue to evolve for both BsAb molecules and analytical technologies available.

Funding: This research received no external funding.

Institutional Review Board Statement: Not applicable.

Informed Consent Statement: Not applicable.

Data Availability Statement: No new data were created or analyzed in this study. Data sharing is not applicable to this article.

Acknowledgments: The authors acknowledge editorial service by Eileen Y. Ivasauskas and review by Dayue Chen for the manuscript.

Conflicts of Interest: The authors declare no conflict of interest.

References

1. Lejeune, M.; Köse, M.C.; Duray, E.; Einsele, H.; Beguin, Y.; Caers, J. Bispecific, T-cell-recruiting antibodies in B-cell malignancies. *Front. Immunol.* **2020**, *11*, 762. [CrossRef] [PubMed]
2. Perez, P.; Hoffman, R.W.; Shaw, S.; Bluestone, J.A.; Segal, D.M. Specific targeting of cytotoxic T cells by anti-T3 linked to anti-target cell antibody. *Nature* **1985**, *316*, 354–356. [CrossRef] [PubMed]
3. Labrijn, A.F.; Janmaat, M.L.; Reichert, J.M.; Parren, P.W.H.I. Bispecific antibodies: A mechanistic review of the pipeline. *Nat. Rev. Drug Discov.* **2019**, *18*, 585–608. [CrossRef]
4. Reichert, J. Bispecific Antibodies Come to the Fore. Available online: https://www.antibodysociety.org/antibody-therapeutics-pipeline/bispecific-antibodies-come-to-the-fore/ (accessed on 15 March 2021).

5. Spiess, C.; Zhai, Q.; Carter, P.J. Alternative molecular formats and therapeutic applications for bispecific antibodies. *Mol. Immunol.* **2015**, *67*, 95–106. [CrossRef] [PubMed]
6. Brinkmann, U.; Kontermann, R.E. The making of bispecific antibodies. *mAbs* **2017**, *9*, 182–212. [CrossRef]
7. Dickopf, S.; Georges, G.J.; Brinkmann, U. Format and geometries matter: Structure-based design defines the functionality of bispecific antibodies. *Comput. Struct. Biotechnol. J.* **2020**, *18*, 1221–1227. [CrossRef] [PubMed]
8. Fabozzi, G.; Pegu, A.; Koup, R.A.; Petrovas, C. Bispecific antibodies: Potential immunotherapies for HIV treatment. *Methods* **2019**, *154*, 118–124. [CrossRef]
9. Wang, Q.; Chen, Y.; Park, J.; Liu, X.; Hu, Y.; Wang, T.; McFarland, K.; Betenbaugh, M.J. Design and production of bispecific antibodies. *Antibodies* **2019**, *8*, 43. [CrossRef]
10. Kontermann, R.E.; Brinkmann, U. Bispecific antibodies. *Drug Discov. Today* **2015**, *20*, 838–847. [CrossRef]
11. Slaga, D.; Ellerman, D.; Lombana, T.N.; Vij, R.; Li, J.; Hristopoulos, M.; Clark, R.; Johnston, J.; Shelton, A.; Mai, E.; et al. Avidity-based binding to HER2 results in selective killing of HER2-overexpressing cells by anti-HER2/CD3. *Sci. Transl. Med.* **2018**, *10*, eaat5775. [CrossRef]
12. Kontermann, R.E. Strategies to extend plasma half-lives of recombinant antibodies. *BioDrugs* **2009**, *23*, 93–109. [CrossRef]
13. Huang, S.; Segués, A.; Hulsik, D.L.; Zaiss, D.M.; Sijts, A.J.A.M.; van Duijnhoven, S.M.J.; van Elsas, A. A novel efficient bispecific antibody format, combining a conventional antigen-binding fragment with a single domain antibody, avoids potential heavy-light chain mis-pairing. *J. Immunol. Methods* **2020**, *483*, 112811. [CrossRef] [PubMed]
14. Atwell, S.; Ridgway, J.B.B.; Wells, J.A.; Carter, P. Stable heterodimers from remodeling the domain interface of a homodimer using a phage display library. *J. Mol. Biol.* **1997**, *270*, 26–35. [CrossRef] [PubMed]
15. Schaefer, W.; Regula, J.T.; Bähner, M.; Schanzer, J.; Croasdale, R.; Dürr, H.; Gassner, C.; Georges, G.; Kettenberger, H.; Imhof-Jung, S.; et al. Immunoglobulin domain crossover as a generic approach for the production of bispecific IgG antibodies. *Proc. Natl. Acad. Sci. USA* **2011**, 201019002. [CrossRef] [PubMed]
16. Krah, S.; Schröter, C.; Eller, C.; Rhiel, L.; Rasche, N.; Beck, J.; Sellmann, C.; Günther, R.; Toleikis, L.; Hock, B.; et al. Generation of human bispecific common light chain antibodies by combining animal immunization and yeast display. *Protein Eng. Des. Sel.* **2017**, *30*, 291–301. [CrossRef] [PubMed]
17. Ahamadi-Fesharaki, R.; Fateh, A.; Vaziri, F.; Solgi, G.; Siadat, S.D.; Mahboudi, F.; Rahimi-Jamnani, F. Single-chain variable fragment-based bispecific antibodies: Hitting two targets with one sophisticated arrow. *Mol. Ther. Oncolytics* **2019**, *14*, 38–56. [CrossRef] [PubMed]
18. Portell, C.A.; Wenzell, C.M.; Advani, A.S. Clinical and pharmacologic aspects of blinatumomab in the treatment of B-cell acute lymphoblastic leukemia. *Clin. Pharm.* **2013**, *5*, 5–11. [CrossRef] [PubMed]
19. Müller, D.; Karle, A.; Meißburger, B.; Höfig, I.; Stork, R.; Kontermann, R.E. Improved pharmacokinetics of recombinant bispecific antibody molecules by fusion to human serum albumin. *J. Biol. Chem.* **2007**, *282*, 12650–12660. [CrossRef] [PubMed]
20. Lum, L.; Davol, P.; Lee, R. The new face of bispecific antibodies: Targeting cancer and much more. *Exp. Hematol.* **2006**, *34*, 1–6. [CrossRef]
21. Hoffmann, P.; Hofmeister, R.; Brischwein, K.; Brandl, C.; Crommer, S.; Bargou, R.; Itin, C.; Prang, N.; Baeuerle, P.A. Serial killing of tumor cells by cytotoxic T cells redirected with a CD19-/CD3-bispecific single-chain antibody construct. *Int. J. Cancer* **2005**, *115*, 98–104. [CrossRef]
22. Ross, S.L.; Sherman, M.; McElroy, P.L.; Lofgren, J.A.; Moody, G.; Baeuerle, P.A.; Coxon, A.; Arvedson, T. Bispecific T cell engager (BiTE®) antibody constructs can mediate bystander tumor cell killing. *PLoS ONE* **2017**, *12*, e0183390. [CrossRef] [PubMed]
23. Bacac, M.; Fauti, T.; Sam, J.; Colombetti, S.; Weinzierl, T.; Ouaret, D.; Bodmer, W.; Lehmann, S.; Hofer, T.; Hosse, R.J.; et al. A Novel carcinoembryonic antigen t-cell bispecific antibody (CEA TCB) for the treatment of solid tumors. *Clin. Cancer Res.* **2016**, *22*, 3286–3297. [CrossRef] [PubMed]
24. Kruse, R.L.; Shum, T.; Legras, X.; Barzi, M.; Pankowicz, F.P.; Gottschalk, S.; Bissig, K.-D. In situ liver expression of HBsAg/CD3-bispecific antibodies for HBV immunotherapy. *Mol. Ther. Methods Clin. Dev.* **2017**, *7*, 32–41. [CrossRef] [PubMed]
25. Laszlo, G.S.; Gudgeon, C.J.; Harrington, K.H.; Dell'Aringa, J.; Newhall, K.J.; Means, G.D.; Sinclair, A.M.; Kischel, R.; Frankel, S.R.; Walter, R.B. Cellular determinants for preclinical activity of a novel CD33/CD3 bispecific T-cell engager (BiTE) antibody, AMG 330, against human AML. *Blood* **2014**, *123*, 554–561. [CrossRef]
26. Junttila, T.T.; Li, J.; Johnston, J.; Hristopoulos, M.; Clark, R.; Ellerman, D.; Wang, B.-E.; Li, Y.; Mathieu, M.; Li, G.; et al. Antitumor efficacy of a bispecific antibody that targets HER2 and activates T cells. *Cancer Res.* **2014**, *74*, 5561–5571. [CrossRef]
27. Li, J.; Ybarra, R.; Mak, J.; Herault, A.; De Almeida, P.; Arrazate, A.; Ziai, J.; Totpal, K.; Junttila, M.R.; Walsh, K.B.; et al. IFNγ-induced chemokines are required for CXCR3-mediated T-cell recruitment and antitumor efficacy of anti-HER2/CD3 bispecific antibody. *Clin. Cancer Res.* **2018**, *24*, 6447–6458. [CrossRef]
28. Meng, W.; Tang, A.; Ye, X.; Gui, X.; Li, L.; Fan, X.; Schultz, R.D.; Freed, D.C.; Ha, S.; Wang, D.; et al. Targeting human-cytomegalovirus-infected cells by redirecting T Cells using an anti-CD3/anti-glycoprotein B bispecific antibody. *Antimicrob. Agents Chemother.* **2018**, *62*, e01717–e01719. [CrossRef]
29. Osada, T.; Patel, S.P.; Hammond, S.A.; Osada, K.; Morse, M.A.; Lyerly, H.K. CEA/CD3-bispecific T cell-engaging (BiTE) antibody-mediated T lymphocyte cytotoxicity maximized by inhibition of both PD1 and PD-L1. *Cancer Immunol. Immunother.* **2015**, *64*, 677–688. [CrossRef]

30. Reusch, U.; Harrington, K.H.; Gudgeon, C.J.; Fucek, I.; Ellwanger, K.; Weichel, M.; Knackmuss, S.H.; Zhukovsky, E.A.; Fox, J.A.; Kunkel, L.A.; et al. Characterization of CD33/CD3 Tetravalent bispecific tandem diabodies (TandAbs) for the treatment of acute myeloid leukemia. *Clin. Cancer Res.* **2016**, *22*, 5829–5838. [CrossRef]
31. Schlereth, B.; Kleindienst, P.; Fichtner, I.; Lorenczewski, G.; Brischwein, K.; Lippold, S.; Silva, A.D.; Locher, M.; Kischel, R.; Lutterbüse, R.; et al. Potent inhibition of local and disseminated tumor growth in immunocompetent mouse models by a bispecific antibody construct specific for Murine CD3. *Cancer Immunol. Immunother.* **2006**, *55*, 785–796. [CrossRef]
32. Shiraiwa, H.; Narita, A.; Kamata-Sakurai, M.; Ishiguro, T.; Sano, Y.; Hironiwa, N.; Tsushima, T.; Segawa, H.; Tsunenari, T.; Ikeda, Y.; et al. Engineering a bispecific antibody with a common light chain: Identification and optimization of an anti-CD3 epsilon and anti-GPC3 bispecific antibody, ERY974. *Methods* **2019**, *154*, 10–20. [CrossRef]
33. Sung, J.A.M.; Pickeral, J.; Liu, L.; Stanfield-Oakley, S.A.; Lam, C.-Y.K.; Garrido, C.; Pollara, J.; LaBranche, C.; Bonsignori, M.; Moody, M.A.; et al. Dual-affinity re-targeting proteins direct T cell–mediated cytolysis of latently HIV-infected cells. *J. Clin. Investig.* **2015**, *125*, 4077–4090. [CrossRef] [PubMed]
34. Sun, L.L.; Ellerman, D.; Mathieu, M.; Hristopoulos, M.; Chen, X.; Li, Y.; Yan, X.; Clark, R.; Reyes, A.; Stefanich, E.; et al. Anti-CD20/CD3 T cell–dependent bispecific antibody for the treatment of B cell malignancies. *Sci. Transl. Med.* **2015**, *7*, 287ra270. [CrossRef] [PubMed]
35. Grosse-Hovest, L.; Hartlapp, I.; Marwan, W.; Brem, G.; Rammensee, H.-G.; Jung, G. A recombinant bispecific single-chain antibody induces targeted, supra-agonistic CD28-stimulation and tumor cell killing. *Eur. J. Immunol.* **2003**, *33*, 1334–1340. [CrossRef]
36. Kroesen, B.J.; Bakker, A.; van Lier, R.A.; The, H.T.; de Leij, L. Bispecific antibody-mediated target cell-specific costimulation of resting T cells via CD5 and CD28. *Cancer Res.* **1995**, *55*, 4409–4415. [PubMed]
37. Li, J.; Stagg, N.J.; Johnston, J.; Harris, M.J.; Menzies, S.A.; DiCara, D.; Clark, V.; Hristopoulos, M.; Cook, R.; Slaga, D.; et al. Membrane-proximal epitope facilitates efficient T cell synapse formation by anti-FcRH5/CD3 and is a requirement for myeloma cell killing. *Cancer Cell* **2017**, *31*, 383–395. [CrossRef]
38. Strohl, W.R.; Naso, M. Bispecific T-cell redirection versus chimeric antigen receptor (CAR)-T cells as approaches to kill cancer cells. *Antibodies* **2019**, *8*, 41. [CrossRef]
39. Piscopo, N.J.; Mueller, K.P.; Das, A.; Hematti, P.; Murphy, W.L.; Palecek, S.P.; Capitini, C.M.; Saha, K. Bioengineering solutions for manufacturing challenges in CAR T cells. *Biotechnol. J.* **2018**, *13*, 1700095. [CrossRef]
40. Shimabukuro-Vornhagen, A.; Gödel, P.; Subklewe, M.; Stemmler, H.J.; Schlößer, H.A.; Schlaak, M.; Kochanek, M.; Böll, B.; von Bergwelt-Baildon, M.S. Cytokine release syndrome. *J. Immunother. Cancer* **2018**, *6*, 56. [CrossRef]
41. Subklewe, M. BiTEs better than CAR T cells. *Blood Adv.* **2021**, *5*, 607–612. [CrossRef]
42. Pahl, J.H.W.; Koch, J.; Götz, J.J.; Arnold, A.; Reusch, U.; Gantke, T.; Rajkovic, E.; Treder, M.; Cerwenka, A. CD16A Activation of NK cells promotes NK cell proliferation and memory-like cytotoxicity against cancer cells. *Cancer Immunol. Res.* **2018**, *6*, 517–527. [CrossRef]
43. Reusch, U.; Burkhardt, C.; Fucek, I.; Le Gall, F.; Le Gall, M.; Hoffmann, K.; Knackmuss, S.H.J.; Kiprijanov, S.; Little, M.; Zhukovsky, E.A. A novel tetravalent bispecific TandAb (CD30/CD16A) efficiently recruits NK cells for the lysis of CD30+ tumor cells. *mAbs* **2014**, *6*, 727–738. [CrossRef] [PubMed]
44. Oberg, H.H.; Kellner, C.; Gonnermann, D.; Sebens, S.; Bauerschlag, D.; Gramatzki, M.; Kabelitz, D.; Peipp, M.; Wesch, D. Tribody [$(HER2)_2$xCD16] is more effective than trastuzumab in enhancing γδ T cell and natural killer cell cytotoxicity against HER2-expressing cancer cells. *Front. Immunol.* **2018**, *9*. [CrossRef] [PubMed]
45. Schmohl, J.U.; Felices, M.; Taras, E.; Miller, J.S.; Vallera, D.A. Enhanced ADCC and NK cell activation of an anticarcinoma bispecific antibody by genetic insertion of a modified IL-15 cross-linker. *Mol. Ther.* **2016**, *24*, 1312–1322. [CrossRef] [PubMed]
46. Li, B.; Xu, L.; Pi, C.; Yin, Y.; Xie, K.; Tao, F.; Li, R.; Gu, H.; Fang, J. CD89-mediated recruitment of macrophages via a bispecific antibody enhances anti-tumor efficacy. *OncoImmunology* **2018**, *7*, e1380142. [CrossRef] [PubMed]
47. Kolumam, G.; Chen, M.Z.; Tong, R.; Zavala-Solorio, J.; Kates, L.; van Bruggen, N.; Ross, J.; Wyatt, S.K.; Gandham, V.D.; Carano, R.A.D.; et al. Sustained brown fat stimulation and insulin sensitization by a humanized bispecific antibody agonist for fibroblast growth factor receptor 1/βKlotho complex. *EBioMedicine* **2015**, *2*, 730–743. [CrossRef]
48. Yu, S.; Liu, Q.; Han, X.; Qin, S.; Zhao, W.; Li, A.; Wu, K. Development and clinical application of anti-HER2 monoclonal and bispecific antibodies for cancer treatment. *Exp. Hematol. Oncol.* **2017**, *6*, 31. [CrossRef] [PubMed]
49. Li, J.Y.; Perry, S.R.; Muniz-Medina, V.; Wang, X.; Wetzel, L.K.; Rebelatto, M.C.; Hinrichs, M.J.M.; Bezabeh, B.Z.; Fleming, R.L.; Dimasi, N.; et al. A biparatopic HER2-targeting antibody-drug conjugate induces tumor regression in primary models refractory to or ineligible for HER2-targeted therapy. *Cancer Cell* **2016**, *29*, 117–129. [CrossRef]
50. Veri, M.-C.; Burke, S.; Huang, L.; Li, H.; Gorlatov, S.; Tuaillon, N.; Rainey, G.J.; Ciccarone, V.; Zhang, T.; Shah, K.; et al. Therapeutic control of B cell activation via recruitment of Fcγ receptor IIb (CD32B) inhibitory function with a novel bispecific antibody scaffold. *Arthritis Rheum.* **2010**, *62*, 1933–1943. [CrossRef]
51. DiGiandomenico, A.; Keller, A.E.; Gao, C.; Rainey, G.J.; Warrener, P.; Camara, M.M.; Bonnell, J.; Fleming, R.; Bezabeh, B.; Dimasi, N.; et al. A multifunctional bispecific antibody protects against Pseudomonas aeruginosa. *Sci. Transl. Med.* **2014**, *6*, 262ra155. [CrossRef]

52. Jimeno, A.; Moore, K.N.; Gordon, M.; Chugh, R.; Diamond, J.R.; Aljumaily, R.; Mendelson, D.; Kapoun, A.M.; Xu, L.; Stagg, R.; et al. A first-in-human phase 1a study of the bispecific anti-DLL4/anti-VEGF antibody navicixizumab (OMP-305B83) in patients with previously treated solid tumors. *Investig. New Drugs* **2019**, *37*, 461–472. [CrossRef] [PubMed]
53. Zheng, S.; Moores, S.; Jarantow, S.; Pardinas, J.; Chiu, M.; Zhou, H.; Wang, W. Cross-arm binding efficiency of an EGFR x c-Met bispecific antibody. *mAbs* **2016**, *8*, 551–561. [CrossRef] [PubMed]
54. Grugan, K.D.; Dorn, K.; Jarantow, S.W.; Bushey, B.S.; Pardinas, J.R.; Laquerre, S.; Moores, S.L.; Chiu, M.L. Fc-mediated activity of EGFR x c-Met bispecific antibody JNJ-61186372 enhanced killing of lung cancer cells. *mAbs* **2017**, *9*, 114–126. [CrossRef]
55. Patel, A.; DiGiandomenico, A.; Keller, A.E.; Smith, T.R.F.; Park, D.H.; Ramos, S.; Schultheis, K.; Elliott, S.T.C.; Mendoza, J.; Broderick, K.E.; et al. An engineered bispecific DNA-encoded IgG antibody protects against Pseudomonas aeruginosa in a pneumonia challenge model. *Nat. Commun.* **2017**, *8*, 637. [CrossRef] [PubMed]
56. Wu, C.; Ying, H.; Grinnell, C.; Bryant, S.; Miller, R.; Clabbers, A.; Bose, S.; McCarthy, D.; Zhu, R.-R.; Santora, L.; et al. Simultaneous targeting of multiple disease mediators by a dual-variable-domain immunoglobulin. *Nat. Biotechnol.* **2007**, *25*, 1290–1297. [CrossRef] [PubMed]
57. Schanzer, J.M.; Wartha, K.; Croasdale, R.; Moser, S.; Künkele, K.P.; Ries, C.; Scheuer, W.; Duerr, H.; Pompiati, S.; Pollman, J.; et al. A novel glycoengineered bispecific antibody format for targeted inhibition of epidermal growth factor receptor (EGFR) and insulin-like growth factor receptor type I (IGF-1R) demonstrating unique molecular properties. *J. Biol. Chem.* **2014**, *289*, 18693–18706. [CrossRef] [PubMed]
58. Godar, M.; Deswarte, K.; Vergote, K.; Saunders, M.; de Haard, H.; Hammad, H.; Blanchetot, C.; Lambrecht, B.N. A bispecific antibody strategy to target multiple type 2 cytokines in asthma. *J. Allergy Clin. Immunol.* **2018**, *142*, 1185–1193.e1184. [CrossRef]
59. Lyman, M.; Lieuw, V.; Richardson, R.; Timmer, A.; Stewart, C.; Granger, S.; Woods, R.; Silacci, M.; Grabulovski, D.; Newman, R. A bispecific antibody that targets IL-6 receptor and IL-17A for the potential therapy of patients with autoimmune and inflammatory diseases. *J. Biol. Chem.* **2018**, *293*, 9326–9334. [CrossRef]
60. Dovedi, S.J.; Elder, M.J.; Yang, C.; Sitnikova, S.I.; Irving, L.; Hansen, A.; Hair, J.; Jones, D.C.; Hasani, S.; Wang, B.; et al. Design and efficacy of a monovalent bispecific PD-1/CTLA-4 antibody that enhances CTLA-4 blockade on PD-1+ activated T cells. *Cancer Discov.* **2021**. [CrossRef]
61. Kitazawa, T.; Igawa, T.; Sampei, Z.; Muto, A.; Kojima, T.; Soeda, T.; Yoshihashi, K.; Okuyama-Nishida, Y.; Saito, H.; Tsunoda, H.; et al. A bispecific antibody to factors IXa and X restores factor VIII hemostatic activity in a hemophilia A model. *Nat. Med.* **2012**, *18*, 1570–1574. [CrossRef]
62. Kitazawa, T.; Esaki, K.; Tachibana, T.; Ishii, S.; Soeda, T.; Muto, A.; Kawabe, Y.; Igawa, T.; Tsunoda, H.; Nogami, K.; et al. Factor VIIIa-mimetic cofactor activity of a bispecific antibody to factors IX/IXa and X/Xa, emicizumab, depends on its ability to bridge the antigens. *Thromb. Haemost.* **2017**, *117*, 1348–1357. [CrossRef] [PubMed]
63. Yu, Y.J.; Atwal, J.K.; Zhang, Y.; Tong, R.K.; Wildsmith, K.R.; Tan, C.; Bien-Ly, N.; Hersom, M.; Maloney, J.A.; Meilandt, W.J.; et al. Therapeutic bispecific antibodies cross the blood-brain barrier in nonhuman primates. *Sci. Transl. Med.* **2014**, *6*, 261ra154. [CrossRef] [PubMed]
64. Yu, Y.J.; Zhang, Y.; Kenrick, M.; Hoyte, K.; Luk, W.; Lu, Y.; Atwal, J.; Elliott, J.M.; Prabhu, S.; Watts, R.J.; et al. Boosting brain uptake of a therapeutic antibody by reducing its affinity for a transcytosis target. *Sci. Transl. Med.* **2011**, *3*, 84ra44. [CrossRef]
65. Niewoehner, J.; Bohrmann, B.; Collin, L.; Urich, E.; Sade, H.; Maier, P.; Rueger, P.; Stracke, J.O.; Lau, W.; Tissot, A.C.; et al. Increased brain penetration and potency of a therapeutic antibody using a monovalent molecular shuttle. *Neuron* **2014**, *81*, 49–60. [CrossRef] [PubMed]
66. Ziegler, M.; Wang, X.; Lim, B.; Leitner, E.; Klingberg, F.; Ching, V.; Yao, Y.; Huang, D.; Gao, X.-M.; Kiriazis, H.; et al. Platelet-targeted delivery of peripheral blood mononuclear cells to the ischemic heart restores cardiac function after ischemia-reperfusion injury. *Theranostics* **2017**, *7*, 3192–3206. [CrossRef] [PubMed]
67. De Goeij, B.E.; Vink, T.; Ten Napel, H.; Breij, E.C.; Satijn, D.; Wubbolts, R.; Miao, D.; Parren, P.W. Efficient payload delivery by a bispecific antibody-drug conjugate targeting HER2 and CD63. *Mol. Cancer Ther.* **2016**, *15*, 2688–2697. [CrossRef]
68. Wec, A.Z.; Nyakatura, E.K.; Herbert, A.S.; Howell, K.A.; Holtsberg, F.W.; Bakken, R.R.; Mittler, E.; Christin, J.R.; Shulenin, S.; Jangra, R.K.; et al. A "Trojan horse" bispecific-antibody strategy for broad protection against ebolaviruses. *Science* **2016**, *354*, 350–354. [CrossRef]
69. Lee, H.Y.; Schaefer, G.; Lesaca, I.; Lee, C.V.; Wong, P.Y.; Jiang, G. "Two-in-One" approach for bioassay selection for dual specificity antibodies. *J. Immunol. Methods* **2017**, *448*, 74–79. [CrossRef] [PubMed]
70. Rajendran, S.; Li, Y.; Ngoh, E.; Wong, H.Y.; Cheng, M.S.; Wang, C.-I.; Schwarz, H. Development of a bispecific antibody targeting CD30 and CD137 on Hodgkin and Reed-Sternberg cells. *Front. Oncol.* **2019**, *9*. [CrossRef]
71. Karlsson, R.; Fridh, V.; Frostell, Å. Surrogate potency assays: Comparison of binding profiles complements dose response curves for unambiguous assessment of relative potencies. *J. Pharm. Anal.* **2018**, *8*, 138–146. [CrossRef]
72. Ritter, N.; Russell, R.; Schofield, T.; Graham, L.; Dillon, P.; Maggio, F.; Bhattacharyya, L.; Schmalzing, D.; Zhou, W.-M.; Miller, K.; et al. Bridging analytical methods for release and stability testing: Technical, quality and regulatory considerations. *BioProcess Int.* **2016**, *14*, 12–23.
73. Brünker, P.; Wartha, K.; Friess, T.; Grau-Richards, S.; Waldhauer, I.; Koller, C.F.; Weiser, B.; Majety, M.; Runza, V.; Niu, H.; et al. RG7386, a novel tetravalent FAP-DR5 antibody, effectively triggers FAP-dependent, avidity-driven DR5 hyperclustering and tumor cell apoptosis. *Mol. Cancer Ther.* **2016**, *15*, 946–957. [CrossRef]

74. Dong, J.; Sereno, A.; Snyder, W.B.; Miller, B.R.; Tamraz, S.; Doern, A.; Favis, M.; Wu, X.; Tran, H.; Langley, E.; et al. Stable IgG-like bispecific antibodies directed toward the type I insulin-like growth factor receptor demonstrate enhanced ligand blockade and anti-tumor activity. *J. Biol. Chem.* **2011**, *286*, 4703–4717. [CrossRef] [PubMed]
75. Macor, P.; Secco, E.; Mezzaroba, N.; Zorzet, S.; Durigutto, P.; Gaiotto, T.; De Maso, L.; Biffi, S.; Garrovo, C.; Capolla, S.; et al. Bispecific antibodies targeting tumor-associated antigens and neutralizing complement regulators increase the efficacy of antibody-based immunotherapy in mice. *Leukemia* **2015**, *29*, 406–414. [CrossRef] [PubMed]
76. Choi, H.-J.; Kim, Y.-J.; Lee, S.; Kim, Y.-S. A heterodimeric Fc-based bispecific antibody simultaneously targeting VEGFR-2 and Met exhibits potent antitumor activity. *Mol. Cancer Ther.* **2013**, *12*, 2748–2759. [CrossRef]
77. FDA. Bispecific Antibody Development Programs: Guidance for Industry: Draft Guidance. Available online: https://r.search.yahoo.com/_ylt=AwrJ7Jz7h1NgnVQA4ltXNyoA;_ylu=Y29sbwNiZjEEcG9zAzEEdnRpZANDMTc1NF8xBHNlYwNzcg--/RV=2/RE=1616115836/RO=10/RU=https%3a%2f%2fwww.fda.gov%2fmedia%2f123313%2fdownload/RK=2/RS=I6KRkNsu63Y7IxvL96a96IT0LUs- (accessed on 15 March 2021).
78. Trivedi, A.; Stienen, S.; Zhu, M.; Li, H.; Yuraszeck, T.; Gibbs, J.; Heath, T.; Loberg, R.; Kasichayanula, S. Clinical pharmacology and translational aspects of bispecific antibodies. *Clin. Transl. Sci.* **2017**, *10*, 147–162. [CrossRef]
79. Jain, T.; Sun, T.; Durand, S.; Hall, A.; Houston, N.R.; Nett, J.H.; Sharkey, B.; Bobrowicz, B.; Caffry, I.; Yu, Y.; et al. Biophysical properties of the clinical-stage antibody landscape. *Proc. Natl. Acad. Sci. USA* **2017**, *114*, 944–949. [CrossRef]
80. Davda, J.; Declerck, P.; Hu-Lieskovan, S.; Hickling, T.P.; Jacobs, I.A.; Chou, J.; Salek-Ardakani, S.; Kraynov, E. Immunogenicity of immunomodulatory, antibody-based, oncology therapeutics. *J. Immunother. Cancer* **2019**, *7*, 105. [CrossRef]
81. FDA. Immunogenicity Testing of Therapeutic Protein Products—Developing and Validating Assays for Anti-Drug Antibody Detection: Guidance for Industry. Available online: https://r.search.yahoo.com/_ylt=A0geK.L9iVNgLn8A6y5XNyoA;_ylu=Y29sbwNiZjEEcG9zAzEEdnRpZANDMTc1NF8xBHNlYwNzcg--/RV=2/RE=1616116349/RO=10/RU=https%3a%2f%2fwww.fda.gov%2fmedia%2f119788%2fdownload/RK=2/RS=bmD0ZLN67iFU.k2iXNU7prdoxY8- (accessed on 15 March 2021).
82. Steiner, G.; Marban-Doran, C.; Langer, J.; Pimenova, T.; Duran-Pacheco, G.; Sauter, D.; Langenkamp, A.; Solier, C.; Singer, T.; Bray-French, K.; et al. Enabling Routine MHC-II-Associated Peptide Proteomics for Risk Assessment of Drug-Induced Immunogenicity. *J. Proteome Res.* **2020**, *19*, 3792–3806. [CrossRef]
83. Tourdot, S.; Hickling, T.P. Nonclinical immunogenicity risk assessment of therapeutic proteins. *Bioanalysis* **2019**, *11*. [CrossRef]
84. Stracke, J.; Emrich, T.; Rueger, P.; Schlothauer, T.; Kling, L.; Knaupp, A.; Hertenberger, H.; Wolfert, A.; Spick, C.; Lau, W.; et al. A novel approach to investigate the effect of methionine oxidation on pharmacokinetic properties of therapeutic antibodies. *mAbs* **2014**, *6*, 1229–1242. [CrossRef] [PubMed]
85. Schlothauer, T.; Rueger, P.; Stracke, J.O.; Hertenberger, H.; Fingas, F.; Kling, L.; Emrich, T.; Drabner, G.; Seeber, S.; Auer, J.; et al. Analytical FcRn affinity chromatography for functional characterization of monoclonal antibodies. *mAbs* **2013**, *5*, 576–586. [CrossRef] [PubMed]
86. Ljungars, A.; Schiött, T.; Mattson, U.; Steppa, J.; Hambe, B.; Semmrich, M.; Ohlin, M.; Tornberg, U.-C.; Mattsson, M. A bispecific IgG format containing four independent antigen binding sites. *Sci. Rep.* **2020**, *10*, 1546. [CrossRef] [PubMed]
87. Jackman, J.; Chen, Y.; Huang, A.; Moffat, B.; Scheer, J.M.; Leong, S.R.; Lee, W.P.; Zhang, J.; Sharma, N.; Lu, Y.; et al. Development of a two-part strategy to identify a therapeutic human bispecific antibody that inhibits IgE receptor signaling. *J. Biol. Chem.* **2010**, *285*, 20850–20859. [CrossRef] [PubMed]
88. Gassner, C.; Lipsmeier, F.; Metzger, P.; Beck, H.; Schnueriger, A.; Regula, J.T.; Moelleken, J. Development and validation of a novel SPR-based assay principle for bispecific molecules. *J. Pharm. Biomed. Anal.* **2015**, *102*, 144–149. [CrossRef] [PubMed]
89. Meschendoerfer, W.; Gassner, C.; Lipsmeier, F.; Regula, J.T.; Moelleken, J. SPR-based assays enable the full functional analysis of bispecific molecules. *J. Pharm. Biomed. Anal.* **2017**, *132*, 141–147. [CrossRef]
90. Kiesgen, S.; Messinger, J.C.; Chintala, N.K.; Tano, Z.; Adusumilli, P.S. Comparative analysis of assays to measure CAR T-cell-mediated cytotoxicity. *Nat. Protoc.* **2021**, *16*, 1331–1342. [CrossRef]
91. Broussas, M.; Broyer, L.; Goetsch, L. Evaluation of antibody-dependent cell cytotoxicity using lactate dehydrogenase (LDH) measurement. In *Glycosylation Engineering of Biopharmaceuticals: Methods and Protocols*; Beck, A., Ed.; Humana Press: Totowa, NJ, USA, 2013; pp. 305–317.
92. Du, K.; Li, Y.; Liu, J.; Chen, W.; Wei, Z.; Luo, Y.; Liu, H.; Qi, Y.; Wang, F.; Sui, J. A bispecific antibody targeting GPC3 and CD47 induced enhanced antitumor efficacy against dual antigen-expressing HCC. *Mol. Ther.* **2021**. [CrossRef]
93. Koopmans, I.; Hendriks, M.A.J.M.; van Ginkel, R.J.; Samplonius, D.F.; Bremer, E.; Helfrich, W. Bispecific antibody approach for improved melanoma-selective PD-L1 immune checkpoint blockade. *J. Investig. Dermatol.* **2019**, *139*, 2343–2351. [CrossRef]
94. Staflin, K.; Zuch de Zafra, C.L.; Schutt, L.K.; Clark, V.; Zhong, F.; Hristopoulos, M.; Clark, R.; Li, J.; Mathieu, M.; Chen, X.; et al. Target arm affinities determine preclinical efficacy and safety of anti-HER2/CD3 bispecific antibody. *JCI Insight* **2020**, *5*. [CrossRef]
95. Lee, H.Y.; Contreras, E.; Register, A.C.; Wu, Q.; Abadie, K.; Garcia, K.; Wong, P.Y.; Jiang, G. Development of a bioassay to detect T-cell-activating impurities for T-cell-dependent bispecific antibodies. *Sci. Rep.* **2019**, *9*, 3900. [CrossRef]
96. Lee, H.Y.; Register, A.; Shim, J.; Contreras, E.; Wu, Q.; Jiang, G. Characterization of a single reporter-gene potency assay for T-cell-dependent bispecific molecules. *mAbs* **2019**, *11*, 1245–1253. [CrossRef] [PubMed]

97. Watanabe, M.; Wallace, P.K.; Keler, T.; Deo, Y.M.; Akewanlop, C.; Hayes, D.F. Antibody dependent cellular phagocytosis (ADCP) and antibody dependent cellular cytotoxicity (ADCC) of breast cancer cells mediated by bispecific antibody, MDX-210. *Breast Cancer Res. Treat.* **1999**, *53*, 199–207. [CrossRef] [PubMed]
98. Syedbasha, M.; Linnik, J.; Santer, D.; O'Shea, D.; Barakat, K.; Joyce, M.; Khanna, N.; Tyrrell, D.L.; Houghton, M.; Egli, A. An ELISA based binding and competition method to rapidly determine ligand-receptor interactions. *J. Vis. Exp.* **2016**, e53575. [CrossRef] [PubMed]
99. Sakamoto, S.; Putalun, W.; Vimolmangkang, S.; Phoolcharoen, W.; Shoyama, Y.; Tanaka, H.; Morimoto, S. Enzyme-linked immunosorbent assay for the quantitative/qualitative analysis of plant secondary metabolites. *J. Nat. Med.* **2018**, *72*, 32–42. [CrossRef] [PubMed]
100. Heinrich, L.; Tissot, N.; Hartmann, D.J.; Cohen, R. Comparison of the results obtained by ELISA and surface plasmon resonance for the determination of antibody affinity. *J. Immunol. Methods* **2010**, *352*, 13–22. [CrossRef] [PubMed]
101. Karlsson, R. Applications of surface plasmon resonance for detection of bispecific antibody activity. *Biopharm. Int.* **2015**, *28*, 38–44.
102. Hadzhieva, M.; Pashov, A.D.; Kaveri, S.; Lacroix-Desmazes, S.; Mouquet, H.; Dimitrov, J.D. Impact of antigen density on the binding mechanism of IgG antibodies. *Sci. Rep.* **2017**, *7*, 3767. [CrossRef]
103. Nguyen, H.H.; Park, J.; Kang, S.; Kim, M. Surface plasmon resonance: A versatile technique for biosensor applications. *Sensors* **2015**, *15*, 10481–10510. [CrossRef] [PubMed]
104. Helmerhorst, E.; Chandler, D.; Nussio, M.; Mamotte, C. Real-time and label-free bio-sensing of molecular interactions by surface plasmon resonance: A laboratory medicine perspective. *Clin. Biochem. Rev. Aust. Assoc. Clin. Biochem.* **2012**, *33*, 161–173.
105. Staffler, R.; Pasternack, R.; Hils, M.; Kaiser, W.; Möller, F.M. Nucleotide binding kinetics and conformational change analysis of tissue transglutaminase with switchSENSE. *Anal. Biochem.* **2020**, *605*, 113719. [CrossRef] [PubMed]
106. Knezevic, J.; Langer, A.; Hampel, P.A.; Kaiser, W.; Strasser, R.; Rant, U. Quantitation of Affinity, Avidity, and Binding Kinetics of Protein Analytes with a Dynamically Switchable Biosurface. *J. Am. Chem. Soc.* **2012**, *134*, 15225–15228. [CrossRef]
107. Agez, M.; Mandon, E.D.; Iwema, T.; Gianotti, R.; Limani, F.; Herter, S.; Mossner, E.; Kusznir, E.A.; Huber, S.; Lauer, M.; et al. Biochemical and biophysical characterization of purified native CD20 alone and in complex with rituximab and obinutuzumab. *Sci. Rep.* **2019**, *9*, 13675. [CrossRef] [PubMed]
108. Bjorkelund, H.; Gedda, L.; Barta, P.; Malmqvist, M.; Andersson, K. Gefitinib Induces Epidermal Growth Factor Receptor Dimers Which Alters the Interaction Characteristics with I-125-EGF. *PLoS ONE* **2011**, *6*, e24739. [CrossRef] [PubMed]
109. Peess, C.; von Proff, L.; Goller, S.; Andersson, K.; Gerg, M.; Malmqvist, M.; Bossenmaier, B.; Schraml, M. Deciphering the Stepwise Binding Mode of HRG1 beta to HER3 by Surface Plasmon Resonance and Interaction Map. *PLoS ONE* **2015**, *10*, e0116870. [CrossRef] [PubMed]
110. Lo, M.; Kim, H.S.; Tong, R.K.; Bainbridge, T.W.; Vernes, J.-M.; Zhang, Y.; Lin, Y.L.; Chung, S.; Dennis, M.S.; Zuchero, Y.J.Y.; et al. Effector-attenuating substitutions that maintain antibody stability and reduce toxicity in mice. *J. Biol. Chem.* **2017**, *292*, 3900–3908. [CrossRef] [PubMed]
111. Couch, J.A.; Yu, Y.J.; Zhang, Y.; Tarrant, J.M.; Fuji, R.N.; Meilandt, W.J.; Solanoy, H.; Tong, R.K.; Hoyte, K.; Luk, W.; et al. Addressing safety liabilities of TfR bispecific antibodies that cross the blood-brain barrier. *Sci. Transl. Med.* **2013**, *5*, 183ra157. [CrossRef]
112. Zhang, H.M.; Li, C.; Lei, M.; Lundin, V.; Lee, H.Y.; Ninonuevo, M.; Lin, K.; Han, G.; Sandoval, W.; Lei, D.; et al. Structural and Functional Characterization of a Hole-Hole Homodimer Variant in a "Knob-Into-Hole" Bispecific Antibody. *Anal. Chem.* **2017**, *89*, 13494–13501. [CrossRef]

International Journal of
Molecular Sciences

MDPI

Review

Antibody Libraries as Tools to Discover Functional Antibodies and Receptor Pleiotropism

Chih-Wei Lin and Richard A. Lerner *

Department of Chemistry, The Scripps Research Institute, La Jolla, CA 92037, USA; cwlin@scripps.edu
* Correspondence: rlerner@scripps.edu

Abstract: Most antibodies currently in use have been selected based on their binding affinity. However, nowadays, antibodies that can not only bind but can also alter the function of cell surface signaling components are increasingly sought after as therapeutic drugs. Therefore, the identification of such functional antibodies from a large antibody library is the subject of intensive research. New methods applied to combinatorial antibody libraries now allow the isolation of functional antibodies in the cellular environment. These selected agonist antibodies have provided new insights into important issues of signal transduction. Notably, when certain antibodies bind to a given receptor, the cell fate induced by them may be the same or different from that induced by natural agonists. In addition, combined with phenotypic screening, this platform allows us to discover unexpected experimental results and explore various phenomena in cell biology, such as those associated with stem cells and cancer cells.

Keywords: combinatorial antibody library; agonist antibody; cell fate; phage display

Citation: Lin, C.-W.; Lerner, R.A. Antibody Libraries as Tools to Discover Functional Antibodies and Receptor Pleiotropism. *Int. J. Mol. Sci.* **2021**, 22, 4123. https://doi.org/10.3390/ijms22084123

Academic Editor: Yong-Seok Heo

Received: 18 March 2021
Accepted: 13 April 2021
Published: 16 April 2021

1. Introduction

Antibodies, also known as immunoglobulins (Ig), are mainly produced by B cells, and can specifically target antigens. After Köhler and Milstein developed hybridoma technology in 1975, the speed of antibody development in both basic and clinical research accelerated markedly [1]. Since the first antibody (muromonab CD3, Orthoclone OKT3) was approved by the Food and Drug Administration (FDA) in 1986, antibodies have become an important category of biopharmaceutical products. To date, more than 80 antibodies have been approved for clinical use in the treatment of various human diseases, including many cancers, autoimmune, metabolic, and infectious diseases [2,3].

Currently, most therapeutic antibodies have been discovered, selected, and developed from animal immunization, B cell cloning, or the use of combinatorial antibody libraries. One of the reasons for the success of combinatorial antibody libraries is that they utilize the characteristics of the natural immune system. Every individual, even before antigen stimulation, carries the genetic information for and the capacity to produce more than 10^7 different antibodies. Moreover, despite an initial low affinity, the antigen binding sites of many of these antibodies can cross-react with a variety of related, but different antigens. The subsequent affinity maturation resulting from repeated stimulation in the continued presence of an antigen leads to higher affinity antibodies capable of binding to the "new" antigen. Thus, an initial naïve repertoire can be expanded many-fold.

Antibody phage display is one aspect of combinatorial antibody library technology, and is the in vitro selection technique most commonly used to select antibodies with high affinity for specific antigens. In 1985, George P. Smith described phage display technology, showing that filamentous bacteriophages can display peptides of interest on their surface after peptide-encoding DNA fragments had been inserted into the bacteriophage coat protein genes. Subsequently, many laboratories developed methods for generating antigen-specific antibodies by creating combinatorial antibody libraries in filamentous phages [4–10]. In general, combinatorial antibody libraries are constructed from mRNA or

RNA extracted from B cells of immunized or naïve donors. Because the variable regions of the heavy chain (VH) and the light chain (VL) representing the immunoglobulin gene-encoding repertoire are known, we can use polymerase chain reaction (PCR), and then specific primers to amplify different VH and VL gene families. These variable regions of antibody repertoires are then ligated to the phage display vector (phagemid), with the net result that the antibody is expressed on the surface of the phage and the gene encoding of the antibody is in the phage genome. The antibody-encoding gene is inserted into a phage coat protein gene causing the antibody fragment to be displayed on the outside of the phage, which results in a connection between genotype and phenotype. Once produced, the antibody library in the phage can be bound to an immobilized antigen. This allows us to use multiple binding and elution cycles for selection of antibodies with high affinity and specificity. Phage binders are screened by ELISA, then DNA sequences are analyzed and cloned into appropriate expression vectors to produce antibodies, or various antibody formats, for functional analysis (Figure 1). The antibody format in the phage display library can be a single-chain variable fragment (scFv) or Fab fragments. Due to the small size and high solubility of phage particles (10^{13} particles/mL), a library size of up to 10^{11} independent clones can be effectively generated, and an extensive antibody diversity can be displayed in a single library. One advantage of combinatorial antibody library technology is the diversity of binders. Another advantage is the ability to directly generate human antibodies in vitro. Since many important therapeutic antibodies are antibodies to self-antigens, which is forbidden by tolerance, in vitro generation allows the by-passing of tolerance and the generation of antibodies to self-antigens such as cell surface proteins, or self-products such as Tumor necrosis factor alpha (TNF-α).

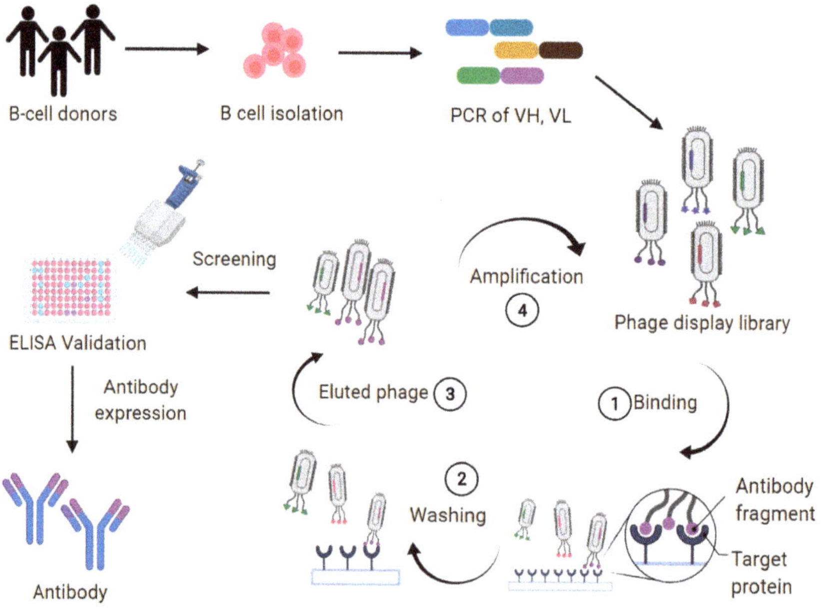

Figure 1. The illustration of phage combinatorial antibody libraries. Lymphocyte cells are collected from humans, e.g., naïve, cancer patients, disease survivors carrying antibodies with unique characteristics, or immunized animals. The RNA of B cells is prepared and transcribed into single-stranded cDNA that is used as the source for PCR amplification of the heavy chain (VH) and the light chain (VL) genes. Variable genes are cloned into phagemid vectors as antibody fragments, then produced to phage combinatorial antibody libraries in *E. coli* bacteria. The target protein is immobilized on immunotubes for selection. Specific binding phages displaying antibodies are enriched over several selection rounds by 1. binding, 2. washing, 3. elution, and 4. phage amplification. After 3–5 rounds of biopanning, the specific phage binders are screened by ELISA, then DNA sequences are analyzed and cloned into appropriate expression vectors to produce antibodies, or various antibody formats for functional analysis.

Currently there are 11 approved antibodies (Table 1) derived from these combinatorial antibody library technologies [11–24]. The majority of these antibodies are originally generated by few companies, Cambridge Antibody Technology (CAT), Dyax and MorphoSys's human combinatorial antibody libraries (HuCAL). The most dominant antibody format of the approved or under clinical investigations phage-derived antibodies is Immunoglobulin G (IgG). The therapeutic antibodies from phage libraries can be successfully screened and isolated to treat cancer and non-cancer medical conditions such as inflammatory, infectious, or immune diseases [25]. Nowadays, combinatorial antibody libraries can be very large, often containing more than 10^{11} members. The sheer number and diversity of antibodies in such libraries increases the likelihood that searches to select binders specific for any one of a wide range of antigens will be successful. In brief, the process usually involves multiple rounds of affinity selection against the desired target, followed by antibody purification, binding analysis, and functional testing. Many antibodies derived from combinatorial libraries that simply bind antigens have been shown to be extremely important. For example, Adalimumab (an antibody that binds to tumor necrosis factor) is the world's best-selling drug [26].

Table 1. FDA-approved antibody-based drugs from combinational antibody library.

Antibody	Brand Name	Target	Indications	Approved	Company	Ref.
Adalimumab	Humira	TNFα	Rheumatoid arthritis	2002	AbbVie	[11]
Belimumab	Benlysta	BLyS	Systemic lupus erythematosus	2011	GlaxoSmithKline/Human Genome Sciences	[12]
Raxibacumab	Abthrax	B. anthrasis PA	Anthrax infection	2012	GlaxoSmithKline/Human Genome Sciences	[13]
Ramucirumab	Cyramza	VEGFR2	Gastric cancer	2014	Eli Lilly/ImClone Systems	[14]
Necitumumab	Portrazza	EGFR	Non-small cell lung cancer	2015	Eli Lilly/ImClone Systems Inc.	[15,16]
Atezolizumab	Tecentriq	PD-L1	Metastatic lung cancer	2016	Genentech	[17,18]
Avelumab	Bavencio	PD-L1	Merkel cell carcinoma	2017	Merck Serono International S.A./Pfizer	[19]
Guselkumab	Tremfya	IL-23	Plaque psoriasis	2017	MorphoSys/Janssen Biotech Inc.	[20]
Lanadelumab	Takhzyro	PKaI	Hereditary angioedema attacks	2018	Dyax Corp/Shire	[21]
Emapalumab	Gamifant	IFNγ	Primary hemophagocytic lymphohistiocytosis	2018	NovImmmune	[22]
Moxetumomab pasudodox	Lumoxiti	CD22	Hairy cell leukemia	2018	MedImmune/AstraZeneca	[23,24]

Abbreviation: TNF-α, tumor necrosis factor-alpha; BLyS, B-lymphocyte stimulator; B. anthrasis PA, protective antigen of Bacillus anthracis; VEGFR2, vascular endothelial growth factor receptor 2; EGFR, epidermal growth factor receptor; PD-L1, programmed death-ligand 1; IL-23, interleukin-23; pKaI, plasma kallikrein; IFN-γ, interferon gamma.

Most antibody libraries are now made in the form of human single-chain variable fragments (scFv) or Fab for the isolation of therapeutic antibodies. Some of the antibody formats, i.e., the single domain antibody fragments (also referred to VHH, sdAb, Nanobodies), have also developed [27–33]. These formats can also be used to find functional antibodies in cell fate, cellular pathways, viral pathways, or G protein-coupled receptor (GPCR) structure. In addition, in respect of the intracellular expression of antibodies in cells, for example, Visintin et al. used the two-hybrid [28] and Cattaneo et al. [34] used intrabody in vivo systems to provide an understanding of individual antigen–antibody fragments that function in cells. The phenotypic screening of nanobody libraries was also used for isolated antiviral VHH that protect human A549 cells from lethal infection with influenza

A virus (IAV) or vesicular stomatitis virus (VSV). This study helps us to understand the viral life pathways [35]. These studies have shown that antibody fragments can efficiently interact with their antigens in vivo. Thanks to the development of new technology, today's researchers can use these 10^{11} binding antibodies in extracellular, intracellular, or cell membrane systems. Antibodies can be secreted, expressed in the cytoplasm, anchored on the plasma membrane, or implanted in the endoplasmic reticulum [36–38]. Using such delivery technology, we can expand the applicability of combinatorial antibody libraries. Like the phage display system, we continue to emphasize the link between genotype and phenotype. However, this time the link is in an animal cell. When the combinatorial antibody library is used to infect eukaryotic cells, the integrated antibody genotype and cell phenotype are permanently connected, and each cell becomes its own selection system. Therefore, we can manipulate antibody libraries to study fundamental biological processes in the cell environment.

Over the years, most antibodies have been screened for molecular targets. Cell-based phenotypic analysis is another new method that can be used to explore biological relevance. This review will highlight recent discoveries using human scFv combinatorial antibody libraries in target-based screening for agonist antibodies, as well as exploring how phenotypic screening can be used to discover functional antibodies that perturb targets involved in cell fate.

2. Using Antibody Libraries to Discover Functional Antibodies and Receptor Pleiotropism

2.1. Target-Based Screening for Agonist Antibodies

In general, most agonist antibodies are obtained by a target-based approach, i.e., by focusing on a specific cellular signal by targeting its receptor. An antibody is then selected that mimics the natural ligand or modulates the effect of the targeted receptor. Previously the initial step in antibody screening was solely based on binding, e.g., hybridomas. The subsequent production, isolation, and identification of clones to obtain functional antibodies was a very laborious and time-consuming process. Now, experimenters are able to directly select antibodies on the basis of their function or mechanism of action, e.g., antibodies with enzyme-like catalytic activity [39] or antibodies with agonist activities capable of binding to desired targets and activating downstream signaling [40,41]. Agonist antibodies directed against cell surface targets have become one of the most effective ways to mimic natural ligands or enhance immune responses, because they can also lead to antibody receptor-mediated downstream signaling in cells. For this purpose, a combinatorial antibody library can be used to screen autoantigens. We can transfer antibody genes to a lentivirus system, with all antibody genes constructed with a membrane anchor sequence, and then use them to infect target animal cells. The integrated antibody genotype and cell phenotype will be permanently connected, and each cell will be available for further selection via fluorescence-activated cell sorting (FACS). If we use known targets, pre-selecting antibodies can improve antibody production efficiency. In 2012, Zhang et al. described a method to screen for erythropoietin (EPO) receptor (EPOR) antibodies from a library of combinatorial antibodies that bind to the EPO receptor with similar activity to the natural ligand, EPO [27]. Based on this concept, many function-based antibodies with high potency and full agonist activity have been developed recently [42–46], and their use in the clinical setting has a number of advantages over present practice. For example, there are several challenges that accompany long-term clinical use of growth factors or cytokines. These include short serum half-life, low bioavailability, dose-limiting toxicity and immunogenicity. An example of an agonist antibody overcoming these issues is the selection of an antibody targeting the leptin receptor, which was shown to be of high potency with full agonist activity and a function similar to leptin (Figure 2a). In this work the leptin antibody was first selectively enriched by phage display and later screened and isolated using leptin receptor reporter cells. This antibody showed identical biochemical properties and cellular profiles as leptin, and rescued leptin-deficiency in ob/ob mice [45].

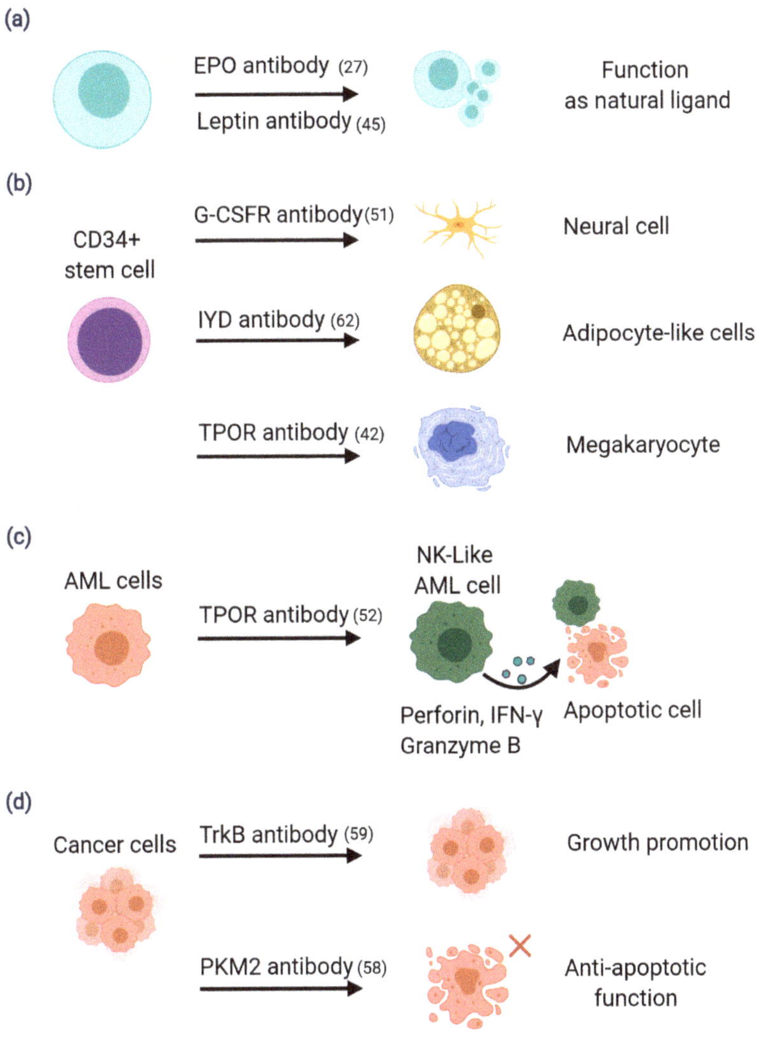

Figure 2. Some examples of antibody libraries as a tool to discover functional antibodies and receptor pleiotropism. Functional antibodies can isolate from target-based or phenotypic-based screening from a combinatorial antibody library. Agonist antibodies that are generated against signaling receptors often induce the same cellular response as the natural agonist ligand for the receptor, or the agonist antibody induces a different cell fate than the natural ligand, even though they both bind to the same receptor. (**a**) The erythropoietin (EPO) agonist or the leptin agonist antibody have the same biological activity as a natural ligand. (**b**) Exposure of CD34+ bone marrow stem cells with different functional agonist antibodies, e.g., Granulocyte Colony Stimulating Factor Receptor (G-CSFR) specific agonist antibody, iodotyrosine deiodinase (IYD) antibody, and thrombopoietin receptor (TPOR) antibody can differentiate into nerve cells, adipocyte-like cells, and megakaryocytes, respectively. (**c**) Exposure of acute myeloid leukemia (AML) cells to TPOR antibody promotes their differentiation into natural killer (NK)-like AML cells that can induce apoptosis in non-differentiated AML cells. (**d**) Exposure of cancer cells to TrkB antibody or PKM2 antibody that promote tumor growth or anti-apoptotic function. Abbreviations: erythropoietin (EPO), Granulocyte Colony Stimulating Factor Receptor (G-CSFR) thrombopoietin receptor (TPOR), acute myeloid leukemia (AML), natural killer (NK), interferon-γ (IFN-γ), iodotyrosine deiodinase (IYD), tropomyosin receptor kinase B (TrkB), pyruvate kinase M2 (PKM2).

Recently, antibodies targeting inhibitory immune checkpoints have been shown to be very effective in cancer immunotherapy. Furthermore, evidence suggests that antibodies targeting stimulatory checkpoints, e.g., OX40, 4-1BB, CD27, and ICOS, may be equally successful in cancer therapy [40]. Many agonist antibodies have been derived from hybridomas, however, they have also been selected from antibody libraries. In one example, the researchers first used a phage library and activated human lymphocytes to generate a large collection of antibodies against 10 immune checkpoints, LAG-3, PD-L1, PD-1, TIM3, BTLA, TIGIT, OX40, 4-1BB, CD27, and ICOS. Through next-generation sequencing and bioinformatics analysis, they identified individual scFvs in each collection and then selected the most enriched antibodies. The antibodies were then further confirmed by assays for lymphocyte proliferation and T-cell function [47].

2.2. Phenotypic Screening for Isolation of Functional Antibodies That Regulate Cell Fate

A large proportion of drugs in clinical use have been developed by first identifying molecules that have the desired effect on the function of a cell, and then subsequently identifying their targets [48]. However, when the goal is to develop antibodies capable of regulating cell phenotype other methods have been used. In these methods the stem cell is the starting point. Stem cells are highly specialized cells with unlimited replication and self-renewal potential. These cells are pluripotent, but may be limited or unlimited (embryonic stem cells, ESC) in terms of their ability to differentiate into a range of somatic cell lineages. Therapies capable of controlling differentiation have long been a goal in the pharmaceutical industry. They would have broad applicability in the fields of tissue regeneration and the treatment of chronic degenerative diseases [49,50], and would be a major advance in the clinical setting. In one study researchers screened an antibody library to find functional antibodies capable of activating specific receptors on bone marrow stem cells. They successfully selected agonist antibodies recognizing the granulocyte colony stimulating receptor (G-CSFR) by anchoring the expressed antibodies to the membrane of a G-CSFR-transfected BaF3 cell line. Importantly, subsequent experiments showed that one of the isolated anti-G-CSFR antibodies was able to induce CD34+ hematopoietic stem cells to differentiate into nerve cells (Figure 2b) [51]. In other experiments, an agonist antibody that functions like a natural ligand specific for the thrombopoietin receptor (TPOR) stimulated bone marrow stem cells to differentiate into megakaryocytes [42]. Interestingly, exposure of acute myeloid leukemia (AML) cells to this same TPOR agonist antibody promoted their differentiation into natural killer (NK)-like AML cells that synthesized large amounts of perforin, granzyme B and interferon-γ, and thereby induced apoptosis in undifferentiated AML (Figure 2c) [52]. This antibody was shown to induce signal transducer and activator of transcription 3 (STAT-3), protein kinase B (AKT), and extracellular signal-regulated kinase (ERK) phosphorylation in CD34+ hematopoietic stem cells. Similarly, in AML cells, the TPOR antibody induced the same signaling in STAT-3 and ERK phosphorylation, but not in AKT. These findings suggest that the ability to use receptor pleiotropism to change the differentiation state of stem cells may open a new route to treating disease [53]. Melidoni et al. reported the selection of antagonist antibodies capable of blocking fibroblast growth factor 4 (FGF4) and its receptor FGFR1β, which control embryonic stem cell differentiation [54]. In addition, antibodies have been shown to be capable of reprogramming differentiated cells into induced pluripotent stem cells (iPSCs), a process that is usually generated by transient expression of Oct4, Sox2, Klf4, and c-Myc in the nucleus. Using the autocrine antibody reprogramming system from an antibody library, multiple antibodies that replaced either Sox2 and c-Myc in combination, or Oct4 alone in generating iPSCs were isolated. Identifying the target of one Sox2 replacement antibody showed that it binds to Basp1, thereby de-repressing nuclear factors WT1, Esrrb, and Lin28a (Lin28) independently of Sox2. This study provides another example whereby an antibody library can be used as a tool for discovery of new biologics, as well as elucidating membrane-to-nucleus signaling pathways that regulate pluripotency and cell fate [55].

As mentioned above, functional antibodies such as agonists can mimic the actions of natural ligands, having the ability to stimulate proliferation and differentiation. However, occasionally these antibodies, in spite of binding the same target, appear to activate a signaling pathway different from the natural ligand, with the consequence that differentiation occurs along a different cell lineage. This indicates a receptor pleiotropism that is like a binary switch, which can regulate a variety of biological activities. Phenotypic screening offers additional opportunities to identify targets and select antibodies that regulate cell fate or affect tumor growth, and combining phenotypic screening with antibody libraries enhances the chance for success. For example, one of the most important phenotypes in biology is cell death. Using a combination of phenotypic screening and combinatorial antibody libraries, researchers were able to select antibodies that protected cell death associated with rhinovirus infection. The target antigen was later identified as the rhinovirus 3C protease [56]. Mammalian cells exposed to disturbances in the intracellular or extracellular microenvironment can activate one of many signal transduction cascades, ultimately leading to their death. Each of these regulated cell death modes is triggered and spread through a different molecular mechanism, all of which exhibit a considerable degree of complexity [57]. In the cancer setting, a current study reported that one anti-apoptotic intrabody was selected from an antibody combinatorial library, and shown to recognize pyruvate kinase M2 (PKM2). This finding helped to identify a new mechanism that allows cells to evade apoptosis [58] (Figure 2d). Two other important phenotypes in biology are cell proliferation and metastasis. In a recent study, two antibodies derived from a combinatorial library, both recognizing tropomyosin receptor kinase B (TrkB) and highly similar in sequence, were shown to have opposite functional activity, one being an agonist while the other was an antagonist. The agonist antibody was shown to increase breast cancer cell growth both in vitro and in vivo, whereas the antagonist antibody inhibited growth. Receptor binding by the agonist antibody triggered the same downstream signaling cascade as the natural ligand, brain-derived neurotrophic factor (BDNF) [59]. This unexpected finding in TrkB represents yet another example showing that the same receptor may have different functions. A platform for phenotypic discovery of antibodies and targets applied on chronic lymphocytic leukemia (CLL) has been reported [60]. The platform utilizes primary patient cells throughout the discovery process and includes methods for differential phage display cell panning, cell-based specificity screening, phenotypic in vitro screening, target deconvolution, and confirmatory in vivo screening. This approach provides another method of discovering potent targets for antibody-based cytotoxicity treatment of CLL, e.g., CD32, CD21, etc.

These antibodies also show promise for the treatment of degenerative diseases. Recent reports have shown that it is possible to select antibodies from a combinatorial library that can induce bone marrow stem cells to differentiate into microglia, which then traffic to the brain where they organize into typical networks. Interestingly, in an Alzheimer's disease mouse model, these induced microglia-like cells were found at sites of plaque formation and significantly reduced their plaque numbers [61].

As we mentioned above, these findings suggest that the use of phenotypic screening with combinatorial antibody libraries shows great promise in terms of allowing identification of receptor pleiotropism, as well as selection of antibodies capable of modulating the differentiation, growth, and function of cells [61–63]. The ultimate goal is to use this new capability to expand treatment options for both cancer patients and patients with degenerative diseases.

3. Antibody Libraries and Emerging Viral Infections

One important advantage of combinatorial antibody libraries is the almost limitless diversity of binding antibodies they contain, potentially greater than that seen in nature. Work focusing on the outbreak of the novel coronavirus disease in 2019 (COVID-19) has shown that this characteristic can be extremely valuable in the development of therapies for emerging viruses [37,64–66]. COVID-19 is the biggest global health threat in many generations. Recently it has been reported that a combinatorial human antibody library, constructed 20 years before the current COVID-19 pandemic, was used to select three highly potent antibodies that specifically bind the severe acute respiratory syndrome coronavirus 2 (SARS-CoV-2) spike protein, and neutralize authentic SARS-CoV-2 virus [67]. This suggests that immunological memory after infection with seasonal human coronaviruses may potentially contribute to cross-protection against SARS-CoV-2 [68,69]. Other researchers have successfully isolated neutralizing antibodies from a phage display library constructed using peripheral lymphocytes collected from patients in the acute phase of the disease. These neutralizing antibodies have been shown to recognize different epitopes on the viral spike receptor-binding domain (RBD). Some subset antibodies exert their inhibitory activity by eliminating the binding of RBD to the human angiotensin-converting enzyme 2 (ACE2) receptor. These papers indicated that antibodies from an antibody library represent a promising basis for an effective treatment design for SARS-CoV-2 infection [70,71]. Perhaps most importantly, the large number of antibodies from such libraries allows one to understand the chemistry of virus neutralization.

4. Summary

This main purpose of this review was to describe current findings and applications of functional antibodies, especially agonist antibodies, selected from combinatorial antibody libraries. The advent of combinatorial antibody library technology has provided scientists with unprecedented control over the output of the acquired immune system. Antibodies can now be generated in test tubes, thus avoiding tolerance. The size of these libraries, combined with a powerful selection system, allows for rapid generation of antibodies and isolation of rare antibodies. In addition to enhancing traditional uses of antibodies in both research and therapeutics, recent advances have identified functional agonist antibodies capable of activating cell signaling cascades, as well as inducing cell differentiation along multiple pathways, suggesting that in the future antibodies may be used as universal operons for cell function.

Author Contributions: C.-W.L. and R.A.L. wrote the manuscript. All authors have read and agreed to the published version of the manuscript.

Funding: This research was funded by The JPB Foundation, grant number 1097.

Institutional Review Board Statement: Not applicable.

Informed Consent Statement: Not applicable.

Data Availability Statement: The data presented in this study are available on request from the corresponding author.

Acknowledgments: We thank Fiona Larmour for manuscript corrections.

Conflicts of Interest: The authors declare no conflict of interest.

References

1. Köhler, G.; Milstein, C. Continuous cultures of fused cells secreting antibody of predefined specificity. *Nature* **1975**, *256*, 495–497. [CrossRef] [PubMed]
2. Kaplon, H.; Muralidharan, M.; Schneider, Z.; Reichert, J.M. Antibodies to watch in 2020. *mAbs* **2020**, *12*, 1703531. [CrossRef] [PubMed]
3. Lu, R.-M.; Hwang, Y.-C.; Liu, I.-J.; Lee, C.-C.; Tsai, H.-Z.; Li, H.-J.; Wu, H.-C. Development of therapeutic antibodies for the treatment of diseases. *J. Biomed. Sci.* **2020**, *27*, 1–30. [CrossRef] [PubMed]
4. Smith, G.P. Filamentous fusion phage: Novel expression vectors that display cloned antigens on the virion surface. *Science* **1985**, *228*, 1315–1317. [CrossRef]
5. Huse, W.; Sastry, L.; Iverson, S.; Kang, A.; Alting-Mees, M.; Burton, D.; Benkovic, S.; Lerner, R. Generation of a large combinatorial library of the immunoglobulin repertoire in phage lambda. *Science* **1989**, *246*, 1275–1281. [CrossRef]
6. McCafferty, J.; Griffiths, A.D.; Winter, G.; Chiswell, D.J. Phage antibodies: Filamentous phage displaying antibody variable domains. *Nature* **1990**, *348*, 552–554. [CrossRef]

7. Barbas, C.F., III; Kang, A.S.; Lerner, R.A.; Benkovic, S.J. Assembly of combinatorial antibody libraries on phage surfaces: The gene III site. *Proc. Natl. Acad. Sci. USA* **1991**, *88*, 7978–7982. [CrossRef]
8. Clackson, T.P.; Hoogenboom, H.R.; Griffiths, A.D.; Winter, G. Making antibody Fragm. using phage display libraries. *Nature* **1991**, *352*, 624–628. [CrossRef]
9. Breitling, F.; Dübel, S.; Seehaus, T.; Klewinghaus, I.; Little, M. A surface expression vector for antibody screening. *Gene* **1991**, *104*, 147–153. [CrossRef]
10. Kang, A.S.; Barbas, C.F.; Janda, K.D.; Benkovic, S.J.; Lerner, R.A. Linkage of recognition and replication functions by assembling combinatorial antibody Fab libraries along phage surfaces. *Proc. Natl. Acad. Sci. USA* **1991**, *88*, 4363–4366. [CrossRef]
11. Jespers, L.S.; Roberts, A.; Mahler, S.M.; Winter, G.; Hoogenboom, H.R. Guiding the Selection of Human Antibodies from Phage Display Repertoires to a Single Epitope of an Antigen. *Nat. Biotechnol.* **1994**, *12*, 899–903. [CrossRef] [PubMed]
12. Edwards, B.M.; Barash, S.C.; Main, S.H.; Choi, G.H.; Minter, R.; Ullrich, S.; Williams, E.; Du Fou, L.; Wilton, J.; Albert, V.R.; et al. The Remarkable Flexibility of the Human Antibody Repertoire; Isolation of Over One Thousand Different Antibodies to a Single Protein, BLyS. *J. Mol. Biol.* **2003**, *334*, 103–118. [CrossRef] [PubMed]
13. Mazumdar, S. Raxibacumab. *mAbs* **2009**, *1*, 531–538. [CrossRef]
14. Lu, D.; Jimenez, X.; Zhang, H.; Bohlen, P.; Witte, L.; Zhu, Z. Selection of high affinity human neutralizing antibodies to VEGFR2 from a large antibody phage display library for antiangiogenesis therapy. *Int. J. Cancer* **2001**, *97*, 393–399. [CrossRef]
15. De Haard, H.J.; van Neer, N.; Reurs, A.; Hufton, S.E.; Roovers, R.C.; Henderikx, P.; de Bruine, A.P.; Arends, J.W.; Hoogenboom, H.R. A large non-immunized human Fab fragment phage library that permits rapid isolation and kinetic analysis of high affinity antibodies. *J. Biol. Chem.* **1999**, *274*, 18218–18230. [CrossRef] [PubMed]
16. Li, S.; Kussie, P.; Ferguson, K.M. Structural Basis for EGF Receptor Inhibition by the Therapeutic Antibody IMC-11F8. *Structure* **2008**, *16*, 216–227. [CrossRef]
17. McDermott, D.F.; Sosman, J.A.; Sznol, M.; Massard, C.; Gordon, M.S.; Hamid, O.; Powderly, J.D.; Infante, J.R.; Fassò, M.; Wang, Y.V.; et al. Atezolizumab, an Anti–Programmed Death-Ligand 1 Antibody, in Metastatic Renal Cell Carcinoma: Long-Term Safety, Clinical Activity, and Immune Correlates from a Phase Ia Study. *J. Clin. Oncol.* **2016**, *34*, 833–842. [CrossRef] [PubMed]
18. Herbst, R.S.; Soria, J.-C.; Kowanetz, M.; Fine, G.D.; Hamid, O.; Gordon, M.S.; Sosman, J.A.; McDermott, D.F.; Powderly, J.D.; Gettinger, S.N.; et al. Predictive correlates of response to the anti-PD-L1 antibody MPDL3280A in cancer patients. *Nature* **2014**, *515*, 563–567. [CrossRef]
19. Boyerinas, B.; Jochems, C.; Fantini, M.C.; Heery, C.R.; Gulley, J.L.; Tsang, K.Y.; Schlom, J. Antibody-Dependent Cellular Cytotoxicity Activity of a Novel Anti–PD-L1 Antibody Avelumab (MSB0010718C) on Human Tumor Cells. *Cancer Immunol. Res.* **2015**, *3*, 1148–1157. [CrossRef]
20. Markham, A. Guselkumab: First Global Approval. *Drugs* **2017**, *77*, 1487–1492. [CrossRef]
21. Kenniston, J.A.; Faucette, R.R.; Martik, D.; Comeau, S.R.; Lindberg, A.P.; Kopacz, K.J.; Conley, G.P.; Chen, J.; Viswanathan, M.; Kastrapeli, N.; et al. Inhibition of Plasma Kallikrein by a Highly Specific Active Site Blocking Antibody. *J. Biol. Chem.* **2014**, *289*, 23596–23608. [CrossRef]
22. Al-Salama, Z.T. Emapalumab: First Global Approval. *Drugs* **2019**, *79*, 99–103. [CrossRef]
23. Salvatore, G.; Beers, R.; Margulies, I.; Kreitman, R.J.; Pastan, I. Improved cytotoxic activity toward cell lines and fresh leukemia cells of a mutant anti-CD22 immunotoxin obtained by antibody phage display. *Clin. Cancer Res.* **2002**, *8*, 995–1002. [PubMed]
24. Alderson, R.F.; Kreitman, R.J.; Chen, T.; Yeung, P.; Herbst, R.; Fox, J.A.; Pastan, I. CAT-8015: A Second-Generation Pseudomonas Exotoxin A–Based Immunotherapy Targeting CD22-Expressing Hematologic Malignancies. *Clin. Cancer Res.* **2009**, *15*, 832–839. [CrossRef] [PubMed]
25. AlFaleh, M.A.; Alsaab, H.O.; Mahmoud, A.B.; Alkayyal, A.A.; Jones, M.L.; Mahler, S.M.; Hashem, A.M. Phage Display Derived Monoclonal Antibodies: From Bench to Bedside. *Front. Immunol.* **2020**, *11*. [CrossRef] [PubMed]
26. Urquhart, L. Market watch: Top drugs and companies by sales in 2017. *Nat. Rev. Drug Discov.* **2018**, *17*, 232. [CrossRef]
27. Zhang, H.; Wilson, I.A.; Lerner, R.A. Selection of antibodies that regulate phenotype from intracellular combinatorial antibody libraries. *Proc. Natl. Acad. Sci. USA* **2012**, *109*, 15728–15733. [CrossRef]
28. Visintin, M.; Tse, E.; Axelson, H.; Rabbitts, T.H.; Cattaneo, A. Selection of antibodies for intracellular function using a two-hybrid in vivo system. *Proc. Natl. Acad. Sci. USA* **1999**, *96*, 11723–11728. [CrossRef]
29. Harmansa, S.; Alborelli, I.; Bieli, D.; Caussinus, E.; Affolter, M. A nanobody-based toolset to investigate the role of protein localization and dispersal in Drosophila. *eLife* **2017**, *6*, e22549. [CrossRef]
30. Moutel, S.; Bery, N.; Bernard, V.; Keller, L.; Lemesre, E.; de Marco, A.; Ligat, L.; Rain, J.C.; Favre, G.; Olichon, A.; et al. NaLi-H1: A universal synthetic library of humanized nanobodies providing highly functional antibodies and intrabodies. *eLife* **2016**, *5*, e16228. [CrossRef] [PubMed]
31. Scholler, P.; Nevoltris, D.; de Bundel, D.; Bossi, S.; Moreno-Delgado, D.; Rovira, X.; Møller, T.C.; El Moustaine, D.; Mathieu, M.; Blanc, E.; et al. Allosteric nanobodies uncover a role of hippocampal mGlu2 receptor homodimers in contextual fear con-solidation. *Nat. Commun.* **2017**, *8*, 1967. [CrossRef]
32. Manglik, A.; Kobilka, B.K.; Steyaert, J. Nanobodies to Study G Protein–Coupled Receptor Structure and Function. *Annu. Rev. Pharmacol. Toxicol.* **2017**, *57*, 19–37. [CrossRef] [PubMed]
33. Cheloha, R.W.; Fischer, F.A.; Woodham, A.W.; Daley, E.; Suminski, N.; Gardella, T.J.; Ploegh, H.L. Improved GPCR ligands from nanobody tethering. *Nat. Commun.* **2020**, *11*, 1–11. [CrossRef] [PubMed]

34. Cattaneo, A.; Biocca, S. The selection of intracellular antibodies. *Trends Biotechnol.* **1999**, *17*, 115–121. [CrossRef]
35. Schmidt, F.I.; Hanke, L.; Morin, B.; Brewer, R.; Brusic, V.; Whelan, S.P.; Ploegh, H.L. Phenotypic lentivirus screens to identify functional single domain antibodies. *Nat. Microbiol.* **2016**, *1*, 1–10. [CrossRef] [PubMed]
36. Marasco, A.W. Intrabodies: Turning the humoral immune system outside in for intracellular immunization. *Gene Ther.* **1997**, *4*, 11–15. [CrossRef] [PubMed]
37. Lerner, R.A. Combinatorial antibody libraries: New advances, new immunological insights. *Nat. Rev. Immunol.* **2016**, *16*, 498–508. [CrossRef]
38. Slastnikova, T.A.; Ulasov, A.V.; Rosenkranz, A.A.; Sobolev, A.S. Targeted Intracellular Delivery of Antibodies: The State of the Art. *Front. Pharmacol.* **2018**, *9*, 1208. [CrossRef]
39. Schultz, P.G.; Lerner, A.R. From molecular diversity to catalysis: Lessons from the immune system. *Science* **1995**, *269*, 1835–1842. [CrossRef]
40. Mayes, P.A.; Hance, K.W.; Hoos, A. The promise and challenges of immune agonist antibody development in cancer. *Nat. Rev. Drug Discov.* **2018**, *17*, 509–527. [CrossRef]
41. Liu, T.; Zhang, Y.; Liu, Y.; Wang, Y.; Jia, H.; Kang, M.; Luo, X.; Caballero, D.; González, J.; Sherwood, L.; et al. Functional human antibody CDR fusions as long-acting therapeutic endocrine agonists. *Proc. Natl. Acad. Sci. USA* **2015**, *112*, 1356–1361. [CrossRef] [PubMed]
42. Zhang, H.; Yea, K.; Xie, J.; Ruiz, D.; Wilson, I.A.; Lerner, R.A. Selecting Agonists from Single Cells Infected with Combinatorial Antibody Libraries. *Chem. Biol.* **2013**, *20*, 734–741. [CrossRef]
43. Zhang, H.; Xie, J.; Lerner, R.A. A proximity based general method for identification of ligand and receptor interactions in living cells. *Biochem. Biophys. Res. Commun.* **2014**, *454*, 251–255. [CrossRef] [PubMed]
44. Merkouris, S.; Barde, Y.-A.; Binley, K.E.; Allen, N.D.; Stepanov, A.V.; Wu, N.C.; Grande, G.; Lin, C.-W.; Li, M.; Nan, X.; et al. Fully human agonist antibodies to TrkB using autocrine cell-based selection from a combinatorial antibody library. *Proc. Natl. Acad. Sci. USA* **2018**, *115*, E7023–E7032. [CrossRef] [PubMed]
45. Tao, P.; Kuang, Y.; Li, Y.; Li, W.; Gao, Z.; Liu, L.; Qiang, M.; Zha, Z.; Fan, K.; Ma, P.; et al. Selection of a Full Agonist Combinatorial Antibody that Rescues Leptin Deficiency In Vivo. *Adv. Sci.* **2020**, *7*, 2000818. [CrossRef] [PubMed]
46. Ren, H.; Li, J.; Zhang, N.; Hu, L.A.; Ma, Y.; Tagari, P.; Xu, J.; Zhang, M.-Y. Function-based high-throughput screening for antibody antagonists and agonists against G protein-coupled receptors. *Commun. Biol.* **2020**, *3*, 1–10. [CrossRef]
47. Sasso, E.; D'Avino, C.; Passariello, M.; D'Alise, A.M.; Siciliano, D.; Esposito, M.L.; Froechlich, G.; Cortese, R.; Scarselli, E.; Zambrano, N.; et al. Massive parallel screening of phage libraries for the generation of repertoires of human immunomodulatory monoclonal antibodies. *mAbs* **2018**, *10*, 1060–1072. [CrossRef] [PubMed]
48. Moffat, J.G.; Vincent, F.; Lee, J.A.; Eder, J.; Prunotto, M. Opportunities and challenges in phenotypic drug discovery: An industry perspective. *Nat. Rev. Drug Discov.* **2017**, *16*, 531–543. [CrossRef]
49. Sidney, L.E.; Branch, M.J.; Dunphy, S.E.; Dua, H.S.; Hopkinson, A. Concise Review: Evidence for CD34 as a Common Marker for Diverse Progenitors. *Stem Cells* **2014**, *32*, 1380–1389. [CrossRef]
50. Watt, F.M.; Hogan, B.L. Out of Eden: Stem cells and their niches. *Science* **2000**, *287*, 1427–1430. [CrossRef]
51. Xie, J.; Zhang, H.; Yea, K.; Lerner, R.A. Autocrine signaling based selection of combinatorial antibodies that transdifferentiate human stem cells. *Proc. Natl. Acad. Sci. USA* **2013**, *110*, 8099–8104. [CrossRef]
52. Yea, K.; Zhang, H.; Xie, J.; Jones, T.M.; Lin, C.-W.; Francesconi, W.; Berton, F.; Fallahi, M.; Sauer, K.; Lerner, R.A. Agonist antibody that induces human malignant cells to kill one another. *Proc. Natl. Acad. Sci. USA* **2015**, *112*, E6158–E6165. [CrossRef]
53. Lerner, R.A.; Grover, R.K.; Zhang, H.; Xie, J.; Han, K.H.; Peng, Y.; Yea, K. Antibodies from combinatorial libraries use functional receptor pleiotropism to regulate cell fates. *Q. Rev. Biophys.* **2015**, *48*, 389–394. [CrossRef]
54. Melidoni, A.N.; Dyson, M.R.; Wormald, S.; McCafferty, J. Selecting antagonistic antibodies that control differentiation through inducible expression in embryonic stem cells. *Proc. Natl. Acad. Sci. USA* **2013**, *110*, 17802–17807. [CrossRef] [PubMed]
55. Blanchard, J.W.; Xie, J.; El-Mecharrafie, N.; Gross, S.; Lee, S.; Lerner, A.R.; Baldwin, K.K. Replacing reprogramming factors with antibodies selected from combinatorial antibody libraries. *Nat. Biotechnol.* **2017**, *35*, 960–968. [CrossRef] [PubMed]
56. Xie, J.; Yea, K.; Zhang, H.; Moldt, B.; He, L.; Zhu, J.; Lerner, R.A. Prevention of Cell Death by Antibodies Selected from Intracellular Combinatorial Libraries. *Chem. Biol.* **2014**, *21*, 274–283. [CrossRef] [PubMed]
57. Galluzzi, L.; Vitale, I.; Aaronson, S.A.; Abrams, J.M.; Adam, D.; Agostinis, P.; Alnemri, E.S.; Altucci, L.; Amelio, I.; Andrews, D.W.; et al. Molecular mechanisms of cell death: Recommendations of the Nomenclature Committee on Cell Death 2018. *Cell Death Differ.* **2018**, *25*, 486–541. [CrossRef]
58. Liu, T.; Kuwana, T.; Zhang, H.; Heiden, M.G.V.; Lerner, R.A.; Newmeyer, D.D. Phenotypic selection with an intrabody library reveals an anti-apoptotic function of PKM2 requiring Mitofusin-1. *PLoS Biol.* **2019**, *17*, e2004413. [CrossRef]
59. Lin, C.-W.; Xie, J.; Zhang, D.; Han, K.H.; Grande, G.; Wu, N.C.; Yang, Z.; Yea, K.; Lerner, R.A. Immunity against cancer cells may promote their proliferation and metastasis. *Proc. Natl. Acad. Sci. USA* **2019**, *117*, 426–431. [CrossRef] [PubMed]
60. Ljungars, A.; Mårtensson, L.; Mattsson, J.; Kovacek, M.; Sundberg, A.; Tornberg, U.-C.; Jansson, B.; Persson, N.; Emruli, V.K.; Ek, S.; et al. A platform for phenotypic discovery of therapeutic antibodies and targets applied on Chronic Lymphocytic Leukemia. *npj Precis. Oncol.* **2018**, *2*, 1–4. [CrossRef] [PubMed]

61. Han, K.H.; Arlian, B.M.; Macauley, M.S.; Paulson, J.C.; Lerner, R.A. Migration-based selections of antibodies that convert bone marrow into trafficking microglia-like cells that reduce brain amyloid beta. *Proc. Natl. Acad. Sci. USA* **2018**, *115*, E372–E381. [CrossRef] [PubMed]
62. Han, K.H.; Arlian, B.M.; Lin, C.-W.; Jin, H.Y.; Kang, G.-H.; Lee, S.; Lee, P.C.-W.; Lerner, R.A. Agonist Antibody Converts Stem Cells into Migrating Brown Adipocyte-Like Cells in Heart. *Cells* **2020**, *9*, 256. [CrossRef] [PubMed]
63. Han, K.H.; Gonzalez-Quintial, R.; Peng, Y.; Baccala, R.; Theofilopoulos, A.N.; Lerner, R.A. An agonist antibody that blocks autoimmunity by inducing anti-inflammatory macrophages. *FASEB J.* **2016**, *30*, 738–747. [CrossRef] [PubMed]
64. Ying, T.; Du, L.; Ju, T.W.; Prabakaran, P.; Lau, C.C.Y.; Lu, L.; Liu, Q.; Wang, L.; Feng, Y.; Wang, Y.; et al. Exceptionally Potent Neutralization of Middle East Respiratory Syndrome Coronavirus by Human Monoclonal Antibodies. *J. Virol.* **2014**, *88*, 7796–7805. [CrossRef]
65. Sui, J.; Hwang, W.C.; Perez, S.; Wei, G.; Aird, D.; Chen, L.-M.; Santelli, E.; Stec, B.; Cadwell, G.; Ali, M.; et al. Structural and functional bases for broad-spectrum neutralization of avian and human influenza A viruses. *Nat. Struct. Mol. Biol.* **2009**, *16*, 265–273. [CrossRef]
66. Kashyap, A.K.; Steel, J.; Oner, A.F.; Dillon, M.A.; Swale, R.E.; Wall, K.M.; Perry, K.J.; Faynboym, A.; Ilhan, M.; Horowitz, M.; et al. Combinatorial antibody libraries from survivors of the Turkish H5N1 avian influenza outbreak reveal virus neutralization strategies. *Proc. Natl. Acad. Sci. USA* **2008**, *105*, 5986–5991. [CrossRef] [PubMed]
67. Qiang, M.; Ma, P.; Li, Y.; Liu, H.; Harding, A.; Min, C.; Liu, L.; Yuan, M.; Ji, Q.; Tao, P.; et al. Potent SARS-CoV-2 neutralizing antibodies selected from a human antibody library constructed decades ago. *bioRxiv* **2020**. [CrossRef]
68. Ng, K.W.; Faulkner, N.; Cornish, G.H.; Rosa, A.; Harvey, R.; Hussain, S.; Ulferts, R.; Earl, C.; Wrobel, A.G.; Benton, D.J.; et al. Preexisting and de novo humoral immunity to SARS-CoV-2 in humans. *Science* **2020**, *370*, 1339–1343. [CrossRef]
69. Yuan, M.; Wu, N.C.; Zhu, X.; Lee, C.C.D.; So, R.T.; Lv, H.; Mok, C.K.P.; Wilson, I.A. A highly conserved cryptic epitope in the receptor binding domains of SARS-CoV-2 and SARS-CoV. *Science* **2020**, *368*, 630–633. [CrossRef]
70. Noy-Porat, T.; Makdasi, E.; Alcalay, R.; Mechaly, A.; Levy, Y.; Bercovich-Kinori, A.; Zauberman, A.; Tamir, H.; Yahalom-Ronen, Y.; Israeli, M.; et al. A panel of human neutralizing mAbs targeting SARS-CoV-2 spike at multiple epitopes. *Nat. Commun.* **2020**, *11*, 4303. [CrossRef]
71. Li, W.; Chen, C.; Drelich, A.; Martinez, D.R.; Gralinski, L.E.; Sun, Z.; Schäfer, A.; Kulkarni, S.S.; Liu, X.; Leist, S.R.; et al. Rapid identification of a human antibody with high prophylactic and therapeutic efficacy in three animal models of SARS-CoV-2 infection. *Proc. Natl. Acad. Sci. USA* **2020**, *117*, 29832–29838. [CrossRef] [PubMed]

International Journal of
Molecular Sciences

MDPI

Review

Antigen Design for Successful Isolation of Highly Challenging Therapeutic Anti-GPCR Antibodies

Man-Seok Ju [1,2] and Sang Taek Jung [1,2,3,4,5,*]

1 Department of Biomedical Sciences, Korea University College of Medicine, Seoul 02841, Korea; seok0801@korea.ac.kr
2 Institute of Human Genetics, Korea University College of Medicine, Seoul 02841, Korea
3 Department of Biomedical Sciences, Graduate School, Korea University, Seoul 02841, Korea
4 BK21 Graduate Program, Department of Biomedical Sciences, Korea University College of Medicine, Seoul 02841, Korea
5 Biomedical Research Center, Korea University Anam Hospital, Seoul 02841, Korea
* Correspondence: sjung@korea.ac.kr; Tel.: +82-2-2286-1422

Received: 12 October 2020; Accepted: 30 October 2020; Published: 3 November 2020

Abstract: G-protein-coupled receptors (GPCR) transmit extracellular signals into cells to regulate a variety of cellular functions and are closely related to the homeostasis of the human body and the progression of various types of diseases. Great attention has been paid to GPCRs as excellent drug targets, and there are many commercially available small-molecule chemical drugs against GPCRs. Despite this, the development of therapeutic anti-GPCR antibodies has been delayed and is challenging due to the difficulty in preparing active forms of GPCR antigens, resulting from their low cellular expression and complex structures. Here, we focus on anti-GPCR antibodies that have been approved or are subject to clinical trials and present various technologies to prepare active GPCR antigens that enable the isolation of therapeutic antibodies to proceed toward clinical validation.

Keywords: G protein-coupled receptor; membrane protein; antigen; therapeutic antibody

1. Introduction

G-protein-coupled receptors (GPCRs), which make up the largest superfamily of human membrane proteins, play pivotal roles in mediating intracellular signaling and inducing cell proliferation, cell growth, and cell motility through the association and subsequent dissociation of G-proteins in response to external stimuli (Figure 1) [1,2]. Many clinical studies have revealed that abnormal functions of GPCRs are highly related to a variety of human diseases and affect the patient survival rate [3–5]. Therefore, GPCRs are crucial drug targets to treat patients with various diseases, and their targeting drugs represent more than 30 percent of all US Food and Drug Administration (FDA)-approved drugs [6–8]. Annual sales of these drugs have increased to about USD 180 billion in 2018 [9].

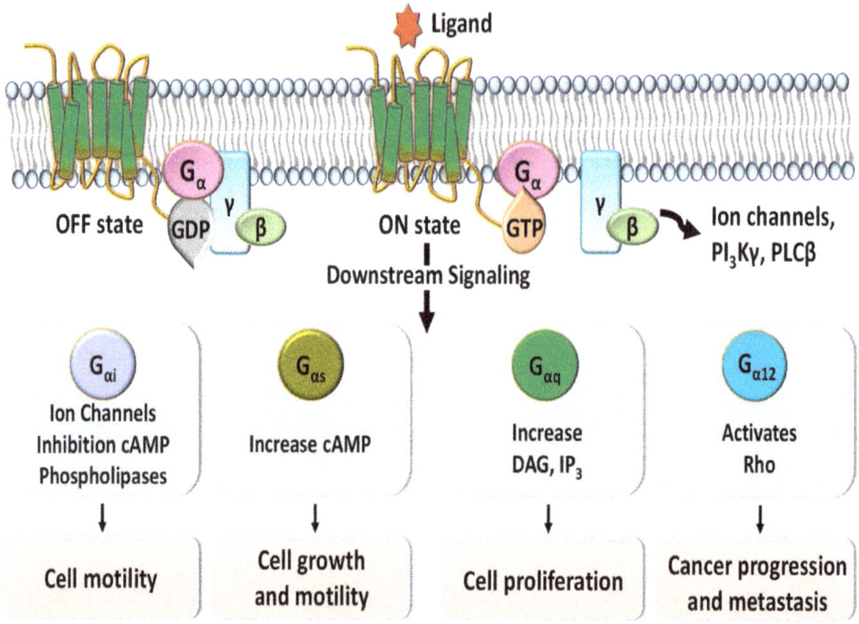

Figure 1. Schematic diagram of G-protein-coupled receptor (GPCR) signaling pathways mediated by G_α protein subunits. Downstream signaling triggered by binding of G proteins changes the concentrations of phospholipase C-beta (PLCβ), phosphoinositide 3-kinases-gamma (PI3Kγ), diacylglycerol (DAG), inositol trisphosphate (IP3), and cyclic adenosine monophosphate (cAMP) and regulates various cellular functions such as cell motility, cell growth, cell proliferation, and cancer progression and metastasis.

Compared to small-molecule chemical drugs and small peptides, therapeutic antibodies have many advantages in terms of higher target specificity, fewer side effects, and superior serum circulating half-life [10]. However, despite clinical and marketing successes of monoclonal antibody products to treat numerous diseases, only two anti-GPCR therapeutic antibody drugs, Amgen's erenumab (trade name: Aimovig), targeting calcitonin gene-related receptor (CGRPR) to treat migraine (Figure 2a) [11] and Kyowa Kirin's mogamulizumab (trade name: Poteligeo), targeting chemokine receptor 4 (CCR4) to treat refractory mycosis fungoides and Sézary syndrome (Figure 2b), have been approved to date [12].

Generally, amenable techniques to isolate therapeutic human antibodies include (1) humanization of candidate antibodies followed by the selection of hybridoma cells derived from immunized animals; (2) screening of the human naïve antibody library displayed on the surface of bacteriophages, bacteria, or yeast, which take advantage of a physical linkage between genotype and phenotype; and (3) hybridoma selection after immunizing an antigen into humanized transgenic animals, referred to as XenoMouse™, which contains the genes for variable regions of the heavy (VH) and light (VL) chains of the human antibody repertoire [13].

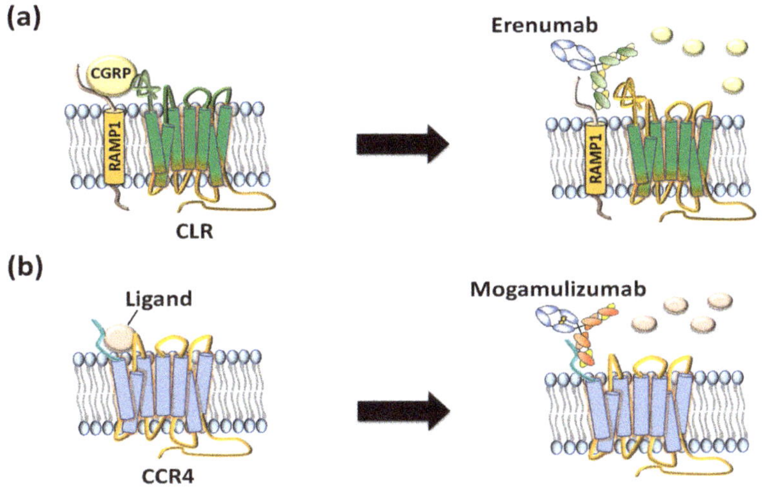

Figure 2. US FDA-approved anti-GPCR antibodies erenumab and mogamulizumab. (**a**) Erenumab is an antagonistic monoclonal antibody against calcitonin gene-related peptide receptor (CGRPR) consisting of calcitonin receptor-like receptor (CLR) and receptor activity-modifying protein 1 (RAMP1) for treatment of chronic migraine. (**b**) Mogamulizumab is an antibody against chemokine receptor 4 (CCR4) for treatment of T-cell leukemia by inactivating the GPCR and clearance of target cells by enhanced antibody-dependent cell-mediated cytotoxicity (ADCC).

Regardless of the antibody isolation technique, preparing pure GPCR antigens with the native conformation of the human in vivo condition is essential for successful isolation of therapeutic functional human anti-GPCR antibodies. In particular, GPCRs containing seven transmembrane α-helices are usually expressed at very low levels in heterologous expression systems; therefore, it is very hard to purify the antigen with a native conformation as a soluble form. Furthermore, the limited surface area of the extracellular region of GPCRs in the whole GPCR structure makes it very difficult to prepare the GPCR antigen as a target for therapeutic anti-GPCR antibodies. Even though antigen preparation is one of the most difficult steps in development of therapeutic anti-GPCR antibodies, two anti-GPCR antibodies have overcome the challenges and have been recently approved. In addition, dozens of anti-GPCR antibodies are under clinical development or are waiting for clinical evaluations of therapeutic efficacy and toxicity. In this review, we focus on therapeutic anti-GPCR antibodies that have been recently approved or those that are subject to clinical trials (Table 1) and how the various types of GPCR antigens are prepared to isolate the highly challenging therapeutic anti-GPCR antibodies that have entered the clinical development phase.

Table 1. Anti-GPCR antibodies approved by the US FDA or subject to clinical trial.

Antigen Type	Antibody Screening Technology	Drug Name	Target	Indication	Status of Clinical Trial	Reference
RAMP1-Fc, CGRPR-Fc	Tg mouse immunization and hybridoma screening	Aimovig™ (Erenumab)	CGRP receptor	Migraine	Approved	[14]
CCR4-KLH	Mouse immunization and hybridoma screening	Poteligeo® (Mogamulizumab)	CCR4	Refractory mycosis fungoides and Sézary disease	Approved	[15]
FZD7-Fc	Synthetic human antibody phage library screening	Vantictumab (OMP-18R5)	FZD7	Non-small cell lung cancer, pancreatic cancer, metastatic breast cancer	Phase I	[16–18]
CCR5 expressing cells	Mouse immunization and hybridoma screening	Leronlimab (Pro 140)	CCR5	HIV infection	Phase III	[19]
CCR2 expressing cells	Mouse immunization and hybridoma screening	Plozalizumab (MLN-1202)	CCR2	Relapsing-remitting multiple sclerosis	Phase II	[20]
CXCR4 expressing cells	Tg mouse immunization and phage library screening	Ulocuplumab (BMS-936564)	CXCR4	Acute myeloid leukemia	Phase I/II	[21]
C5Aa1 expressing cells	Tg mouse immunization and hybridoma screening	Avdoralimab (IPH5401)	C5aR1	Non-small cell lung cancer, liver cancer	Phase I	[22]
Membrane fraction of GLP1R expressing cells	Tg mouse immunization and hybridoma screening	Glutazumab (GMA102)	GLP1R	Type 2 diabetes	Phase II	[23]
Membrane fraction of GCGR expressing cells	Tg mouse immunization and hybridoma screening	Volagidemab (REMD-477)	GCGR	Diabetes mellitus	Phase II	[24]
Reconstituted CNR1 GLB complex	Mouse immunization and hybridoma/phage library screening	Namacizumab (RYI-018)	CNR1	Non-alcoholic fatty liver disease	Phase I	[25]

2. GPCR Extracellular Region Fusion Proteins as GPCR Antigens

Interaction between the extracellular region of GPCRs and their ligands triggers conformational changes in the intracellular region of the protein, resulting in the association of G-proteins and the transmission of extracellular signals into cells [26]. GPCRs consist of seven transmembrane α-helical bundles, four extracellular regions: N-terminal, extracellular loop 1 (ECL1), extracellular loop 2 (ECL2), and extracellular loop 3 (ECL3), and four intracellular regions: intracellular loop 1 (ICL1), intracellular loop 2 (ICL2), intracellular loop 3 (ICL3), and C-terminal. The unique three-dimensional structure of each GPCR determines its ligand specificity to elicit its characteristic cellular responses. To isolate antibodies that recognize the extracellular region of a GPCR, a simple strategy is to chemically conjugate or genetically fuse a designed peptide comprising the part of the GPCR extracellular region with a carrier protein (Figure 3a). The prepared antigen can be used to immunize animals or screen antibodies from a human naïve antibody library [27]. Although the extracellular region peptide prepared with a carrier protein is unable to perfectly mimic the extracellular peptide conformation of a native GPCR, some human GPCR extracellular region polypeptides containing post-translational modifications such as glycosylation can be expressed in mammalian cells [28]. A mimic GPCR extracellular loop was fused with a carrier protein and employed to isolate erenumab, targeting calcitonin gene-related peptide receptor (CGRPR) [29], mogamulizumab, targeting chemokine receptor 4 (CCR4) [30], and vantictumab, targeting Frizzled-7 (FZD7) [31].

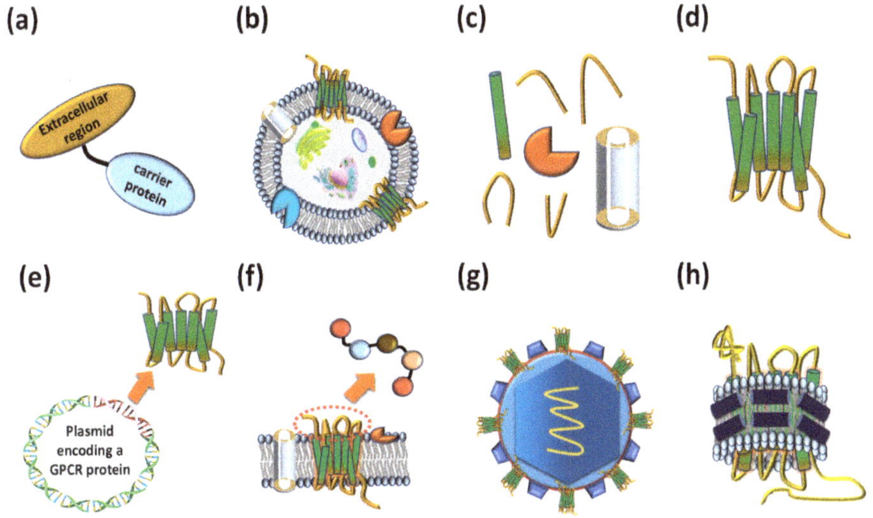

Figure 3. Various types of antigens that have been employed to isolate anti-GPCR antibodies. (**a**) Extracellular region fused proteins. (**b**) Whole cells expressing GPCRs on their cellular membrane. (**c**) Membrane factions expressing GPCRs. (**d**) Purified whole GPCRs. (**e**) DNA molecules encoding GPCRs. (**f**) Extracellular region peptides. (**g**) Virus-like particles (VLPs) displaying GPCRs on the surface. (**h**) Reconstituted GPCR–lipid–belt protein (GLB) complexes.

Erenumab is an antibody developed to treat patients with chronic migraine. It regulates the function of calcitonin receptor-like receptor (CLR), interacting with the receptor activity-modifying protein (RAMP) family. The single transmembrane domain has selectivity for three types of ligands: calcitonin gene-related peptide (CGRP), adrenomedullin 1, and adrenomedullin 2 [32]. The calcitonin gene-related peptide receptor (CGRPR), comprising CLR and RAMP1, is mainly distributed in the peripheral and central nervous systems.

Moreover, it is closely related to migraine through vasodilation following $G_{\alpha s}$ protein release and the activation of adenylyl cyclase [33,34]. Based on the finding that the CGRP binding site spans the extracellular regions of CLR and RAMP1 [35], a heterodimeric Fc (fragment crystallizable) fusion protein consisting of an ectodomain of RAMP and an N-terminal extracellular region of CLR was designed as an antigen to isolate CGRPR antagonistic antibodies (Figure 4a). In addition, the prepared heterodimeric Fc fusion was immunized into XenoMouse to generate erenumab, followed by hybridoma screening [36,37] (Figure 4b). Erenumab showed a high binding affinity to CGRPR (K_D = 56 pM) and excellent inhibition of cAMP production (IC_{50} = 2.3 nM) [38]. Additionally, structural analysis of the CGRPR-CGRP complex confirmed that erenumab directly blocks the conformation of CGRP into CGRPR [39]. In the phase III clinical trial, patients treated with 70 mg and 140 mg of erenumab once a month for at least 6 months showed 43.3% and 50% reductions of number of days of migraine [40], respectively, and these efficacy results enabled the antibody to be the first anti-GPCR antibody approved by the US FDA in May 2018 and by the European Medicines Agency (EMA) in July 2018.

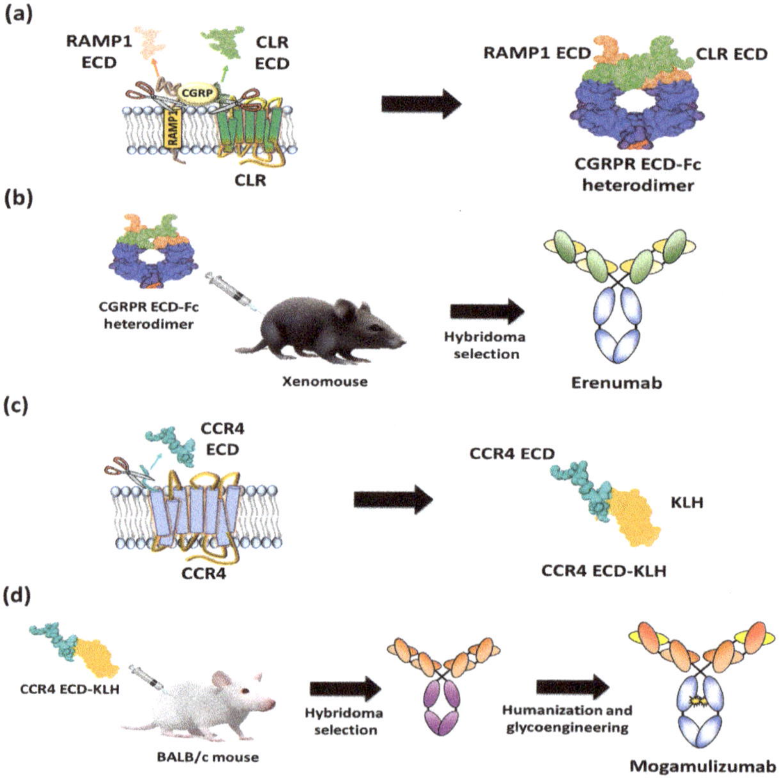

Figure 4. Schematic diagrams of antigen preparation and overall procedure for discovery of US FDA-approved anti-GPCR antibody. (**a**) A heterodimer CGRPR Fc protein prepared by Fc fusion constructs of N-terminal extracellular regions of CLR and ectodomain of RAMP1. (**b**) Immunization of heterodimeric CGRPR Fc proteins into XenoMouse hybridoma selection to isolate erenumab. (**c**) The N-terminal region of CCR4 (28 amino acids: N2-C29) fused with keyhole limpet hemocyanin (KLH). (**d**) Injection of the N-terminal region of CCR4-KLH into BALB/c mice and hybridoma selection, humanization, and defucosylation of N-inked glycans of Fc to generate mogamulizumab.

Mogamulizumab is a humanized monoclonal antibody targeting chemokine receptor 4 (CCR4) with a glyco-engineered Fc region to enhance the antibody-dependent cellular cytotoxicity (ADCC) for the clearance of adult t-cell leukemia (ATL). The protein CCR4 is overexpressed on the surface of FOXP3+ regulatory T (Treg) cells of ATL patients and is involved in the evasion of immune surveillance against tumors [41,42]. To isolate anti-CCR4 antibodies, extracellular partial N-terminal peptide (28 amino acids: N2-C29) was fused to a carrier protein, keyhole limpet hemocyanin (KLH) (Figure 4c), and injected into mice for the screening of antigen-specific antibodies (Figure 4d) [43]. After humanization of the candidate antibodies, glycol engineering was performed to defucosylate the N-linked glycan of Fc to enhance FcγIIIa binding and Natural Killer (NK) cell-mediated ADCC activity [44–47]. The resulting mogamulizumab (KW-0761) exhibited significant efficacy in 50% of ATL patients treated in clinical trials, leading to successful commercialization in 2012 in Japan and in 2019 in the US for the treatment of mycosis fungoides (MF) and Sézary syndrome (SS) [12,48].

Uncontrolled cell signaling in the Wnt/β-catenin pathway affects various types of tumors [49]. Vantictumab (anti-FZD7), a Wnt/β-catenin pathway-blocking antibody, was isolated by screening the human naïve Fab antibody library displayed on bacteriophages using the Fc-fused extracellular N-terminal domain of the GPCR as an antigen. The resulting antibody (vantictumab) could inhibit Wnt pathway signaling through specific binding to five kinds of Frizzled receptors: FZD1, FZD2, FZD5, FZD7, and FZD8 [31]. In human phase 1 clinical examination, vantictumab significantly inhibited the growth of pancreatic, colon, and breast cancer cells in combination with other chemotherapeutic agents [50].

3. GPCR-Expressing Cells or Membrane Fractions as GPCR Antigens

The use of GPCR-expressing cells (Figure 3b) or their membrane fractions as antigens containing integral and associated proteins (Figure 3c) has been limited due to difficulty in overexpressing a target GPCR on the cell surface due to the presence of numerous other membrane components. In addition, a very advanced handling technique is necessary to apply the fragile whole cells as antigens for repeated rounds of antibody screening. Alternatively, the membrane fraction from cells displaying a target GPCR has been used as a type of antigen. The biggest advantage of using GPCR-expressing cells or membrane fractions is their native conformation that allows for the isolation of a desired anti-GPCR antibody capable of recognizing the native structure of GPCR compared to using other GPCR mimetic antigens.

Representative examples of therapeutic anti-GPCR antibodies that have been isolated using animal immunization with GPCR-overexpressing cells or their membranes fraction as antigens are glutazumab, targeting glucagon-like peptide-1 receptor (GLP1R) [51,52], volagidemab, targeting glucagon receptor (GCGR) [53], plozalizumab, targeting chemokine receptor type 2 (CCR2) [54], leronlimab (Pro 140), targeting C-C chemokine receptor type 5 (CCR5) [55], ulocuplumab (BMS-936564), targeting C-X-C chemokine receptor type 4 (CXCR4) [56], and avdoralimab (IPH5401), targeting C5a receptor (C5aR) [57].

Glutazumab is an agonist antibody targeting GLP1R for the treatment of type 2 diabetes resulting from an abnormal cellular response to insulin. It was developed by hybridoma selection from mice that were immunized with GLP1R-expressing mammalian cells, humanization, and genetic fusion of the GLP1 (29 amino acids: H7-G35), a ligand of GLP1R, at the N-terminus of the variable light chain of IgG [51,58]. Glutazumab was efficacious in suppressing the interaction between GLP-1 and GLP1R and showed significant efficacy in suppressing glucagon secretion in a human phase II clinical trial in Australia and New Zealand [23].

Leronlimab (Pro 140) is a humanized monoclonal antibody targeting CCR5, which is expressed on the surface of T lymphocytes and is essential for the fusion of HIV with immune cells. Anti-CCR5 antibodies were isolated by immunizing mice with CCR5-expressing mammalian cells, and humanization of the resulting antibodies enabled the development of leronlimab (Pro 140) [55]. The antibody inhibits HIV infection pathways by selectively binding to the N-terminus and extracellular loop 2 of CCR5, and a human phase III clinical trial is ongoing [19,59].

4. Purified Whole GPCR Proteins as GPCR Antigens

For preparative production of whole GPCR proteins (Figure 3d) that mimic the native GPCR structure, several strategies, including the optimization of expression conditions, detergents to extract the complicated membrane proteins, and purification, have been attempted. Despite reports of the successful production of functional GPCRs in mammalian, insect, and Escherichia coli host cells, their preparation techniques are highly variable depending on the type of GPCR. In addition, the same ligand binding affinity and specificity for purified GPCRs as those on cellular membranes are not guaranteed because the structures extracted from cellular membranes are likely to be different from those of native GPCRs. Nevertheless, the use of purified whole GPCR proteins as antigens enables the exclusion of a number of unrelated components on the cellular membrane, which may improve the isolation of GPCR target-specific antibodies. For the efficient production of functional native-like GPCRs, significant efforts have aimed to resolve issues including the (i) low expression level of GPCR on the cell membrane surface, (ii) low solubility and stability of expressed GPCRs, and (iii) complicated reconstitution steps to maintain the active conformation of GPCRs.

To improve the expression level of endothelin receptor type A (ET_A) in *E. coli*, Lee et al. fused the N-terminus of a GPCR with the P9 peptide derived from an envelope protein of Pseudomonas phage Φ6 (Phi6). The P9 peptide fusion significantly increased ET_A expression in *E. coli*, and the purified ET_A showed binding affinity to both its native ligand (ET-1 peptide) and G_α protein [60]. Corin et al. added non-ionic detergents in a commercial cell-free translation system to successfully express and purify 13 GPCRs. Human vomeronasal receptor 1 (hVN1R1), prepared through its modified cell-free translation system, showed similar ligand binding affinity compared to the hVN1R1 counterpart produced in HEK293 cells [61]. For enhanced expression of GPCRs, Sarkar et al. optimized the conditions to enhance outer membrane permeability for the access of additional small ligands to the GPCRs expressed on the *E. coli* inner membrane. Using the screening of an error-prone PCR library for rat neurotensin receptor-1 (NTR1), they successfully isolated NTR1 variants exhibiting an improved fluorescence signal upon binding to fluorescent dye-conjugated ligands in the flow cytometric analysis. The resulting GPCR variants showed enhanced stability and were successfully purified in *E. coli*, yeast, and mammalian cells [62]. A. James Link et al. fused Green Fluorescent Protein (GFP) to the C-terminus of GPCRs and monitored the effect of co-expression of a panel of selected *E. coli* proteins on GPCR expression. They found that co-expression of membrane-anchored AAA+ protease FtsH could significantly improve the expression levels of full-length cannabinoid receptors (CB_1, CB_2) and bradykinin receptor 2 (BR2) in *E. coli* [63]. Vukoti et al. examined the effect of detergents on the solubility of recombinant purified cannabinoid receptor 2 (CB_2) using the *E. coli* expression system and optimized conditions for the reconstitution of CB_2 from mixed n-dodecyl-ß-D-maltopyranoside (DDM), 3-[(3-cholamidopropyl) dimethylammonio]-1-propanesulfonate (CHAPS), and cholesteryl hemisuccinate (CHS) micelles. The reconstituted CB2 exhibited an equivalent binding affinity to ligands (CP-55,940 or SR-144,528) and $G_{\alpha i1}$ compared to the CB2 expressed in Chinese Hamster Ovary (CHO) cells [64].

5. Other Types of Prepared GPCR Antigens

In addition to the previously mentioned types of antigens, other types of prepared GPCR antigens such as DNA (Figure 3e), peptide (Figure 3f), virus-like particles (VLP) (Figure 3g), and the GPCR-lipid-belt protein (GLB) complex (Figure 3h) have been harnessed to isolate therapeutic anti-GPCR antibodies. The biggest advantage of using GPCR-coding DNAs as antigens is to bypass production of complex GPCR membrane proteins or GPCR-overexpressing cells. When the DNA encoding the GPCR antigen is cloned into a vector optimized for GPCR protein expression and injected into an animal host, it produces heterologous GPCR protein antigen and GPCR overexpressing cells. The resulting GPCR antigen enables to isolate GPCR antigen specific antibodies through the immune response of the animal host [65,66] However, injected DNAs are highly labile to decomposition by the immune responses of animals. In addition, it is hard to isolate a desired target-specific anti-GPCR antibody in the case of low antigenic GPCR expression. Peptide antigens can be effectively used when the structures of the antigen proteins are complex or protein production is very difficult. And GPCR-specific antibodies can be discovered using peptides consisting of the sequence of the extracellular loop of the GPCR [67,68]. However, it is not easy to prepare the peptide antigens that mimic the native GPCR extracellular loop structure, and the short-length peptide antigen may be labile to be degraded in the host when it is immunized into an animal. VLPs are divided into two main types, non-enveloped VLPs and enveloped VLPs, depending on the presence of a lipid bilayer on the VLP surface displaying antigens [69]. Enveloped VLP containing a lipid bilayer structure can display complex membrane proteins on the cell surface and has been used to isolate anti-GPCR antibodies [70,71]. However, it is possible that the conformation and topology of GPCRs displayed on the surface of VLP differ from those of natural GPCR expressed on cellular membrane.

Similarly, the GPCR-lipid-belt protein (GLB) complex prepared by reconstituting solubilized GPCR proteins, lipids, and belt proteins has been used as an antigen to isolate various anti-GPCR antibodies [72,73]. Namacizumab, a therapeutic antibody for treatment of non-alcoholic fatty liver disease (NAFLD), was isolated using the prepared GLB complex reconstituted with belt protein, lipid, and cannabinoid 1 receptor (CNR1) [74]. CNR1 is a main receptor for anandamide and 2-arachidonoyl glycerol and is involved in energy metabolism [75,76]. Previous research results indicate that overexpression and dysfunction of CNR1 cause obesity and hepatic steatosis (fatty liver disease) in a diet-induced obesity mouse model [77]. The anti-CNR1 antibody was isolated by injecting reconstituted CNR1 GLB complex particles into mice [74,78], and a phase I human clinical trial of its humanized antibody was conducted [25].

6. Conclusions

In contrast to small-molecule drugs, monoclonal antibodies have many advantages, including high target specificity, much reduced side effects, prolonged serum half-life, and the ability to harness immune effector functions mediated by a variety of leukocytes. Due to these unique characteristics possessed by antibodies, they are the fastest growing sector in drug development. GPCRs are crucial for regulating the cell growth, motility, proliferation, progression, and metastasis of cancer. Although many small-molecule drugs targeting GPCRs are commercially available, only two anti-GPCR therapeutic antibody drugs have been approved by the US FDA as of 16 September 2020. One of the main reasons for the slow speed of development of therapeutic antibodies against the attractive drug target is the difficulty in preparing functional (native or native-like) GPCR antigens. It is evident that GPCRs are highly challenging antigens for which to isolate therapeutic antibodies because of their complex structure. However, as noted above, various strategies to prepare homogeneous and more native-like GPCR antigens have been developed. In keeping pace with the development of GPCR antigen preparation methods, various cutting-edge antibody isolation platforms have emerged. Our research group also discovered novel anti-GPCR antibodies for cancer treatment through the innovative methods described in this manuscript, and the results will be reported soon. In combination with efficient GPCR antigen preparation methods and advanced antibody screening techniques, many advances have been achieved and will soon be able to exploit a variety of anti-GPCR therapeutic antibodies with new mechanisms of action, which may be used for the treatment of a variety of diseases related to GPCR signaling.

Author Contributions: M.-S.J. and S.T.J. designed and wrote the paper. All authors have read and agreed to the published version of the manuscript.

Funding: This work was supported by grants from the Bio & Medical Technology Development Program (2020M3E5E2037775) and the Basic Science Research Programs (2019R1F1A1059834, 2019R1A4A1029000, and 2019R1A6A3A01097279) through the National Research Foundation of Korea, funded by the Ministry of Science and ICT and by the Ministry of Education, and by a Korea National Institute of Health fund (2020-ER5311-00).

Conflicts of Interest: The authors declare no conflict of interest.

References

1. Wu, J.; Xie, N.; Zhao, X.; Nice, E.C.; Huang, C. Dissection of aberrant GPCR signaling in tumorigenesis—A systems biology approach. *Cancer Genom Proteom.* **2012**, *9*, 37–50.
2. New, D.C.; Wong, Y.H. Molecular mechanisms mediating the G protein-coupled receptor regulation of cell cycle progression. *J. Mol. Signal.* **2007**, *2*, 2. [CrossRef] [PubMed]
3. Zougman, A.; Hutchins, G.G.; Cairns, D.A.; Verghese, E.; Perry, S.L.; Jayne, D.G.; Selby, P.J.; Banks, R.E. Retinoic acid-induced protein 3: Identification and characterisation of a novel prognostic colon cancer biomarker. *Eur. J. Cancer.* **2013**, *49*, 531–539. [CrossRef] [PubMed]
4. Sriram, K.; Moyung, K.; Corriden, R.; Carter, H.; Insel, P.A. GPCRs show widespread differential mRNA expression and frequent mutation and copy number variation in solid tumors. *PLoS Biol.* **2019**, *17*, e3000434. [CrossRef] [PubMed]
5. Feigin, M.E.; Xue, B.; Hammell, M.C.; Muthuswamy, S.K. G-protein–coupled receptor GPR161 is overexpressed in breast cancer and is a promoter of cell proliferation and invasion. *Proc. Natl. Acad. Sci. USA* **2014**, *111*, 4191–4196. [CrossRef] [PubMed]
6. Santos, R.; Ursu, O.; Gaulton, A.; Bento, A.P.; Donadi, R.S.; Bologa, C.G.; Karlsson, A.; Al-Lazikani, B.; Hersey, A.; Oprea, T.I.; et al. A comprehensive map of molecular drug targets. *Nat. Rev. Drug Discov.* **2017**, *16*, 19–34. [CrossRef]
7. Rask-Andersen, M.; Masuram, S.; Schioth, H.B. The druggable genome: Evaluation of drug targets in clinical trials suggests major shifts in molecular class and indication. *Annu. Rev. Pharmacol. Toxicol.* **2014**, *54*, 9–26. [CrossRef] [PubMed]
8. Hauser, A.S.; Attwood, M.M.; Rask-Andersen, M.; Schioth, H.B.; Gloriam, D.E. Trends in GPCR drug discovery: New agents, targets and indications. *Nat. Rev. Drug Discov.* **2017**, *16*, 829–842. [CrossRef] [PubMed]
9. Hauser, A.S.; Chavali, S.; Masuho, I.; Jahn, L.J.; Martemyanov, K.A.; Gloriam, D.E.; Babu, M.M. Pharmacogenomics of GPCR Drug Targets. *Cell* **2018**, *172*, 41–54. [CrossRef]
10. Igawa, T.; Tsunoda, H.; Kuramochi, T.; Sampei, Z.; Ishii, S.; Hattori, K. Engineering the variable region of therapeutic IgG antibodies. In *MAbs*; Taylor & Francis: Abingdon, UK, 2011; Volume 3, pp. 243–252. [CrossRef]
11. Dolgin, E. First GPCR-directed antibody passes approval milestone. *Nat. Rev. Drug Discov.* **2018**, *17*, 457–459. [CrossRef]
12. Kasamon, Y.L.; Chen, H.; de Claro, R.A.; Nie, L.; Ye, J.; Blumenthal, G.M.; Farrell, A.T.; Pazdur, R. FDA Approval Summary: Mogamulizumab-kpkc for Mycosis Fungoides and Sezary Syndrome. *Clin. Cancer Res.* **2019**, *25*, 7275–7280. [CrossRef]
13. Hoogenboom, H.R. Selecting and screening recombinant antibody libraries. *Nat. Biotechnol.* **2005**, *23*, 1105–1116. [CrossRef] [PubMed]
14. Amgen Inc. Erenumab (Aimovig™): US Prescribing Information. 2018. Available online: https://www.accessdata.fda.gov/drugsatfda_docs/label/2018/761077s000lbl.pdf (accessed on 13 October 2020).
15. Kyowa Kirin Inc. Mogamulizumab (POTELIGEO®): US Prescribing Information. 2018. Available online: https://www.accessdata.fda.gov/drugsatfda_docs/label/2018/761051s000lbl.pdf (accessed on 13 October 2020).
16. OncoMed Pharmaceuticals Inc. A Study of Vantictumab (OMP-18R5) in Combination with Docetaxel in Patients with Previously Treated NSCLC. 2013. Available online: https://clinicaltrials.gov/ct2/show/NCT01957007 (accessed on 13 October 2020).
17. OncoMed Pharmaceuticals Inc. A Study of Vantictumab (OMP-18R5) in Combination with Paclitaxel in Locally Recurrent or Metastatic Breast Cancer. 2013. Available online: https://clinicaltrials.gov/ct2/show/NCT01973309 (accessed on 13 October 2020).
18. OncoMed Pharmaceuticals Inc. A Study of Vantictumab (OMP-18R5) in Combination with Nab-Paclitaxel and Gemcitabine in Previously Untreated Stage IV Pancreatic Cancer. 2013. Available online: https://clinicaltrials.gov/ct2/show/NCT02005315 (accessed on 13 October 2020).
19. CytoDyn Inc. PRO 140 in Treatment-Experienced HIV-1 Subjects. 2019. Available online: https://clinicaltrials.gov/ct2/show/NCT03902522 (accessed on 13 October 2020).

20. Millennium Pharmaceuticals Inc. Study of the Safety and Efficacy of MLN1202 in Patients in Multiple Sclerosis. 2010. Available online: https://clinicaltrials.gov/ct2/show/NCT01199640?cond=plozalizumab&draw=2&rank=3 (accessed on 13 October 2020).
21. Bristol-Myers Squibb. An Investigational Immuno-therapy Study of Ulocuplumab in Combination with Low Dose Cytarabine in Patients with Newly Diagnosed Acute Myeloid Leukemia. 2014. Available online: https://clinicaltrials.gov/ct2/show/NCT02305563?cond=Ulocuplumab&draw=2&rank=4 (accessed on 13 October 2020).
22. Innate Pharma. IPH5401 (Anti-C5aR) in Combination with Durvalumab in Patients with Advanced Solid Tumors (STELLAR-001). 2018. Available online: https://clinicaltrials.gov/ct2/show/NCT03665129 (accessed on 13 October 2020).
23. Gmax Biopharm LLC. First Patient Dose of Glutazumab (GMA102) in the Phase II Clinical Trial for Treatment of Type 2 Diabetes. 2017. Available online: http://www.gmaxbiopharm.com/newng2_detail/id/15.html (accessed on 13 October 2020).
24. REMD Biotherapeutics Inc. Multiple Dose Study to Evaluate the Efficacy, Safety and Pharmacodynamics of REMD-477 in Subjects with Type 1 Diabetes Mellitus. 2017. Available online: https://clinicaltrials.gov/ct2/show/NCT03117998 (accessed on 13 October 2020).
25. Bird Rock Bio Inc. Safety tolerability, and PK of RYI-018 after Repeat Dosing in Subjects with Non-Alcoholic Fatty Liver Disease (NAFLD). 2017. Available online: https://clinicaltrials.gov/ct2/show/NCT03261739 (accessed on 13 October 2020).
26. Lefkowitz, R.J.; Shenoy, S.K. Transduction of receptor signals by beta-arrestins. *Science* **2005**, *308*, 512–517. [CrossRef]
27. Webb, D.R.; Handel, T.M.; Kretz-Rommel, A.; Stevens, R.C. Opportunities for functional selectivity in GPCR antibodies. *Biochem. Pharmacol.* **2013**, *85*, 147–152. [CrossRef]
28. Soto, A.G.; Smith, T.H.; Chen, B.; Bhattacharya, S.; Cordova, I.C.; Kenakin, T.; Vaidehi, N.; Trejo, J. N-linked glycosylation of protease-activated receptor-1 at extracellular loop 2 regulates G-protein signaling bias. *Proc. Natl. Acad. Sci. USA* **2015**, *112*, E3600–E3608. [CrossRef]
29. Markham, A. Erenumab: First Global Approval. *Drugs* **2018**, *78*, 1157–1161. [CrossRef]
30. Subramaniam, J.M.; Whiteside, G.; McKeage, K.; Croxtall, J.C. Mogamulizumab: First global approval. *Drugs* **2012**, *72*, 1293–1298. [CrossRef]
31. Smith, D.C.; Rosen, L.S.; Chugh, R.; Goldman, J.W.; Xu, L.; Kapoun, A.; Brachmann, R.K.; Dupont, J.; Stagg, R.J.; Tolcher, A.W.; et al. First-in-human evaluation of the human monoclonal antibody vantictumab (OMP-18R5; anti-Frizzled) targeting the WNT pathway in a phase I study for patients with advanced solid tumors. *J. Clin. Oncol.* **2013**, *31*, 2540. [CrossRef]
32. Brain, S.D.; Grant, A.D. Vascular actions of calcitonin gene-related peptide and adrenomedullin. *Physiol. Rev.* **2004**, *84*, 903–934. [CrossRef] [PubMed]
33. Hay, D.L.; Pioszak, A.A. Receptor Activity-Modifying Proteins (RAMPs): New Insights and Roles. *Annu. Rev. Pharmacol. Toxicol.* **2016**, *56*, 469–487. [CrossRef]
34. Kee, Z.; Kodji, X.; Brain, S.D. The Role of Calcitonin Gene Related Peptide (CGRP) in Neurogenic Vasodilation and Its Cardioprotective Effects. *Front. Physiol.* **2018**, *9*, 1249. [CrossRef]
35. Liang, Y.L.; Khoshouei, M.; Deganutti, G.; Glukhova, A.; Koole, C.; Peat, T.S.; Radjainia, M.; Plitzko, J.M.; Baumeister, W.; Miller, L.J.; et al. Cryo-EM structure of the active, Gs-protein complexed, human CGRP receptor. *Nature* **2018**, *561*, 492–497. [CrossRef]
36. King, C.T.; Gegg, C.V.; Hu, S.N.-Y.; Sen Lu, H.; Chan, B.M.; Berry, K.A.; Brankow, D.W.; Boone, T.J.; Kezunovic, N.; Kelley, M.R.; et al. Discovery of the Migraine Prevention Therapeutic Aimovig (Erenumab), the First FDA-Approved Antibody against a G-Protein-Coupled Receptor. *ACS Pharmacol. Transl. Sci.* **2019**, *2*, 485–490. [CrossRef]
37. Booe, J.M.; Walker, C.S.; Barwell, J.; Kuteyi, G.; Simms, J.; Jamaluddin, M.A.; Warner, M.L.; Bill, R.M.; Harris, P.W.; Brimble, M.A.; et al. Structural Basis for Receptor Activity-Modifying Protein-Dependent Selective Peptide Recognition by a G Protein-Coupled Receptor. *Mol. Cell* **2015**, *58*, 1040–1052. [CrossRef] [PubMed]
38. Shi, L.; Lehto, S.G.; Zhu, D.X.; Sun, H.; Zhang, J.; Smith, B.P.; Immke, D.C.; Wild, K.D.; Xu, C. Pharmacologic Characterization of AMG 334, a Potent and Selective Human Monoclonal Antibody against the Calcitonin Gene-Related Peptide Receptor. *J. Pharmacol. Exp. Ther.* **2016**, *356*, 223–231. [CrossRef]

39. Garces, F.; Mohr, C.; Zhang, L.; Huang, C.S.; Chen, Q.; King, C.; Xu, C.; Wang, Z.L. Molecular Insight into Recognition of the CGRPR Complex by Migraine Prevention Therapy Aimovig (Erenumab). *Cell Rep.* **2020**, *30*, 1714–1723. [CrossRef]
40. Goadsby, P.J.; Reuter, U.; Hallstrom, Y.; Broessner, G.; Bonner, J.H.; Zhang, F.; Sapra, S.; Picard, H.; Mikol, D.D.; Lenz, R.A. A Controlled Trial of Erenumab for Episodic Migraine. *N. Engl. J. Med.* **2017**, *377*, 2123–2132. [CrossRef]
41. Ishida, T.; Ueda, R. CCR4 as a novel molecular target for immunotherapy of cancer. *Cancer Sci.* **2006**, *97*, 1139–1146. [CrossRef]
42. Sugiyama, D.; Nishikawa, H.; Maeda, Y.; Nishioka, M.; Tanemura, A.; Katayama, I.; Ezoe, S.; Kanakura, Y.; Sato, E.; Fukumori, Y.; et al. Anti-CCR4 mAb selectively depletes effector-type FoxP3+CD4+ regulatory T cells, evoking antitumor immune responses in humans. *Proc. Natl. Acad. Sci. USA* **2013**, *110*, 17945–17950. [CrossRef] [PubMed]
43. Shitara, K.; Hanai, N.; Shoji, E.; Sakurada, M.; Furuya, A.; Nakamura, K.; Niwa, R.; Shibata, K.; Yamasaki, M. Method for producing recombinant antibody and antibody fragment thereof. U.S. Patent 8,632,996, 21 January 2014.
44. Niwa, R.; Shoji-Hosaka, E.; Sakurada, M.; Shinkawa, T.; Uchida, K.; Nakamura, K.; Matsushima, K.; Ueda, R.; Hanai, N.; Shitara, K. Defucosylated chimeric anti-CC chemokine receptor 4 IgG1 with enhanced antibody-dependent cellular cytotoxicity shows potent therapeutic activity to T-cell leukemia and lymphoma. *Cancer Res.* **2004**, *64*, 2127–2133. [CrossRef]
45. Niwa, R.; Sakurada, M.; Kobayashi, Y.; Uehara, A.; Matsushima, K.; Ueda, R.; Nakamura, K.; Shitara, K. Enhanced natural killer cell binding and activation by low-fucose IgG1 antibody results in potent antibody-dependent cellular cytotoxicity induction at lower antigen density. *Clin. Cancer Res.* **2005**, *11*, 2327–2336. [CrossRef]
46. Yano, H.; Ishida, T.; Inagaki, A.; Ishii, T.; Ding, J.; Kusumoto, S.; Komatsu, H.; Iida, S.; Inagaki, H.; Ueda, R. Defucosylated anti CC chemokine receptor 4 monoclonal antibody combined with immunomodulatory cytokines: A novel immunotherapy for aggressive/refractory Mycosis fungoides and Sezary syndrome. *Clin. Cancer Res.* **2007**, *13*, 6494–6500. [CrossRef]
47. Yoshie, O.; Matsushima, K. CCR4 and its ligands: From bench to bedside. *Int. Immunol.* **2014**, *27*, 11–20. [CrossRef]
48. Ishida, T.; Joh, T.; Uike, N.; Yamamoto, K.; Utsunomiya, A.; Yoshida, S.; Saburi, Y.; Miyamoto, T.; Takemoto, S.; Suzushima, H.; et al. Defucosylated anti-CCR4 monoclonal antibody (KW-0761) for relapsed adult T-cell leukemia-lymphoma: A multicenter phase II study. *J. Clin. Oncol.* **2012**, *30*, 837–842. [CrossRef]
49. Clevers, H.; Nusse, R. Wnt/beta-catenin signaling and disease. *Cell* **2012**, *149*, 1192–1205. [CrossRef] [PubMed]
50. Gurney, A.; Axelrod, F.; Bond, C.J.; Cain, J.; Chartier, C.; Donigan, L.; Fischer, M.; Chaudhari, A.; Ji, M.; Kapoun, A.M.; et al. Wnt pathway inhibition via the targeting of Frizzled receptors results in decreased growth and tumorigenicity of human tumors. *Proc. Natl. Acad. Sci. USA* **2012**, *109*, 11717–11722. [CrossRef]
51. Li, C.; Yang, M.; Wang, X.; Zhang, H.; Yao, C.; Sun, S.; Liu, Q.; Pan, H.; Liu, S.; Huan, Y.; et al. Glutazumab, a novel long-lasting GLP-1/anti-GLP-1R antibody fusion protein, exerts anti-diabetic effects through targeting dual receptor binding sites. *Biochem. Pharmacol.* **2018**, *150*, 46–53. [CrossRef] [PubMed]
52. Yan, H.; Gu, W.; Yang, J.; Bi, V.; Shen, Y.; Lee, E.; Winters, K.A.; Komorowski, R.; Zhang, C.; Patel, J.J.; et al. Fully human monoclonal antibodies antagonizing the glucagon receptor improve glucose homeostasis in mice and monkeys. *J. Pharmacol. Exp. Ther.* **2009**, *329*, 102–111. [CrossRef]
53. Pettus, J.; Reeds, D.; Cavaiola, T.S.; Boeder, S.; Levin, M.; Tobin, G.; Cava, E.; Thai, D.; Shi, J.; Yan, H.; et al. Effect of a glucagon receptor antibody (REMD-477) in type 1 diabetes: A randomized controlled trial. *Diabetes Obes. Metab.* **2018**, *20*, 1302–1305. [CrossRef]
54. Gilbert, J.; Lekstrom-Himes, J.; Donaldson, D.; Lee, Y.; Hu, M.; Xu, J.; Wyant, T.; Davidson, M.; MLN1202 Study Group. Effect of CC chemokine receptor 2 CCR2 blockade on serum C-reactive protein in individuals at atherosclerotic risk and with a single nucleotide polymorphism of the monocyte chemoattractant protein-1 promoter region. *Am. J. Cardiol.* **2011**, *107*, 906–911. [CrossRef]

55. Olson, W.C.; Rabut, G.E.; Nagashima, K.A.; Tran, D.N.; Anselma, D.J.; Monard, S.P.; Segal, J.P.; Thompson, D.A.; Kajumo, F.; Guo, Y.; et al. Differential inhibition of human immunodeficiency virus type 1 fusion, gp120 binding, and CC-chemokine activity by monoclonal antibodies to CCR5. *J. Virol.* **1999**, *73*, 4145–4155. [CrossRef] [PubMed]
56. Kuhne, M.R.; Mulvey, T.; Belanger, B.; Chen, S.; Pan, C.; Chong, C.; Cao, F.; Niekro, W.; Kempe, T.; Henning, K.A.; et al. BMS-936564/MDX-1338: A fully human anti-CXCR4 antibody induces apoptosis in vitro and shows antitumor activity in vivo in hematologic malignancies. *Clin. Cancer Res.* **2013**, *19*, 357–366. [CrossRef] [PubMed]
57. Massard, C.; Cassier, P.; Bendell, J.C.; Marie, D.B.; Blery, M.; Morehouse, C.; Ascierto, M.; Zerbib, R.; Mitry, E.; Tolcher, A.W. 1203P—Preliminary results of STELLAR-001, a dose escalation phase I study of the anti-C5aR, IPH5401, in combination with durvalumab in advanced solid tumours. *Ann. Oncol.* **2019**, *30*, v492. [CrossRef]
58. Zhang, C.; Jing, S.; Zhang, H.; Wang, X.; Chenjiang, Y.A.O. Antibody Specifically Binding to GLP-1 R and Fusion Protein thereof with GLP-1 Patent. U.S. Patent 10,059,773, 28 August 2018.
59. Trkola, A.; Ketas, T.J.; Nagashima, K.A.; Zhao, L.; Cilliers, T.; Morris, L.; Moore, J.P.; Maddon, P.J.; Olson, W.C. Potent, broad-spectrum inhibition of human immunodeficiency virus type 1 by the CCR5 monoclonal antibody PRO 140. *J. Virol.* **2001**, *75*, 579–588. [CrossRef]
60. Lee, K.; Jung, Y.; Lee, J.Y.; Lee, W.K.; Lim, D.; Yu, Y.G. Purification and characterization of recombinant human endothelin receptor type A. *Protein Expr. Purif.* **2012**, *84*, 14–18. [CrossRef]
61. Corin, K.; Baaske, P.; Ravel, D.B.; Song, J.; Brown, E.; Wang, X.; Geissler, S.; Wienken, C.J.; Jerabek-Willemsen, M.; Duhr, S.; et al. A robust and rapid method of producing soluble, stable, and functional G-protein coupled receptors. *PLoS ONE* **2011**, *6*, e23036.
62. Sarkar, C.A.; Dodevski, I.; Kenig, M.; Dudli, S.; Mohr, A.; Hermans, E.; Pluckthun, A. Directed evolution of a G protein-coupled receptor for expression, stability, and binding selectivity. *Proc. Natl. Acad. Sci. USA* **2008**, *105*, 14808–14813. [CrossRef] [PubMed]
63. Link, A.J.; Skretas, G.; Strauch, E.M.; Chari, N.S.; Georgiou, G. Efficient production of membrane-integrated and detergent-soluble G protein-coupled receptors in Escherichia coli. *Protein Sci.* **2008**, *17*, 1857–1863. [CrossRef]
64. Vukoti, K.; Kimura, T.; Macke, L.; Gawrisch, K.; Yeliseev, A. Stabilization of functional recombinant cannabinoid receptor CB(2) in detergent micelles and lipid bilayers. *PLoS ONE* **2012**, *7*, e46290.
65. Liu, S.; Wang, S.; Lu, S. DNA immunization as a technology platform for monoclonal antibody induction. *Emerg. Microbes Infect.* **2016**, *5*, 1–12. [CrossRef]
66. Van der Woning, B.; De Boeck, G.; Blanchetot, C.; Bobkov, V.; Klarenbeek, A.; Saunders, M.; Waelbroeck, M.; Laeremans, T.; Steyaert, J.; Hultberg, A.; et al. DNA immunization combined with scFv phage display identifies antagonistic GCGR specific antibodies and reveals new epitopes on the small extracellular loops. In *MAbs*; Taylor & Francis: Abingdon, UK, 2016; Volume 8, pp. 1126–1135. [CrossRef]
67. Heimann, A.S.; Gupta, A.; Gomes, I.; Rayees, R.; Schlessinger, A.; Ferro, E.S.; Unterwald, E.M.; Devi, L.A. Generation of G protein-coupled receptor antibodies differentially sensitive to conformational states. *PLoS ONE* **2017**, *12*, e0187306. [CrossRef]
68. Boshuizen, R.S.; Marsden, C.; Turkstra, J.; Rossant, C.J.; Slootstra, J.; Copley, C.; Schwamborn, K. A combination of in vitro techniques for efficient discovery of functional monoclonal antibodies against human CXC chemokine receptor-2 (CXCR2). In *MAbs*; Taylor & Francis: Abingdon, UK, 2014; Volume 6, pp. 1415–1424. [CrossRef]
69. Kushnir, N.; Streatfield, S.J.; Yusibov, V. Virus-like particles as a highly efficient vaccine platform: Diversity of targets and production systems and advances in clinical development. *Vaccine* **2012**, *31*, 58–83. [CrossRef]
70. O'Rourke, J.P.; Peabody, D.S.; Chackerian, B. Affinity selection of epitope-based vaccines using a bacteriophage virus-like particle platform. *Curr. Opin. Virol.* **2015**, *11*, 76–82. [CrossRef]
71. Ho, T.T.; Nguyen, J.T.; Liu, J.; Stanczak, P.; Thompson, A.A.; Yan, Y.G.; Chen, J.; Allerston, C.K.; Dillard, C.L.; Xu, H.; et al. Method for rapid optimization of recombinant GPCR protein expression and stability using virus-like particles. *Protein Expr. Purif.* **2017**, *133*, 41–49. [CrossRef]
72. Rouck, J.E.; Krapf, J.E.; Roy, J.; Huff, H.C.; Das, A. Recent advances in nanodisc technology for membrane protein studies (2012–2017). *FEBS Lett.* **2017**, *591*, 2057–2088. [CrossRef]
73. Denisov, I.G.; Sligar, S.G. Nanodiscs in Membrane Biochemistry and Biophysics. *Chem. Rev.* **2017**, *117*, 4669–4713. [CrossRef]

74. Kretz-Rommel, A.; Shi, L.; Ferrini, R.; Yang, T.; Xu, F.; Campion, B. Antibodies That Bind Human Cannabinoid 1 (CB1) Receptor. U.S. Patent 16/257,511, 17 October 2019.
75. Mallat, A.; Lotersztajn, S. Endocannabinoids and liver disease. I. Endocannabinoids and their receptors in the liver. *Am. J. Physiol. Gastrointest. Liver Physiol.* **2008**, *294*, G9–G12. [CrossRef]
76. Di Marzo, V. Targeting the endocannabinoid system: To enhance or reduce? *Nat. Rev. Drug Discov.* **2008**, *7*, 438–455. [CrossRef] [PubMed]
77. Osei-Hyiaman, D.; DePetrillo, M.; Pacher, P.; Liu, J.; Radaeva, S.; Bátkai, S.; Harvey-White, J.; Mackie, K.; Offertáler, L.; Wang, L.; et al. Endocannabinoid activation at hepatic CB1 receptors stimulates fatty acid synthesis and contributes to diet-induced obesity. *J. Clin. Investig.* **2005**, *115*, 1298–1305. [CrossRef]
78. Dodd, R.B.; Wilkinson, T.; Schofield, D.J. Therapeutic Monoclonal Antibodies to Complex Membrane Protein Targets: Antigen Generation and Antibody Discovery Strategies. *Biodrugs* **2018**, *32*, 339–355. [CrossRef] [PubMed]

International Journal of
Molecular Sciences

MDPI

Review

Targeted Molecular Therapeutics for Bladder Cancer—A New Option beyond the Mixed Fortunes of Immune Checkpoint Inhibitors?

Olga Bednova [1] **and Jeffrey V. Leyton** [1,2,*]

[1] Departément de Medécine Nucléaire et Radiobiologie, Faculté de Medécine et des Sciences de la Santé, Université de Sherbrooke, Sherbrooke, QC J1H5N4, Canada; olga.bednova@usherbrooke.ca

[2] Centre d'Imagerie Moleculaire, Centre de Rechcerche, Centre Hospitalier Universitaire de Sherbrooke (CHUS), Sherbrooke, QC J1H5N4, Canada

[*] Correspondence: jeffrey.leyton@usherbrooke.ca; Tel.: +1-819-346-1110

Received: 24 August 2020; Accepted: 30 September 2020; Published: 1 October 2020

Abstract: The fact that there are now five immune checkpoint inhibitor (ICI) monoclonal antibodies approved since 2016 that target programmed cell death protein 1 or programmed death ligand-1 for the treatment of metastatic and refractory bladder cancer is an outstanding achievement. Although patients can display pronounced responses that extend survival when treated with ICIs, the main benefit of these drugs compared to traditional chemotherapy is that they are better tolerated and result in reduced adverse events (AEs). Unfortunately, response rates to ICI treatment are relatively low and, these drugs are expensive and have a high economic burden. As a result, their clinical efficacy/cost-value relationship is debated. Long sought after targeted molecular therapeutics have now emerged and are boasting impressive response rates in heavily pre-treated, including ICI treated, patients with metastatic bladder cancer. The antibody-drug conjugates (ADCs) enfortumab vedotin (EV) and sacituzumab govitecan (SG) have demonstrated the ability to provide objective response rates (ORRs) of 44% and 31% in patients with bladder tumor cells that express Nectin-4 and Trop-2, respectively. As a result, EV was approved by the U.S. Food and Drug Administration for the treatment of patients with advanced or metastatic bladder cancer who have previously received ICI and platinum-containing chemotherapy. SG has been granted fast track designation. The small molecule Erdafitinib was recently approved for the treatment of patients with advanced or metastatic bladder cancer with genetic alterations in fibroblast growth factor receptors that have previously been treated with a platinum-containing chemotherapy. Erdafitinib achieved an ORR of 40% in patients including a proportion who had previously received ICI therapy. In addition, these targeted drugs are sufficiently tolerated or AEs can be appropriately managed. Hence, the early performance in clinical effectiveness of these targeted drugs are substantially increased relative to ICIs. In this article, the most up to date follow-ups on treatment efficacy and AEs of the ICIs and targeted therapeutics are described. In addition, drug price and cost-effectiveness are described. For best overall value taking into account clinical effectiveness, price and cost-effectiveness, results favor avelumab and atezolizumab for ICIs. Although therapeutically promising, it is too early to determine if the described targeted therapeutics provide the best overall value as cost-effectiveness analyses have yet to be performed and long-term follow-ups are needed. Nonetheless, with the arrival of targeted molecular therapeutics and their increased effectiveness relative to ICIs, creates a potential novel paradigm based on 'targeting' for affecting clinical practice for metastatic bladder cancer treatment.

Keywords: bladder cancer; antibodies; immune checkpoint inhibitors; antibody-drug conjugates; sacituzumab govitecan; enfortumab vedotin; erdafitinib; cost-effectiveness

1. Introduction

Urothelial cancer typically arises from the transitional cells in the urothelium of the bladder, renal pelvis, ureter, and urethra and is commonly referred to as bladder cancer. According to the World Health Organization, bladder cancer represents the 10th most diagnosed and 13th most deadly malignancy worldwide [1]. Bladder cancer is a particular challenge to treat as it is most frequent (>50%) within the elderly and these patients often have underlying comorbidities and reduced functional status [2]. Bladder cancer is a heterogeneous disease, with 70% of cases diagnosed with superficial (non-invasive) tumors and 20% and 10% present as muscle-invasive bladder cancer (MIBC) and metastatic disease, respectively [3]. Importantly, 50–70% of superficial tumors will recur and 10–20% will progress to MIBC [3]. Despite therapy, MIBC progresses to incurable metastatic disease in about half of cases [4]. Cisplatin-containing chemotherapy regimens are the current standard-of-care for the treatment of metastatic bladder cancer. Unfortunately, the 5-year survival rate of metastatic patients treated with regimens consisting of cisplatin plus gemcitabine and methotrexate/vinblastine/doxorubicin/cisplatin is poor [5]. Chemotherapy is also related to high toxicity and has caused adverse events (AEs) of grade ≥3 in up to 82% of cases [6]. In addition, treatment related death occurs in 3–4% of cases [7]. Due to the frailty of many elderly patients, there are significant proportions of cases that are ineligible for platinum-containing chemotherapy. In these patients, carboplatin-based regimens are typically used. However, carboplatin-based chemotherapy is considered limited as the overall survival (OS) rate for these patients is approximately 9 months [5,8]. Patients who relapse after platinum-containing chemotherapy and are treated with second-line chemotherapy, have even more limited responses and poor survival [9,10]. Thus, there are unmet needs for effective and tolerable therapies for patients that are cisplatin-ineligible or for those with metastatic tumor recurrences after receiving platinum-containing chemotherapy.

In concept, precision-based therapy is the systemic administration of a drug that specifically targets tumors and, as a result, reduces nonspecific toxicities while maximizing tumor killing. Although the paradigm of targeted therapeutics has been effective and part of the standard of care for certain tumor types, it has been a challenge to accomplish in the clinic for bladder cancer [11–13]. The inability of targeted therapeutics to provide patients with robust patient responses or significant responses relative to chemotherapy is the major reason why chemotherapy has been the primary option for systemically treating advanced or metastatic bladder cancer for the past three decades, until the approval of immunotherapy and targeted therapeutics starting in 2016.

The advent of immunotherapies in the form of immune checkpoint inhibitors (ICIs), which are monoclonal antibodies (mAbs) that target specific factors that regulate the immune response, has dramatically changed the landscape of bladder cancer treatment. In general, ICIs work well—but only for a minority of patients providing them with long-lasting immunologic memory [14]. However, the majority of patients treated with ICIs fail to ever respond, and those that initially respond eventually develop resistance and disease progression. Unlike targeted therapeutics, there remains no predictive molecular biomarker to determine the patients who are most likely to benefit from ICI therapy.

In other tumor types, ICIs have been incredibly successful and have helped patients who have previously received not only traditional chemotherapy, but also targeted therapies [15–17]. A unique aspect of bladder cancer, ICIs have provided benefit in a tumor type where targeted therapy is inexistent. Bladder cancer is a unique case study because it is now targeted therapies that are coming to the rescue of patients who have previously received ICIs. Many of the ICIs have now provided results with follow-up periods that provide data with increased insight on important phase II/III trials. Thus, we provide a timely analysis of the latest clinical effectiveness of the five ICIs that are currently approved by the U.S. Food and Drug Administration (FDA). We also describe AEs, drug price, and cost-effectiveness in order to integrate important health economic insight. We found that, with some exceptions, the clinical effectiveness of ICIs is marginal and if it is worth paying a high price is justifiably questionable. In essence, the current paradigm of ICIs for bladder cancer is somewhat of a mixed fortune.

In contrast, our review of the key trials for the targeted therapeutics enfortumab vedotin (EV), sacituzumab govitecan (SG), and erdafitinib show these agents are proving more effective than the current ICIs. EV and erdafitinib are (SG has only fast track designation) approved and now available. However, the cost of these targeted therapeutics is significantly more expensive, than the already high cost of ICIs. We also caution that these clinical results are early. This review hopes to provide clinicians and patients with the up-to-date facts in order to help decide on the best-value option for treating patients with advanced or metastatic bladder cancer. The approval process timeline is shown in Figure 1.

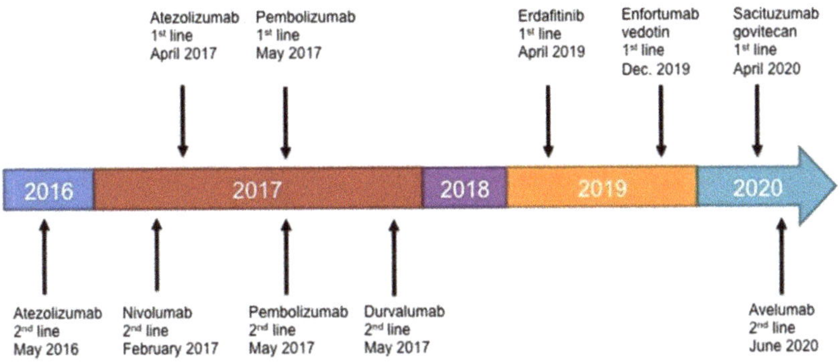

Figure 1. FDA approval timeline for ICIs, EV, and Erdafitinib against bladder cancer.

2. Up-to-Date Clinical Benefit of the Current ICI Paradigm

The five approved ICI mAbs target either programmed cell death protein 1 (PD-1) or programmed death ligand-1 (PD-L1). The rationale for targeting the PD-1/PD-L1 axis with mAbs is multi-fold. First, blocking the interaction of PD-1 and PD-L1 increases the likelihood that the immune system, if active against malignant cells, remains active. Second, levels of PD-L1 expression have been shown to correlate with bladder cancer aggressiveness and outcome. Third, the tumor mutation burden (TMB) is high, which suggests that ICIs could have significant clinical impact because of a greater T-cell-mediated antitumor immune response elicited by invasive bladder cancer [18]. Briefly, the TMB is defined as the total number of somatic mutations per DNA megabase. A thorough review on the evolution of the PD-1/PD-L1 axis in bladder cancer is reviewed in Bellmunt et al. [19].

Approvals were based on key endpoints such as objective response rate (ORR), OS and, duration of response (DOR) for locally advanced or metastatic bladder cancer. We highlight the most up-to-date clinically relevant information. AEs were also important parameters and, closely monitored and are described in a focused subsequent section.

2.1. *Atezolizumab (Tecentriq; Genentech; South San Francisco, CA, USA)*

2.1.1. IMvigor210 Trial Cohort 2

On 18 May 2016, the FDA granted accelerated approval to atezolizumab, a PD-L1-targeting mAb, for use in patients with bladder cancer with locally advanced or metastatic bladder cancer who have disease progression during or following platinum-containing chemotherapy or within 12 months of receiving neoadjuvant or adjuvant platinum-containing chemotherapy [20]. Approval was based on this single-arm phase II trial. This cohort contained 310 patients with inoperable locally advanced or metastatic bladder cancer that had previously received cisplatin-containing chemotherapy [21]. Immunohistochemistry (IHC) staining evaluated the number of PD-L1-positive tumor-infiltrating immune cells (IC) and categorized patients into IC0, IC1, or IC2/3 groups. IC0, IC1, IC2, and IC3 scoring was proportional to tumors containing <1%, ≥1% and <5%, ≥5% and <10%, and ≥10% ICs within a given microscopic field of view, respectively. This PD-L1 scoring system was determined using the diagnostic assay SP142 (Ventana Medical Systems Inc. Tucson, AZ, USA). The scoring method first identifies a defined tumor area that contains at least 50 viable tumor cells [22]. For example, a score of IC3 is given when a tumor tissue shows either ≥50% of tumor cells that stain for PD-L1 or ≥10% of the tumor area is occupied with ICs that stain for PD-L1 [22]. Thus, PD-L1 scoring can be determined solely by the percentage of tumor cells or ICs that express PD-L1 and a combined score is not taken into account. The scoring for atezolizumab in patients with bladder cancer was reliant on ICs and not on tumor cells [21].

At the initial follow-up time of 11.7 months, the ORRs were 26% (95% CI, 18–36%) in the IC2/3 group, 18% (95% CI, 13–24%) in the IC1 and IC2/3 combined group, and 15% (95% CI, 11–19%) in all patients [21]. There were ongoing responses in 85% of responding patients and the median DOR was not reached (2.0–13.7 months). The median OS was 11.4 months (95% CI, 9.0—not reached) in the IC2/3 group, 8.8 months (95% CI, 7.1–10.6) for the combined IC1 and IC2/3 groups, and 7.9 months (95%, 6.6–9.3) in all patients. At the median follow-up of 33 months, the median ORR, OS, and DOR were 16%, 7.9 months, and 24.8 months (Table 1).

Table 1. Updated clinical trial ORR, OS, and DOR for ICIs and targeted agents as monotherapies.

ICIs	Trial and Updated (Ref)	ORR (95% CI)	OS (95% CI; Months)	DOR (95% CI; Months)
Atezolizumab [1]	IMvigor210 Phase II [23] June 2018	Cohort 1: 24% Cohort 2: 16%	16.2 (10.4–24.5) 7.9 (6.7–9.3)	NR (30.4-NR) 24.8 (13.8–30.4)
Atezolizumab [2]	IMvigor211 Phase III [24] December 2017	13.4%	8.6 (7.8–9.6)	21.7 (13.0–21.7)
Atezolizumab [3]	IMvigor130 Phase III [25] May 2020	23%	15.7 (13.1–17.8)	NR (15.9-NR)
Pembrolizumab [1]	KEYNOTE-045 Phase III [26,27] September 2019	21.1%	10.1 (8.0–12.3)	29.7 (1.6–42.7)
Pembrolizumab [2]	KEYNOTE-052 Phase II [28] June 2020	28.6%	11.3 (9.7–13.1)	30.1 (18.1-NR)
Nivolumab	CheckMate 275 Phase II [29] June 2020	20.7%	8.6 (6.1–11.3)	20.3 (11.5–31.3)
Durvalumab	Study 1108 Phase I/II [30,31] July 2018	17.8%	10.5 (6.9–15.7)	NR (2.7–25.7+)
Avelumab	JAVELIN Bladder 100 Phase III [32] June 2020	17%	21.4 (18.9–26.1) [33]	NR (10.5-NR)
ADCs				
Enfortumab vedotin [4]	EV-201 Phase II [34] July 2019	44%	11.7 (9.1-NR)	7.6 (1.0–11.3)
Sacituzumab govitecan [4,5]	IMMU-132 Phase I/II [35] February 2019	31%	18.9	12.6 (7.5–24.0)
Small molecule				
Erdafitinib [4,6]	BLC2001 Phase II [36] July 2019	40%	13.8 (9.8-NR)	5.6 (4.2–7.2)

ICIs = Immune checkpoint inhibitor; ADCs = Antibody-drug conjugates; ORR = Objective response rate; OS = Median overall survival; DOR = Median duration of response; NR = Not reached. [1] For first-line treatment (cisplatin-ineligible). [2] For second-line treatment. [3] For first-line treatment (cisplatin-eligible). [4] Patient population included those who had previously received ICI therapy. [5] Not approved. Has been granted fast track designation by the FDA. [6] For patients with prespecified *FGFR* alterations.

2.1.2. IMvigor 210 Trial Cohort 1

On 17 April 2017, the FDA granted accelerated approval for atezolizumab in patients who are cisplatin-ineligible. This cohort consisted of 119 patients with a median age of 73 years old. The most common reason for cisplatin ineligibility was impaired kidney function. At a median follow-up time of 14.2 months the ORR was 23.5% (95% CI, 16.2–32.2%) in all treated patients [23]. Based on PD-L1 status, the ORRs were 28% (95% CI, 14–47%) and 21% (95% CI, 10–35%) for PD-L1 expression of ≥5% and <5% groups, respectively. The DOR was not reached in either subgroup. Responses were ongoing for 82% and 29% of responding patients at 5 months and 1 year, respectively. At the median follow-up of 29 months, the median ORR, OS, and DOR were 24%, 16.2 months, and not reached (95% CI: 30.4—N) (Table 1).

2.1.3. IMvigor211 Trial

The phase III IMvigor211 trial compared atezolizumab with physician's choice of chemotherapy in patients with metastatic bladder cancer who had progressed after platinum-containing chemotherapy [24]. Again, patients were stratified based on PD-L1 expression. Unfortunately, patients with the greatest relative PD-L1 expression did not significantly survive longer when treated with atezolizumab (11.1 months) relative to chemotherapy (10.6 (8.4–12.2) months) [24]. There was also no significant difference in ORR. Thus, other patient cohorts were not evaluated. The most recent results are listed in Table 1.

2.1.4. IMvigor130 Trial

This randomized trial enrolled 1213 patients with locally advanced or metastatic bladder cancer who were newly diagnosed or had received neoadjuvant or adjuvant chemotherapy more than 12 months prior to commencement of atezolizumab treatment [25]. The goal was to determine the therapeutic effectiveness of atezolizumab alone or in combination with chemotherapy versus chemotherapy alone. In addition, patients were stratified by PD-L1 status as previously described. Chemotherapy was gemcitabine with cisplatin and carboplatin for cisplatin-eligible and cisplatin-ineligible patients, respectively. Although cisplatin-ineligible patients were only originally recruited, the trial was amended to include cisplatin-eligible patients. Cisplatin-ineligible and eligible patients were randomized into three treatment arms: group A—atezolizumab plus open-label chemotherapy, group B—open-label atezolizumab monotherapy, or group C—masked placebo plus open-label chemotherapy. The two primary efficacy endpoints were OS and progression-free survival (PFS).

The most up-to-date results of the trial as reported by Galsky et al., did not statistically show that atezolizumab improved OS in all intention-to-treat patients [25]. The proportions (53–58%) of cisplatin-ineligible patients were similar among the three groups. At the median follow-up at 11.8 (6.1–17.2) months, the median OS among groups A and C were 16.0 (13.9–18.9) and 13.1 (11.7–15.1) months, respectively. This result did not cross the prespecified interim efficacy boundary for statistical significance. Group A did meet the co-primary PFS endpoint. Patients in group A had a statistically significant increased PFS of 8.2 (95% CI, 6.5–8.3) months. In contrast, patients in group C had a PFS of 6.3 (95% CI, 6.2–7.0) months. Unfortunately, the ORR for groups A and C were similar (47% (95% CI, 43–52%) and 44% (95% CI, 39–49%), respectively).

When evaluating atezolizumab alone versus chemotherapy alone, the results were not favorable. In all patients, the OS values for atezolizumab and chemotherapy alone were 15.7 (13.1–17.8) and 13.1 (11.7–15.1) months, respectively. Although significance for OS between groups B and C were not tested, the survival curves appear to show marginal benefit with atezolizumab alone. The median ORR for group B was 23% (95% CI, 19–28%), which was much lower than the previously described ORR values for groups A and C. The PFS was not reported.

For PD-L1 subgroups, atezolizumab alone and atezolizumab plus chemotherapy improved OS relative to chemotherapy alone in patients with PD-L1 expression IC2/3. The OS for the patients treated with atezolizumab and chemotherapy was 23.6 months versus 15.9 months for chemotherapy alone. The OS for the patients treated with atezolizumab alone was not estimable (17.7—not estimable) versus 17.8 (10.0—not estimable) months for chemotherapy alone. There were no survival advantages for both groups A and B relative to C in patients with PD-L1 expression scores of IC0 or IC1. Although OS was improved ORR was not. In patients with PD-L1 IC2/3 treated with atezolizumab or chemotherapy alone were 34% (95% CI, 28–50%) and 37% (95% CI, 33–55%), respectively.

IMvigor130 group B and IMvigor210 cohort 1 were the key trials that demonstrated a decreased response among patients with a PD-L1 status of <5% (i.e., IC0/1) when treated with atezolizumab alone, versus patients with the same PD-L1 status but who received cisplatin- or carboplatin-containing chemotherapy alone. Based on these results the FDA and the European Medicines Agency revised the indication for atezolizumab. Atezolizumab is now restricted for use in patients with locally advanced or metastatic bladder cancer who (i) are not eligible for cisplatin-containing chemotherapy, and whose tumors express PD-L1 ≥5% (based on the Ventana assay) and, (ii) are not eligible for any platinum-containing therapy regardless of PD-L1 status [37,38]. Notably, because atezolizumab did not reach its endpoints in the IMvigor211 trial, it is not indicated for cisplatin-eligible patients in the first-line regardless of PD-L1 tumor status.

2.2. *Pembrolizimab (Keytruda; Merck; Kenilworth, NJ, USA)*

2.2.1. KEYNOTE-045 Trial

On 18 May 2017, the FDA granted accelerated approval to pembrolizumab, a PD-1-targeting mAb, for use in patients with bladder cancer who have either received platinum-containing chemotherapy or who are cisplatin-ineligible [39]. The phase III KEYNOTE-045 clinical trial enrolled patients with advanced or metastatic bladder cancer previously treated with any platinum-containing chemotherapy [40]. Patients (542) were randomly assigned to receive pembrolizumab or the investigator's choice of chemotherapy containing paclitaxel, docetaxel, or vinflunine. PD-L1 expression status was assessed using the Agilent PD-L1 IHC22C3 pharmDx assay. PD-L1 expression scores were defined as a 'tumor proportion score' (TPS), which is defined as the combined positive score determined from the percentage of PD-L1-expressing tumor cells and ICs relative to the total number of tumor cells. TPS values of <1%, 1–49%, ≥50% corresponding to PD-L1 expression of no expression, 'positive' expression, and 'high' expression [41].

In all patients treated with pembrolizumab the ORR was 21.1% (95% CI, 16.4–26.4%). In contrast patients treated with chemotherapy the ORR was 11.4% (95% CI, 7.9–15.8%). Pembrolizumab treatment also extended the median OS to 10.3 months (95% CI, 8.0–11.8). In comparison, the OS for patients in the chemotherapy-alone group was 7.4 (95% CI, 6.1–8.3) months. When focusing on patients whose tumor biopsies had a TPS ≥ 10%, the median OS was 8.0 (95% CI, 5.0–12.3) months compared to 5.2 (95% CI, 4.0–7.4) months for chemotherapy alone. The ORRs for the PD-L1-positive and chemotherapy alone groups were 21.6% (95% CI, 12.9–32.7%) and 6.7% (95% CI, 2.5–13.9%). Hence, there was a significant therapeutic response advantage for patients whose tumors with PD-L1 TPS ≥ 10%.

Necchi et al. and Fradet et al., recently reported the most up-to-date follow-ups of the KEYNOTE-045 trial [26,27]. The median ORR, OS, and DOR values were 21.1%, 10.1, and 29.7 months for patients treated with pembrolizumab (Table 1). In comparison, the updated median ORR, DOR, and OS values for patients in the chemotherapy group were 11%, 7.3, and 4.4 months [26]. In contrast to the earlier reported findings, patients with PD-L1 tumor TPS ≥ 10 had a lower ORR (20.3%) compared to all patients. When the effectiveness of both pembrolizumab and chemotherapy were evaluated in patients who did respond to treatment, the OS increased to 39.6 versus 17.7 months, respectively. This indicated that in patients who had been heavily pretreated with prior platinum-containing chemotherapy, have a clear increased benefit by being treated with pembrolizumab versus chemotherapy, and if responding to pembrolizumab, can survive out to >3-years. However, benefit from pembrolizumab appeared to be independent of PD-L1 expression status [40].

2.2.2. KEYNOTE-052 Trial

This phase II trial was a single-arm study designed to evaluate the efficacy of pembrolizumab in patients (370) with advanced bladder cancer who were ineligible for cisplatin-containing chemotherapy [42]. The up-to-date ORR in all treated patients was 28.6% (95% CI, 24.1–33.5%) (Table 1). Responses remained ongoing in 84% of patients. Patients in the PD-L1-high expression subgroup responded better to pembrolizumab compared to the PD-L1-low subgroup. Specifically, the ORR was 47% (95% CI, 38–57%) and 21% (95%, 16–26%) in patients with PD-L1 expression TPS $\geq$ 10 and <10, respectively. The median DOR for both subgroups was not reached. Among all responding patients, 52% and 7% continued responding at 6 months and at 1 year. Thus, these results strengthen the use of pembrolizumab in the first-line setting for cisplatin-ineligible patients with locally advanced and unresectable or metastatic bladder cancer.

2.2.3. KEYNOTE-361 Trial

This current phase III trial (NCT02853305) is a randomized evaluation to verify the first-line effectiveness of pembrolizumab from the KEYNOTE-052 trial. Patients were stratified by their tumors either having ≥10 or <10 PD-L1 score. Unfortunately, pembrolizumab did not meet its two primary endpoints of OS or PFS [43]. As of 9 June 2020, patients receiving pembrolizumab and whose tumors were PD-L1-low had decreased survival compared to patients receiving cisplatin- or carboplatin-containing chemotherapy. We have not found any reports providing additional information on other patient cohorts.

Based on KEYNOTE-052 and KEYNOTE-361 results, the FDA issued an alert to health care professionals and oncology clinical investigators due to the substantial uncertainty concerning efficacy as a monotherapy to treat bladder cancer patients whose tumor express low (TPS < 10%) amounts of PD-L1 [44]. Cisplatin-ineligible patients should receive pembrolizumab only if their tumors express PD-L1 TPS $\geq$ 10. However, if patients are not eligible for any platinum containing chemotherapy, pembrolizumab can be used regardless of PD-L1 tumor status.

2.3. *Nivolumab (Opdivo; Bristol-Myers Squibb; New York, NY, USA)*

Checkmate 275 Trial

Nivolumab is a PD-1 blocking mAb that was approved in 2017 based on its performance in the multicenter, single-arm phase II Checkmate 275 clinical trial [45,46]. The trial evaluated Nivolumab in 270 patients with metastatic or surgically unresectable locally advanced bladder cancer, or with progression or recurrence after at least one platinum-based regimen, or within 12 months of perioperative platinum treatment for muscle-invasive disease. [46] PD-L1 expression was assessed using the Dako PD-L1 IHC 28-8 pharmDx kit [47]. PD-L1-positive staining is defined as complete and/or partial plasma membrane staining of tumor cells at any intensity. A minimum number of 100 viable tumor cells should be present in the PD-L1 stained tumor slide. Notably, infiltrating ICs that may stain positive for PD-L1 are not included in the scoring for the determination of PD-L1 positivity.

At the median follow-up of 7 (3.0–8.8) months, nivolumab treatment resulted in an ORR of 19.6%, (95% CI, 15.0–24.9%). Regarding, PD-L1 status: PD-L1 expression scores of ≥5%, ≥1% and <5%, and <1% of tumor cells, ORR values were 24.8% (95% CI, 18.9–39.5%), 23.8% (95% CI, 16.5–32.3%) and 16.1% (95% CI, 10.5–23.1%) respectively. The median OS was 8.7 months (95% CI, 6.1 to not reached) in the overall population, 11.3 (8.7 to not reached) months in the patients with PD-L1 expression of ≥1% and 6.0 (95% CI, 4.3–8.1%) months in patients with tumors with low PD-L1 expression of <1%. DOR was not reached (7.4—NR) in all patients at the moment of the publication of these results.

Based on these results, the FDA granted accelerated approval to durvalumab for the treatment of patients with locally advanced or metastatic bladder cancer who have disease progression during or following platinum-containing chemotherapy or have disease progression within 12 months of neoadjuvant or adjuvant treatment with platinum-based chemotherapy [45].

The most recent follow-up reported in Galsky et al., reported on the effectiveness of nivolumab [29]. At 33.7 months minimum follow-up, the ORR was 20.7% (Table 1), with complete responses in 6.7% of patients. Importantly, when the efficacy of nivolumab was evaluated in patients whose PD-L1 status was either <1% (n = 146) or ≥1% (n = 124), the ORR values were 16.4% (95% CI, 10.8–23.5%) and 25.8% (95% CI, 18.4–34.4%), respectively. When PD-L1 expression was evaluated at <5% (n = 187) and ≥5% (n = 83) the ORR values were 16.0% (95% CI, 11.1–22.1%) and 31.3% (95% CI, 21.6–42.4%), respectively. Out of the responding population, 73.2% (41/56) and 58.9% (33/56) had responses lasting ≥6- and ≥12-months, respectively. At the time of the evaluation, 25% of patients had ongoing responses.

Importantly, TMB was an important factor for successful patient response. A 'high' TMB was defined as ≥170 mutations per tumor. Low and medium TMB was defined as <85 and 85–169 mutations per tumor, respectively. Cox proportional hazards regression models were used to assess the dependence of PFS and OS on TMB alone and in combination with PD-L1 scoring. The ORR was 13.0%, 19.6%, and 31.9% in patients with low, medium, and high TMBs. High TMB tumors showed a positive association with ORR (odds ratio (95% CI): 2.13 (1.26–3.60), $p < 0.05$) regardless of PD-L1 scoring. However, futher evaluation including sufficiently large numbers of patients will be needed to determine the nuances if there is a benefit in ORR with subgroups evaluating combinations of low, medium, high TMB ≥1% and <1% PD-L1. PFS and OS were longer in patients with high TMB values compared to low and medium TMB tumors. Interestingly, when TMB was analyzed in combination with PD-L1 status there were diverging trends with PFS and OS. For PFS, there was approximately a 1 month increase in patients with ≥1% PD-L1 with tumors that were both low and high TMB. However, patients with ≥1% PD-L1 had poorer OS compared to patients with <1% PD-L1 for low, medium, and high TMB.

This study at almost 3-years of minimum follow-up indicated that nivolumab is not only effective for treating metastatic bladder cancer, but high TMB was strongly associated with improved outcomes relative to all treated patients. Moreover, TMB and PD-L1 could be used in combination as biomarkers for predicting PFS and OS. As a result this study is the first to show for ICI treatment of bladder cancer, TMB may prove a superior biomarker than PD-L1. For example, patients can be grouped into low, medium, and high TMB levels as opposed to the 1% cutoff for PD-L1.

2.4. Durvalumab (Imfinzi; AstraZeneca;Cambridge, United Kingdom)

2.4.1. Trial

Durvalumab is a human mAb that binds PD-L1 and also provided encouraging results on clinical response with respect to the tumor expression status of PD-L1 and was approved in 2017. The phase I/II 1108 trial evaluated patients who had received prior platinum-based chemotherapy [48]. At the median follow-up time point of 4.3 months, the ORR was 31% (95% CI, 17.6–47.1%) in all patients. PD-L1 expression was performed using the Ventana PD-L1 (SP263) assay. The proportion of tumor cells with PD-L1 membrane staining was partitioned based on defined intervals of <1%, 1–4%, 5–9%, 10–14%, ... , 90–99%, 100%. [49] Strikingly, patients in the PD-L1-positive cohort, defined as ≥25%, had an ORR of 46.4% (95% CI, 27.5–66.1%). In contrast, patients with a score of <25% were considered as PD-L1- negative cohort and had an ORR of 0% (95% CI, 0.0–23.2%).

However, updated results with a median follow-up of 5.8 (0.4–25.9) months showed that the ORR was now 17.8% (95% CI, 12.7–24.0%) in all patients [31], much lower than previously reported in the trial that led to its approval (Table 1) [48]. In addition, the ORR in the PD-L1-positive cohort dropped from 46.4% to 27.6% (95% CI, 19.0–37.5%). Nonetheless, PD-L1-positive patient ORR was still notably higher than in patients that were PD-L1-negative 5.1% (95% CI, 1.4–12.5%). The median OS was 18.2 (8.1—not estimable) months in the total population. The OS was 20.0 (11.6—not estimable) months and 8.1 (3.1—not estimable) months for the PD-L1-high and PD-L1-negative expressing cohorts, respectively. The 1-year survival rate was 55% (44–65%) in all patients. Survival rates for PD-L1-expression subgroups were 63% and 41% for PD-L1-high and PD-L1 low/negative groups respectively. Based on these first results, the FDA granted accelerated approval to durvalumab for the same indication as described for nivolumab [50]. This study was significant as, for the first time, the results indicated that patient tumors should most likely contain substantially high levels of PD-L1. PD-L1 expression cut-offs at 1–10% may be insufficient for identifying patients who will respond to ICI therapy.

Durvalumab is currently being investigated in combination with the ICI mAb tremelimumab that targets CTLA-4 (another immune checkpoint receptor) in a few different clinical trials and is reviewed in [51]. Unfortunately, in one significant trial, the phase III DANUBE trial evaluating durvalumab plus tremelimumab in unresectable, metastatic bladder cancer patients did not meet the primary endpoints for improving OS versus standard-of-care chemotherapy [52]. The trial is evaluating the efficacy of durvalumab in the first-line treatment of both cisplatin-eligible and -ineligible patients with metastatic bladder cancer. The trial arms are durvalumab monotherapy, durvalumab plus tremelimumab, and cisplatin and gemcitabine or carboplatin and gemcitabine chemotherapy. In addition, patients whose tumors were PD-L1-positive did not benefit from durvalumab plus tremelimumab. This was surprising since high PD-L1 was set at the high cut-off of ≥25% of only tumor cells expressing PD-L1. Taken together, these results are puzzling. On one hand, durvalumab effectiveness is associated with PD-L1 expression as a monotherapy in the second-line but not in combination with an additional non-overlapping ICI in patients with metastatic bladder cancer in a first-line setting. The DANUBE trial is a post-approval commitment from AstraZeneca in agreement with the FDA from the accelerated 2017 approval, and it is unclear what actions regarding its approval and/or use will follow. Result details have yet to be published or presented at the time of this review.

2.5. *Avelumab (Bavencio; Pfizer; New York, NY, USA)*

2.5.1. JAVELIN Solid Tumor Trial

Avelumab is another fully human mAb that targets PD-L1. In the phase Ib JAVELIN clinical trial [33], avelumab was studied in 249 patients with metastatic bladder cancer previously treated with platinum-containing chemotherapy. PD-L1 expression was assessed using the Dako PD-L1 IHC 28-8 pharm Dx assay. The scoring system was similar to the Dako 28-8 assay used for nivolumab. Notably, scoring only accounted for PD-L1 expression on tumor cells only. At 6 months follow-up, the ORR was 17% (95% CI, 11–24%). In PD-L1-positive (≥5% of tumor cells) patients, the ORR was 24% (95% CI, 14–36%). In patients whose tumors had a PD-L1 status of <5% tumor cells, the ORR was 13% (95% CI, 7–23%). The median DOR for all patients was not reached (95% CI, 42.1 weeks to not estimable). Median OS was 6.5 (95% CI, 4.8–9.5) months in all patients. Patients in the PD-L1 status ≥5% and <5% subgroups, the median OS values were 11.9 (6.1–18.0) and 6.1 (5.9–8.0) months, respectively.

2.5.2. JAVELIN Bladder 100 Trial

This was followed with the phase III JAVELIN Bladder 100 trial that evaluated 700 patients given gemcitabine with either first-line cisplatin or carboplatin with and without maintenance avelumab plus best supportive care (BSC; n = 350) or BSC alone (n = 350) [32]. At the median follow-up time of approximately 19 months, avelumab plus BSC significantly prolonged OS versus BSC alone. The median OS for avelumab plus BSC was 21.4 months compared to 14.3 months for BSC alone. Of note, patients with PD-L1-positive tumors had a median OS that was not reached versus 17.1 months for BSC alone. The ORR of 17% and 24.1% in all patients and PD-L1 ≥5% ICs, respectively, obtained from the phase Ib study is the only available ORR (Table 1) as no ORR for the phase III study has been reported as of submission of our findings. Nonetheless, avelumab has thus far reached its primary objective in a large-scale randomized trial. Based on these results, the FDA approved avelumab on

June 20, 2020 for the treatment of patients with locally advanced or metastatic bladder cancer that has not progressed with first-line platinum-containing chemotherapy [53].

Avelumab is currently being studied in the GCISAVE trial (NCT03324282) that will assess the effectiveness of avelumab in combination with gemcitabine/cisplatin in the first-line treatment of locally advanced metastatic bladder cancer. Avelumab is also currently being evaluated in combination with Bacille Calmette-Guerin in patients with non-muscle invasive bladder cancer (NCT03892642), radiation (NCT03747419), and KHK2455 (a indoleamine 2,3-dioxygenase inhibitor; NCT03915405) in patients with advanced bladder cancer. These findings indicate that avelumab is very promising as maintenance therapy in patients who respond after receiving first-line platinum-containing chemotherapy. In addition, we look forward to ORR results from the Bladder 100 trial and the results of the multiple combination strategies currently being evaluated in the clinic.

2.6. Comparative Nuances between Studies for PD-L1 Expression as a Biomarker

- Atezolizumab: PD-L1 expression scoring was based solely on ICs and not tumor cells. In patients who previously received platinum-containing chemotherapy, the IMvigor210 (cohort 2) trial showed patients achieved ORRs of 26% in the IC2/3 (≥5%) group compared to 18% in the IC0/1 group. Unfortunately, in the IMvigor211 trial patients with the greatest relative PD-L1 expression did not significantly survive longer when treated with atezolizumab. However, the Imvigor210 (cohort 1) patients with who were cisplatin-ineligible, the ORRs were 28% and 21% for PD-L1 expression of ≥5% and <5% groups, respectively. The IMvigor130 trial did show an improved OS in patients with PD-L1 IC2/3. However, patients with PD-L1 IC2/3 actually had poorer relative ORR values.
- Pembrolizumab: PD-L1 expression scoring was based on a combination of both tumor cells and ICs. Although initial reports from the KEYNOTE-045 trial demonstrated increased ORR for patients with high PD-L1 expression, longer follow-up reports did not show an outcome advantage for patients with high expression levels of PD-L1. In cisplatin-ineligible patients (KEYNOTE-052), there was an association with PD-L1 expression and patient outcome. However, the phase III KEYNOTE-361 trial showed that patients in the PD-L1 high group did not have improved PFS or OS.
- Nivolumab: PD-L1 expression scoring was based solely on tumor cells and not ICs. Although clear differences in ORR were observed when patients were grouped into ≥1% (25.8%) versus ≥5% (31.3%) PD-L1 expression, TMB provided the best predictor of response. An additional complication is when TMB was combined with <1% or ≥1% PD-L1 expression, OS was dramatically reduced indicating PD-L1 was a negative predictor in this context.
- Durvalumab: PD-L1 expression scoring was based solely on tumor cells and not ICs. The 1108 trial has demonstrated differences in ORR and OS based on PD-L1 expression levels. One potential explanation is the much higher expression threshold of 25%. ORR and OS were 27.6% and 20.0 months for patients with ≥25% PD-L1 expression. In contrast, ORR and OS were 5.1% and 8.1 months for patients with <25% PD-L1 expression. This indicates, that much higher levels of PD-L1 expression cutoffs may provide improved prediction of patient outcomes.
- Avelumab: PD-L1 expression scoring was based solely on tumor cells and not ICs. At a threshold of 5%, patients in the ≥5% group had ORR and OS values of 24% and 11.9 months, respectively. In contrast, the ORR and OS for patients in the <5% group were 13% and 6.1 months, respectively.

3. Antibody-Drug Conjugates

Antibody-drug conjugates (ADCs) are the most mature offshoot of unmodified mAb therapeutics [54]. ADCs are mAbs conjugated to a small molecule chemotherapeutic via a chemical crosslinker. Although ADCs are considered biological therapeutic agents, the concept can also be viewed as 'targeted chemotherapy'. ADC therapeutic efficacy is reliant on the ability to efficiently internalize and accumulate the delivered cytotoxic drug inside diseased cells. Cells constantly internalize extracellular ligands via receptor-mediated endocytosis. Often, these internalized ligand-receptor complexes are encapsulated inside endosomes and trafficked to lysosomes for enzymatic degradation. Mechanistically, ADCs exert their cytotoxic activity by binding to target antigen receptors on the surface of tumor cells where they are internalized by a process known as receptor-mediated internalization and are entrapped inside endosomes in the intracellular space. Motor proteins then naturally traffic endosomes to lysosomes for membrane fusion and transfer of the encapsulated contents. Lysosomal proteases digest the antibody backbone or cleave the chemical crosslinker and liberate functional chemotherapeutic metabolites. The metabolites are able to permeate the lysosomal membrane and diffuse and bind their target and inhibit their function [54]. We highlight two recent clinically successful ADCs for bladder cancer.

3.1. *Enfortumab Vedotin (Padcev; Astellas; Tokyo, Japan; and Seattle Genetics; Bothell, WA, USA)*

EV is an ADC that targets Nectin-4 that is overexpressed on the surface of bladder tumor cells. EV is conjugated to the microtubule inhibitor monomethyl auristatin E that causes G2/M cell cycle arrest and results in apoptosis. [55] Nectins are involved in cellular adhesion, migrations and polarization [56]. IHC analysis showed Nectin-4 to be overexpressed in 93% of metastatic urothelial tumor specimens [55]. In contrast, 294 normal tissue specimens representing 36 human organs showed homogeneous weak to moderate staining. Nectin-4 expression via IHC staining was determined by the H-score. The H-score was calculated by summing the products of the staining intensity (score of 0–3) multiplied by the percentage of cells (0–100) stained in a given field of tumor tissue [55]. Specimens were then classified as negative (H-score 0–14), weak (H-score 15–99), moderate (H-score 100–199), and strong (H-score 200–300). Thus, Nectin-4 is an attractive target due to its preferential overexpression in bladder cancer relative to normal tissues.

3.1.1. EV-101 Trial

EV was approved in the United States in December 2019 based on the results from the phase I and II EV-101 and EV-201 clinical trials, respectively (extensively reported in [57]) (Table 1) [58]. Of note, patients in the EV-101 study who had previously received ICI therapy had an ORR of 42% (95% CI, 31.2–52.5%). In addition, patients with high tumor burdens such as liver metastases had a 36% (95% CI, 20.4–54.9%) ORR [59].

3.1.2. EV-201 Trial

In the phase II EV-201 trial, 125 patients with locally advanced or metastatic bladder cancer who were previously treated with platinum-containing chemotherapy or ICI therapy were treated with EV. Tumor expression levels of Nectin-4 and PD-L1 were evaluated. Nectin-4 expression levels were evaluated and scored as previously described [55]. The median Nectin-4 expression level was H-score = 290 (14–300) and, hence, all patient tumors evaluated were positive for Nectin-4 and, they were considered as having 'strong' expression. PD-L1 expression was scored as previously performed for pembrolizumab with tumors being classified as positive with a score ≥10 [42]. The proportion of patients with <10 and ≥10 PD-L1 scores was 65% and 35%, respectively.

At the median follow-up time point of 10.2 (0.5–16.5) months the ORR was 44% (95% CI, 35.1–53.2%), including 12% with complete responses regardless of PD-L1 status (Table 1) [34]. The median DOR was 7.6 (4.9–7.5) months. The median OS was 11.7 (9.1—not reached) months. Hence, these patient outcomes are reflective for tumors that had 'strong' Nectin-4 expression. In contrast, in the PD-L1 subgroups the ORRs were 47% (95% CI, 36–59.1%) and 36% (95% CI, 21.6–52%) for TPS < 10 and TPS ≥ 10 PD-L1 expression scores, respectively. This indicated that patients responded regardless of PD-L1 expression. This study demonstrated, (i) the importance of Nectin-4 as a biological target for bladder cancer, relative to PD-L1, and (ii) EV has the potential to significantly extend the lives of patients, including those who failed ICI treatment.

EV is currently being evaluated in the phase III EV-301 clinical trial (NCT02091999). In this global study, approximately 550 patients are being randomized to receive EV or investigator's choice of docetaxel, paclitaxel, or vinflunine [60]. There is also currently active recruitment for a phase II study (NCT03288545) to evaluate EV alone and in combination with various anticancer therapies, including the ICI pembrolizumab [61,62]. Preliminary results have shown an ORR of 71% with the combination of EV plus pembrolizumab in 45 cisplatin-ineligible patients. The available data for DOR, PFS, and OS are not yet mature. Taken together, these clinical studies reveal EV has the potential to significantly extend the lives of patients who fail ICI treatment and has the potential to synergize patient response with ICI therapy.

3.2. *Sacituzumab Govitecan (Trodelvy; Immunomedics; Morris Plains, NJ, USA)*

SG is an ADC that targets Trop-2 that is overexpressed on the surface of bladder tumor cells. SG is conjugated to the topoisomerase I inhibitor SN-38 [63]. It is currently approved for use in patients with triple-negative breast cancer who have received at least two prior forms of chemotherapy. Trop-2 is a transmembrane glycoprotein, which participates in cellular self-renewal, invasion, proliferation and survival and overexpressed in multiple solid tumors, including bladder cancer [64]. An IHC analysis showed Trop-2 was generally overexpressed in bladder tumor tissue with little expression detected in the corresponding normal tissue [65]. The method in which Trop-2 expression level was determined was not provided.

IMMU-132 Trial

SG was evaluated in the phase I/II IMMU-132 clinical trial in patients with advanced bladder cancer that received prior platinum-based treatment (Table 1) [35]. Patient tumors were determined as positive if >10% of tumor cells had anti-Trop-2 staining. Expression was scored as 3+ (strong), 2+ (moderate), and 1+ (weak) [35]. Tumors with <10% tumor cells that stained for Trop-2 were considered Trop-2-negative tumors. SG treatment resulted in an ORR of 31%, with two complete and 12 partial responses out of 45 patients. In a patient cohort previously treated with ICIs, the ORR was 23% (4/17). A single-arm, open-label, global TROPHY U-01 phase II trial is currently ongoing to evaluate SG in advanced bladder cancer (NCT03547973). Interim results from 35 patients from the 100-patient cohort of cisplatin-eligible patients who have also previously received ICI therapy and platinum-containing chemotherapy showed an ORR of 28% [66]. Based on these results, the FDA granted Immunomedics request for fast track designation in order to make SG available as rapidly as possible. It is not known whether there was a correlation in patient responses with respect to Trop-2 expression levels.

4. Erdafitinib (Balversa; Janssen Pharmaceuticals; Beerse, Belgium)

Bladder cancer is the third most common mutated malignancy and has the strongest association to fibroblast growth factor receptors (FGFRs) 1–4 gene mutations relative to all other cancer types [67,68]. Moreover, FGFR mutational aberrations occur in >50% of all bladder cancer cases [68]. Interestingly, FGFR3 mutations occur in 60% of invasive bladder tumors and it is a poor prognostic marker [69].

FGFRs represent a family of tyrosine kinases found on the surface of normal cells. There are currently four recognized receptor isoforms, which bind corresponding ligands, and leads to receptor dimerization and phosphorylation [68]. Ligand binding and dimerization results in downstream signaling and expression of several gene products that function to promote cell survival and proliferation. Gene mutations including gene amplification combine to promote cell growth beyond normal limits and results in the development of cancer. Further abnormal FGFR mechanisms that promote bladder cancer is nicely reviewed in Roubal et al. [70].

BLC2001 Trial

Erdafitinib is a pan-FGFR inhibitor and exerts is action by binding to and blocking FGFR phosphorylation and signaling, which decreases cell viability, particularly in tumor cells with FGFR genetic alterations. It was approved on 12 April 2019 for use in patients with locally advanced or metastatic bladder cancer, with susceptible FGFR3 or FGFR2 genetic alterations, that has progressed during or following platinum-containing chemotherapy, including within 12 months of neoadjuvant or adjuvant platinum-containing chemotherapy [71]. Approval was based on its performance in the phase II BLC2001 clinical trial (Table 1) [36]. Patients with locally advanced and unresectable or metastatic bladder cancer, with prespecified FGFR alterations, and who had been previously treated with platinum-containing chemotherapy were enrolled into the study. Importantly, a proportion of enrolled patients also received prior ICI therapy. Erdafitinib treatment resulted in an impressive ORR of 40% (95% CI, 31–50%). The median OS was 13.8 (9.8—not reached) months. In addition, at 1 year, 19% (11–29%) of patients continued to respond to treatment. Interestingly, Patients with FGFR3 mutations had the highest ORR at 49%. In contrast, patients with FGFR fusions had the lowest ORR at 16%. This indicates that erdafitinib can serve patients more effectively with tumors that contain FGFR mutations as opposed to fusions. In addition, erdafitinib can improve the outcomes of patients who previously received ICI therapy.

These targeted drugs, finally, are clinical breakthroughs that demonstrate molecular targets can result in precision therapeutics that are highly effective against metastatic bladder cancer. In addition, these drugs can also improve outcomes of patients that don't respond or relapse after receiving ICI therapy.

5. Adverse Events

Comparative percentages between the described ICIs and targeted therapeutics for % any AE, % grade ≥3 AE, % discontinued due to AE, and % treatment related deaths are listed in Table 2. The median % any AE was 64% (60.7–69.3%) among the key ICI clinical trials described in this review. For the ICIs, fatigue was the most commonly observed AE. Other observed AEs specifically related to ICI therapy were asthenia, infusion-related reactions, diarrhea, anorexia, peripheral edema, pruritus and rash. Severe AEs of grade ≥3 were fatigue, anemia, hepatitis, increased lipase and amylase, diarrhea, and asthenia. Grade 5 treatment-related pneumonitis that resulted in death, occurred in patients treated with durvalumab, nivolumab, and avelumab [31,33,46]. Nivolumab caused a death due to respiratory failure. Durvalumab caused a death due to autoimmune hepatitis. Pembrolizumab caused death due to sepsis and myositis [28].

For EV, SG, and erdafitinib, the most common treatment-related AEs was also fatigue. Other AEs common for the targeted therapeutics were diarrhea, nausea, any peripheral neuropathy, neutropenia, alopecia, any rash, decreased appetite and dysgeusia, hyperphosphatemia, and stomatitis. Severe AEs of grade ≥3 were neutropenia, anemia, hypophosphatemia, fatigue, leukopenia, hyponatremia, stomatitis, and asthenia. The most common reason for treatment discontinuation were retinal pigment epithelium, hand-foot syndrome, dry mouth, and skin or nail events [35,36,72]. Notably, thus far there have been no treatment-related deaths. However, a note of caution is that there were increased proportions of patients that discontinued treatment relative to ICIs. The median % discontinued due to AE was 6% (1.6–9.2%). In contrast, EV, SG and erdafitinib had % discontinued due to AE of 1.5–2.2-fold higher. In addition, the % grade ≥3 AE category the targeted therapeutics was increased by a factor of 2.6–3.4. Although the targeted therapeutics appear to be sufficiently tolerated or AEs are appropriately managed, they are more toxic than ICIs and thus the safety of patients should be closely monitored.

Table 2. Treatment-related adverse events (AEs) from ICIs and targeted therapeutics.

AEs	Atezolizumab [21,23]	Nivolumab [29]	Pembrolizumab [26–28]	Avelumab [33]	Durvalumab [31]	Enfortumab Vedotin [34]	Sacituzumab Govitecan [66]	Erdafitinib [73]
% of any AE	69% [1]/60% [2]	69.3%	62% [1]/64% [2]	67%	60.7%	94%	NR [3]	93%
% grade ≥3 AE	16%/15%	24.8%	16.9%/16%	8%	6.8%	54%	NR [3]	46%
% discontinued due to AE	4%/6%	10%	6.8%/9.2%	6%	1.6%	12%	9%	13%
% treatment related deaths	0/1%	1.1%	0.8%/0.3%	0.6%	1%	0	0	0

[1] Second-line setting. [2] First-line setting. [3] NR = not reported. Tagawa et al. [66], reports that the AE profile for sacituzumab govitecan in patients with bladder cancer was consistent with prior reports for breast cancer. Thus, the % of any AE and % grade ≥3 AE are from the reported clinical trial of sacituzumab govitecan in patients with metastatic triple-negative breast cancer, which was the basis for its approval for this cancer type [72], should be taken with caution.

6. Health Economic Factors

The innovative therapeutic approach brought by ICIs has undoubtedly ushered a new paradigm for treating patients with metastatic bladder cancer. ICIs have provided physicians the ability to control tumor growth, extend survival, and can be administered with a better safety profile compared to traditional chemotherapy. This is a major advancement for a disease that afflicts patients that are typically elderly and are frail or have co-morbidities, and cannot tolerate harsh chemotherapy. However, the exorbitant cost of these ICIs combined with the latest follow-up results (Table 1) demonstrating either less than hoped for patient responses or failure to meet endpoints in critical phase III trials that were a condition of their accelerated approval, their high economic burden and cost-effectiveness is now widely debated [74–76].

6.1. Drug Costs

Table 3 shows the current price ($US)/mg of ICI, a typical dose, and the price/dose. The current attitude is that these drugs cost too much [74]. Renner et al., has pointed out that ICIs may reduce toxicity but they are financially toxic and high costs limit their access in many countries inside and outside the U.S. [77]. A potential drawback for targeted therapeutics, the ADCs EV and SG and, the small molecule erdafitinib are more expensive than the listed ICIs. Unlike ICIs, ADCs are composed of three key components (antibody, chemical crosslinker, and cytotoxic payload). ADC construction involves chemical conjugation steps that can be complicated and make production and purification difficult.

Table 3. Pricing for ICIs and targeted therapeutics.

Drugs	$ [1]/mg	Dose	$/Dose	CE [2]
Pembrolizumab	$51.79	200 mg/3 weeks	$10,358	Difficult to justify [4,5]
Nivolumab	$28.78	3 mg/kg/2 weeks	$7770 [3]	No
Atezolizumab	$8.00	1200 mg/3 weeks	$9611	No [4]/Likely [5]
Durvalumab	$7.85	10 mg/kg/2 weeks	$7065 [3]	No
Avelumab	$6.63	10 mg/kg/2 weeks	$5967	Yes
Enfortumab vedotin	$110	125 mg/kg/days 1, 8, 15 (28-day cycle)	$37,125 [3]	Unknown
Sacituzumab govitecan	$11.20	10 mg/kg/days 1 and 8 (3-week cycle)	$20,120 [3]	Unknown
Erdafitinib	$90	8 mg/day	$20,160 [6]	Unknown

CE = Cost-effective. [1] Prices in U.S. currency. [2] At a $100,000 willing-to-pay threshold. [3] Calculated for 90 kg person. [4] For 'after platinum-containing chemotherapy'. [5] For 'cisplatin-ineligible'. [6] For 28-day supply.

6.2. Cost-Effectiveness

6.2.1. Pembrolizumab for Patients Who Have Progressed within 12 Months of Neoadjuvant or Adjuvant Platinum-Containing Chemotherapy Regardless of PD-L1 Expression

The National Comprehensive Cancer Network and the European Society for Medical Oncology recommend pembrolizumab in their treatment guidelines for patients who relapse after any platinum-containing chemotherapy [18,78]. This was due to the evidence from the KEYNOTE-045 trial and pembrolizumab is the only one of the five approved ICIs to demonstrate increased survival compared to standard chemotherapy after progression on platinum-containing chemotherapy.

However, there appears to be uncertainty in the cost-effectiveness of pembrolizumab. A 2018 analysis by Sarfaty et al., based off data from KEYNOTE-045 determined that for this indication relative to chemotherapy pembrolizumab did not produce the quality-adjusted life years (QALY) gains at a willingness-to-pay threshold of $100,000 in the U.S. [79]. QALY is a measure of the incremental health improvement provided by a new treatment compared to previous treatment options. The cost-effectiveness ratio for pembrolizumab was calculated at $122,557/QALY in the U.S. The author's did find that pembrolizumab was cost-effective in Canada, Australia, and the United Kingdom (UK), as the costs were below the $100,000 threshold. This finding was reliant on short-term data obtained from the trial. In comparison, Slater et al. analyzed results from the KEYNOTE-045 study at a median follow-up of >2-years [80]. The study reported that at a willingness-to-pay threshold of $100,000, pembrolizumab is a cost-effective option ($93,481/QALY gained) compared to chemotherapy in the U.S.

Unlike in the U.S., many countries have cost-effectiveness assessment agencies. In March 2020, the UKs National Institute for Health and Care Excellence (NICE) Evidence Review Group (ERG) recommended against the use of pembrolizumab for this indication based on cost-effectiveness estimates (Table 3) [81]. The current list price for pembrolizumab in the UK is £26.30/mg [82]. As a single treatment course is 200 mg this amounts to approximately £5260 for a single administration. Administration of pembrolizumab is recommended at 200 mg each 3 weeks until disease progression, unacceptable toxicity, or up to 24 months without disease progression. NICE projected that pembrolizumab will cost well beyond £50,000/QALY, which is NICE's limit threshold for a drug that can extend life ≥3 months in patients suffering from a disease with a life expectancy of <2-years. We believe, these results reveal that cost-effectiveness for pembrolizumab is difficult to justify.

6.2.2. Pembrolizumab for Patients Who Are Cisplatin-Ineligible

NICE's ERG did recommend the use of pembrolizumab for use in patients who are cisplatin-ineligible. NICE projected the cost-effectiveness of pembrolizumab for this indication will be £67,068/QALY ($U.S. ~87,000) [83]. Merck Sharp & Dohme economic modeling projected a cost of £37,081/QALY ($U.S. ~49,000). NICE did acknowledge that there was a level of uncertainty in the calculated cost-effectiveness projections as the data was from the KEYNOTE-052 phase II study and not a randomized phase III study. This meant that the extrapolation of OS and PFS in patients treated with pembrolizumab were compared to an independent comparator arm that received gemcitabine plus carboplatin reported by De Santis et al. [8]. In the U.S., Merck Sharp & Dohme calculated that the cost-effectiveness of pembrolizumab in this setting will be $81,493/QALY at a willingness-to-pay threshold of $100,000. [84] However, it is unknown if the cost-effectiveness in the UK or the U.S. of pembrolizumab has changed since the announcement that it did not reach its primary endpoints in the critical phase III KEYNOTE-361 trial [43]. Thus, we believe the cost-effectiveness for pembrolizumab is currently difficult to justify and will most likely be deemed not cost-effective.

6.2.3. Atezolizumab for Patients Who Have Progressed within 12 Months of Neoadjuvant or Adjuvant Platinum-Containing Chemotherapy Regardless of PD-L1 Expression

As pembrolizumab and atezolizumab are the only ICIs evaluated in randomized controlled trial for this bladder cancer treatment setting, Slater et al., performed a cost-effective evaluation comparative study [80]. The analysis compared a >2-year follow-up for pembrolizumab's KEYNOTE-045 trial with the data from atezolizumab's IMvigor211 trial. The study found because atezolizumab was less effective at extending the lives of patients, it use would increase costs by $26,458 in the U.S. for the same QALY-gained with pembrolizumab. Pembrolizumab had a cost-effective ratio of $93,481/QALY-gained. Thus, at a willingness-to-pay threshold of $100,000, the increased costs for using atezolizumab make it non cost-effective option for treating bladder cancer for this indication. The Scottish Medicines Consortium also determined that atezolizumab was not cost-effective for use within its healthcare system [85]. The primary reason was the small numerical increase in median OS compared with chemotherapy.

6.2.4. Atezolizumab for Patients Who Are Cisplatin-Ineligible

NICE's ERG performed an analysis of the cost-effectiveness of atezolizumab for cisplatin-ineligible patients. NICE recommended atezolizumab as an option for untreated advanced or metastatic bladder cancer in patients who are ineligible for cisplatin-containing chemotherapy [86]. However, the ERG did note that although atezolizumab appears to be an effective treatment, it is difficult to establish the size of the clinical benefit compared with current treatments. Clinicians invited to comment during the review commented that atezolizumab therapy was not favorable over current treatments. The ERG further notes that they are awaiting data from the IMvigor130 trial. The trial has shown that the addition of atezolizumab to chemotherapy was associated with a significant prolongation of PFS and able to improve OS particularly in patients with a relative high PD-L1 expression status. NICE has not updated its findings or recommendation. We believe atezolizumab is likely cost-effective in this setting for patients with high PD-L1 status.

6.2.5. Avelumab

Avelumab has been studied and deemed that its use would have a cost-neutral impact within a US commercial and a Medicare health plan [87]. Based on that it is the lowest priced drug on the list (Table 3), and the positive data from the phase III JAVELIN Bladder 100 trial, avelumab is a relatively affordable and a cost-effective option.

6.2.6. Nivolumab and Durvalumab

NICE did not recommend nivolumab as an option for treating locally advanced, unresectable or metastatic bladder cancer who have had platinum-containing therapy [88]. The cost-effectiveness was not better than cisplatin plus gemcitabine. Nivolumab was also shown to not be cost-effective in the US economic healthcare system [76]. This may be due to nivolumab having the highest relative toxicity profile among the ICIs. For durvalumab, AstraZeneca advised that they would not be pursuing a licensing application from the European Medicines Agency for a bladder cancer indication and, thus, NICE has suspended its cost-effectiveness appraisal [89].

6.2.7. ADCs and Erdafitinib

There are currently no cost-effective appraisals for EV or for SG (for its current approval for use in triple-negative breast cancer). For erdafitinib, NICE is currently appraising its cost-effectiveness and results are to come [90].

7. Discussion

Patients with metastatic or advanced bladder cancer once had limited options after failed chemotherapy leading to disease progression and death. Active application and examination of immune checkpoint inhibition has provided new therapeutic possibilities for patients with metastatic bladder cancer. Today, patients typically receiving ICI therapy do not have to withstand the severe toxicity associated with chemotherapy. In addition, patients who respond typically have long-lasting responses and increased survival. However, the median ORR from the clinical trials evaluating the described ICIs was 20.9% (13.4–28.6%). In contrast for the two approved targeted therapeutics, EV and erdafitinib, the ORR values were increased by factors of 2.1 and 1.9, respectively. In addition, ICI affordability, not only for patients, but also for national health care systems threatens patient access to these drugs. However, the targeted therapeutics are even more expensive than the ICIs. The findings that avelumab and atezolizumab (for cisplatin-ineligible patients only) are most likely the only cost-effective ICIs provides a wake-up call to develop strategies to make these drugs more affordable and/or how to improve patient responses.

As described in this review, in general, it is difficult for physicians to identify patient groups that will benefit from ICI therapy based on PD-L1 tumor expression and has previously been discussed [91]. Some patients have demonstrated strong responses under ICI therapy whose tumors express relative 'high' levels of PD-L1, such as in the JAVELIN Solid Tumor (avelumab) and in the Checkmate 275 (nivolumab) trials. However, in general PD-L1-specific responses were not better than in patients regardless of PD-L1 expression, or PD-L1 associated responses were not reproducible in larger randomized trials or when responses were evaluated at longer follow-up periods. The major reason for these scattered results, in the context of PD-L1 expression, is that PD-L1 is an unreliable marker to predict treatment response. One major challenge for PD-L1 as a biomarker is the different assays and expression scoring systems used, as described in the above ICI clinical trials. Currently, different IHC assays have different PD-L1 expression cutoffs and scoring is either only on tumor cells (nivolumab, durvalumab, avelumab), only on tumor-infiltrating ICs (atezolizumab), or on the combination of tumor cells and ICs (pembrolizumab). Attempts to standardize PD-L1 expression evaluation using IHC are underway. Preliminary harmonization studies have indicated that the assays 22C3, SP263 and, 28–8 (used for pembrolizumab, durvalumab and avelumab, respectively) can be comparable, additional research is needed regarding the interchangeability of the assays as it pertains to response and once a universal assays is in place, what will be the PD-L1 expression thresholds required to achieve robust responses [92].

ADCs and small molecules have given another life-saving chance to patients with advanced and metastatic bladder cancer, and have demonstrated a higher ORR in clinical trials, compared to ICI therapies, but increased frequency of any-grade treatment-related AE (Table 2) and high cost (Table 3) remain a serious barrier for mainstream application in patients. In addition, these results are early and longer follow-up analyses are needed. Nonetheless, EV and erdafitinib are effective for treating bladder cancer and, hence, inaugurated the era of targeted therapy for bladder cancer.

8. Future

8.1. Improved Biomarkers

Biomarkers are needed that will be able to identify patients for treatment-specific responses. Unlike, other tumor types, there remains no biomarker in the clinic that allows physicians to determine which patients are most likely to benefit from immuno- or targeted therapeutics. As described in the Checkmate 275 trial, TMB appears to be a promising biomarker. There are active investigations for developing bladder cancer-specific biomarkers and reviewed in [12,93].

The antigens Nectin-4 and Trop-2 as biomarkers to identify patients to respond to EV and SG, respectively, appear promising. Specifically, the fact that all patients were positive for Nectin-4 and that the majority of these patients had 'strong' expression is highly encouraging. Although, the EV-201 trial performed many subgroup analyses, it did not report patient responses based on 'low', 'moderate', and 'high' Nectin-4 expression. [34] This was most likely because the majority of patients had 'high' Nectin-4 expression and there may have been too few patients with 'low' and 'moderate' expression. A larger phase II EV-202 trial (NCT04225117) is currently recruiting and estimates to enrol 240 patients and perhaps they will determine patient responses based on Nectin-4 tumor expression.

8.2. Additional Targeted Therapeutics in the Pipeline

Emerging targeted therapies that have reached the clinic include inhibitors against angiogenesis, FGFR, HER2, phosphoinositide 3 kinase, protein kinase B, mammalian target of rapamycin, and epigenetic targets and are nicely described by Mendiratta and Grivas [12]. Notably, many of the investigational drugs have not shown significant activity reinforcing the difficulty with the targeted therapy approach for bladder cancer.

MAbs make up a large portion of these investigational drugs. For example, mAbs such as bevacizumab and ramucirumab that target vascular endothelial growth factor (VEGF) have been evaluated. Bevacizumab failed to improve OS relative to placebo in a phase III study, and caused grade ≥3 AEs in 83.4% of patients [94]. In the RANGE phase III trial, ramucirumab did not significantly improve OS in patients who had previously been treated with platinum-containing chemotherapy and/or ICI therapy [95]. The mAb trastuzumab that targets HER2 has also been extensively evaluated in the clinic against bladder cancer. Unfortunately, trastuzumab has also not had any significant clinical impact. One of the great examples of antibody-targeted therapy for cancer is the story of HER2 [54]. Trastuzumab in combination with paclitaxel is standard practice for patients with HER2-positive breast cancer. Initially, a phase II study showed a remarkable ORR of 70% in patients with advanced bladder cancer treated with trastuzumab plus chemotherapy [96]. However, a larger trial that evaluated chemotherapy with and without trastuzumab did not show a difference between the two arms for bladder cancer patients [97].

ADCs may be the best option for antibody-based therapies relative to unmodified mAbs. The ICIs and the above described mAbs targeting VEGF and HER2, and mAbs in general, that are reliant on an antagonistic (blockade or receptor-ligand or receptor-receptor interactions) mechanism of action may show some therapeutic potency—the effects tend to be various and ultimately not curative [98]. The strategy of conjugating chemotherapy drugs to mAbs to generate ADCs appears to be the more clinically successful approach for antibody-based treatment of metastatic bladder cancer. Hence, future research directions should discover additional antigens that are overexpressed on the surface of bladder cancer, and for the development of ADCs that deliver highly cytotoxic payloads. One example is the discovery of the interleukin-5 receptor α-subunit (CD125) as being preferentially overexpressed in MIBC tumors but not on superficial bladder tumors or normal urothelium [99]. An anti-CD125 ADC has potent cytotoxicity against MIBC cells [99]. Additional target with accompanying ADCs that have shown promise in preclinical models of bladder cancer include The Slit- and Trk-like receptor family, transmembrane glycoprotein epithelial cell-adhesion molecule, and Thomsen-Fridenreich antigen and are described in further detail in [100].

9. Conclusions

ICIs have greatly reduced AEs compared to traditional chemotherapy. However, their relatively low response rates make it unclear on their ability to increase the therapeutic window relative to traditional chemotherapy remains unclear. In addition, their high cost makes ICIs, with the exception of avelumab and atezolizumab (for cisplatin-ineligible patients), not cost-effective. Based on the evidence described in this review, newly diagnosed patients with advanced bladder cancer will most likely significantly benefit from avelumab plus cisplatin-containing or carboplatin-containing chemotherapy. The targeted therapeutics EV, SG, and erdafitinib still have to demonstrate their worth in randomized phase III testing. If successful, it is likely patients who have relapsed after traditional chemotherapy or ICI therapy will benefit from these targeted therapeutics. Bladder cancer therapy has advanced tremendously in a short period of time since the first ICI approval, and the future looks hopeful as science will increase knowledge to make responses more robust to ICI therapy or new targetable biomarkers will be discovered.

Author Contributions: O.B. carried our literature studies and wrote the manuscript. J.V.L. conceived of the review topic and helped in drafting the manuscript. All authors have read and agreed to the published version of the manuscript.

Funding: This research was funded by the Canadian Institutes of Health Research, grant number 201610PJT-378389-PJT-CFDA-190713 and Fonds de recherche Quebec—Santé.

Conflicts of Interest: The authors declare no conflict of interest.

References

1. Bladder Cancer Fact Sheet. Available online: https://gco.iarc.fr/today/data/factsheets/cancers/30-Bladder-fact-sheet.pdf (accessed on 24 July 2020).
2. Bellmunt, J.; Mottet, N.; De Santis, M. Urothelial carcinoma management in elderly or unfit patients. *Eur. J. Cancer Suppl.* **2016**, *14*, 1–20. [CrossRef] [PubMed]
3. Kaufman, D.S.; Shipley, W.U.; Feldman, A.S. Bladder cancer. *Lancet* **2009**, *374*, 239–249. [CrossRef]
4. Ghatalia, P.; Zibelman, M.; Geynisman, D.M.; Plimack, E.R. Approved checkpoint inhibitors in bladder cancer: Which drug should be used when? *Ther. Adv. Med Oncol.* **2018**, *10*, 1758835918788310. [CrossRef] [PubMed]
5. Kamat, A.M.; Hahn, N.M.; Efstathiou, J.A.; Lerner, S.P.; Malmström, P.U.; Choi, W.; Guo, C.C.; Lotan, Y.; Kassouf, W. Bladder cancer. *Lancet* **2016**, *388*, 2796–2810. [CrossRef]

6. Von der Maase, H.; Hansen, S.; Roberts, J.; Dogliotti, L.; Oliver, T.; Moore, M.; Bodrogi, I.; Albers, P.; Knuth, A.; Lippert, C.; et al. Gemcitabine and Cisplatin Versus Methotrexate, Vinblastine, Doxorubicin, and Cisplatin in Advanced or Metastatic Bladder Cancer: Results of a Large, Randomized, Multinational, Multicenter, Phase III Study. *J. Clin. Oncol.* **2000**, *18*, 3068–3077. [CrossRef]
7. Sternberg, C.N.; Pizzocaro, G.; Marini, L.; Schnetzer, S.; Sella, A.; Calabrò, F. Chemotherapy with an every-2-week regimen of gemcitabine and paclitaxel in patients with transitional cell carcinoma who have received prior cisplatin-based therapy. *Cancer* **2001**, *92*, 2993–2998. [CrossRef]
8. De Santis, M.; Bellmunt, J.; Mead, G.; Kerst, J.M.; Leahy, M.; Maroto, P.; Gil, T.; Marreaud, S.; Daugaard, G.; Skoneczna, I.; et al. Randomized Phase II/III Trial Assessing Gemcitabine/Carboplatin and Methotrexate/Carboplatin/Vinblastine in Patients With Advanced Urothelial Cancer Who Are Unfit for Cisplatin-Based Chemotherapy: EORTC Study 30986. *J. Clin. Oncol.* **2012**, *30*, 191–199. [CrossRef]
9. Galsky, M.D.; Mironov, S.; Iasonos, A.; Scattergood, J.; Boyle, M.G.; Bajorin, D.F. Phase II trial of pemetrexed as second-line therapy in patients with metastatic urothelial carcinoma. *Investig. New Drugs* **2006**, *25*, 265–270. [CrossRef]
10. Vaughn, D.J.; Broome, C.M.; Hussain, M.; Gutheil, J.C.; Markowitz, A.B. Phase II trial of weekly paclitaxel in patients with previously treated advanced urothelial cancer. *J. Clin. Oncol.* **2002**, *20*, 937–940. [CrossRef]
11. Fassan, M.; Trabulsi, E.J.; Gomella, L.G.; Baffa, R. Targeted therapies in the management of metastatic bladder cancer. *Biologics* **2007**, *1*, 393–406.
12. Mendiratta, P.; Grivas, P. Emerging biomarkers and targeted therapies in urothelial carcinoma. *Ann. Transl. Med.* **2018**, *6*, 250. [CrossRef] [PubMed]
13. Pilie, P.G.; Lorusso, P.M.; Yap, T.A. Precision Medicine: Progress, Pitfalls, and Promises. *Mol. Cancer Ther.* **2017**, *16*, 2641–2644. [CrossRef] [PubMed]
14. Jenkins, R.W.; Barbie, D.A.; Flaherty, K.T. Mechanisms of resistance to immune checkpoint inhibitors. *Br. J. Cancer* **2018**, *118*, 9–16. [CrossRef] [PubMed]
15. Chen, R.; Zinzani, P.L.; Lee, H.J.; Armand, P.; Johnson, N.A.; Brice, P.; Radford, J.; Ribrag, V.; Molin, D.; Vassilakopoulos, T.P.; et al. Pembrolizumab in relapsed or refractory Hodgkin lymphoma: 2-year follow-up of KEYNOTE-087. *Blood* **2019**, *134*, 1144–1153. [CrossRef] [PubMed]
16. Scherpereel, A.; Mazieres, J.; Greillier, L.; Lantuejoul, S.; Dô, P.; Bylicki, O.; Monnet, I.; Corre, R.; Audigier-Valette, C.; Locatelli-Sanchez, M.; et al. Nivolumab or nivolumab plus ipilimumab in patients with relapsed malignant pleural mesothelioma (IFCT-1501 MAPS2): A multicentre, open-label, randomised, non-comparative, phase 2 trial. *Lancet Oncol.* **2019**, *20*, 239–253. [CrossRef]
17. Zhu, A.X.; Finn, R.S.; Edeline, J.; Cattan, S.; Ogasawara, S.; Palmer, D.; Verslype, C.; Zagonel, V.; Fartoux, L.; Vogel, A.; et al. Pembrolizumab in patients with advanced hepatocellular carcinoma previously treated with sorafenib (KEYNOTE-224): A non-randomised, open-label phase 2 trial. *Lancet Oncol.* **2018**, *19*, 940–952. [CrossRef]
18. Flaig, T.W. NCCN Guidelines Updates: Management of Muscle-Invasive Bladder Cancer. *J. Natl. Compr. Cancer Netw.* **2019**, *17*, 591–593.
19. Bellmunt, J.; Powles, T.; Vogelzang, N.J. A review on the evolution of PD-1/PD-L1 immunotherapy for bladder cancer: The future is now. *Cancer Treat. Rev.* **2017**, *54*, 58–67. [CrossRef]
20. Ning, Y.M.; Suzman, D.; Maher, V.E.; Zhang, L.; Tang, S.; Ricks, T.; Palmby, T.; Fu, W.; Liu, Q.; Goldberg, K.B.; et al. FDA Approval Summary: Atezolizumab for the Treatment of Patients with Progressive Advanced Urothelial Carcinoma after Platinum-Containing Chemotherapy. *Oncologist* **2017**, *22*, 743–749. [CrossRef]
21. Rosenberg, J.E.; Hoffman-Censits, J.; Powles, T.; Van Der Heijden, M.S.; Balar, A.V.; Necchi, A.; Dawson, N.; O'Donnell, P.H.; Balmanoukian, A.; Loriot, Y.; et al. Atezolizumab in patients with locally advanced and metastatic urothelial carcinoma who have progressed following treatment with platinum-based chemotherapy: A single-arm, multicentre, phase 2 trial. *Lancet* **2016**, *387*, 1909–1920. [CrossRef]
22. Vennapusa, B.; Baker, B.; Kowanetz, M.; Boone, J.; Menzl, I.; Bruey, J.-M.; Fine, G.; Mariathasan, S.; McCaffery, I.; Mocci, S.; et al. Development of a PD-L1 Complementary Diagnostic Immunohistochemistry Assay (SP142) for Atezolizumab. *Appl. Immunohistochem. Mol. Morphol.* **2019**, *27*, 92–100. [CrossRef]
23. Balar, A.V.; Dreicer, R.; Loriot, Y.; Perez-Gracia, J.L.; Hoffman-Censits, J.H.; Petrylak, D.P.; Van Der Heijden, M.S.; Ding, B.; Shen, X.; Rosenberg, J.E. Atezolizumab (atezo) in first-line cisplatin-ineligible or platinum-treated locally advanced or metastatic urothelial cancer (mUC): Long-term efficacy from phase 2 study IMvigor210. *J. Clin. Oncol.* **2018**, *36*, 4523. [CrossRef]

24. Powles, T.; Durán, I.; Van Der Heijden, M.S.; Loriot, Y.; Vogelzang, N.J.; De Giorgi, U.; Oudard, S.; Retz, M.M.; Castellano, D.; Bamias, A.; et al. Atezolizumab versus chemotherapy in patients with platinum-treated locally advanced or metastatic urothelial carcinoma (IMvigor211): A multicentre, open-label, phase 3 randomised controlled trial. *Lancet* **2018**, *391*, 748–757. [CrossRef]
25. Galsky, M.D.; Arija, J.; Ángel, A.; Bamias, A.; Davis, I.D.; De Santis, M.; Kikuchi, E.; Garcia-Del-Muro, X.; De Giorgi, U.; Mencinger, M.; et al. Atezolizumab with or without chemotherapy in metastatic urothelial cancer (IMvigor130): A multicentre, randomised, placebo-controlled phase 3 trial. *Lancet* **2020**, *395*, 1547–1557. [CrossRef]
26. Fradet, Y.; Bellmunt, J.; Vaughn, D.J.; Lee, J.L.; Fong, L.; Vogelzang, N.J.; Climent, M.A.; Petrylak, D.P.; Choueiri, T.K.; Necchi, A.; et al. Randomized phase III KEYNOTE-045 trial of pembrolizumab versus paclitaxel, docetaxel, or vinflunine in recurrent advanced urothelial cancer: Results of >2 years of follow-up. *Ann. Oncol.* **2019**, *30*, 970–976. [CrossRef] [PubMed]
27. Necchi, A.; Fradet, Y.; Bellmunt, J.; de Wit, R.; Lee, J.L.; Fong, L.; Vozelgang, N.J.; Climent, M.A.; Petrylak, D.P.; Choueiri, T.K.; et al. Three-year follow-up from the phase 3 KEYNOTE-045 trial: Pembrolizumab (Pembro) versus investigator's choice (paclitaxel, docetaxel, or vinflunine) in recurrent, advanced urothelial cancer (UC). In Proceedings of the ESMO 2019 Congress, Barcelona, Spain, 27 September–1 October 2019.
28. Vuky, J.; Balar, A.V.; Castellano, D.; O'Donnell, P.H.; Grivas, P.; Bellmunt, J.; Powles, T.; Bajorin, D.; Hahn, N.M.; Savage, M.J.; et al. Long-Term Outcomes in KEYNOTE-052: Phase II Study Investigating First-Line Pembrolizumab in Cisplatin-Ineligible Patients With Locally Advanced or Metastatic Urothelial Cancer. *J. Clin. Oncol.* **2020**, *38*, 2658–2666. [CrossRef]
29. Galsky, M.; Saci, A.; Szabo, P.M.; Han, G.C.; Grossfeld, G.D.; Collette, S.; Siefker-Radtke, A.O.; Necchi, A.; Sharma, P. Nivolumab in Patients with Advanced Platinum-resistant Urothelial Carcinoma: Efficacy, Safety, and Biomarker Analyses with Extended Follow-up from CheckMate 275. *Clin. Cancer Res.* **2020**. [CrossRef]
30. O'Donnell, P.; Massard, C.; Keam, B.; Kim, S.-W.; Friedlander, T.; Ahn, M.-J.; Ong, M.; Gordon, M.; Butler, M.; Antonia, S.; et al. Abstract CT031: Updated efficacy and safety profile of durvalumab monotherapy in urothelial carcinoma. *Clin. Trials* **2018**, *78*, CT031. [CrossRef]
31. Powles, T.; O'Donnell, P.H.; Massard, C.; Arkenau, H.-T.; Friedlander, T.W.; Hoimes, C.J.; Lee, J.L.; Ong, M.; Sridhar, S.S.; Vogelzang, N.J.; et al. Efficacy and Safety of Durvalumab in Locally Advanced or Metastatic Urothelial Carcinoma. *JAMA Oncol.* **2017**, *3*, e172411. [CrossRef]
32. Powles, T.; Park, S.H.; Voog, E.; Caserta, C.; Valderrama, B.; Gurney, H.; Kalofonos, H.; Radulovic, S.; Demey, W.; Ullén, A.; et al. Maintenance avelumab + best supportive care (BSC) versus BSC alone after platinum-based first-line (1L) chemotherapy in advanced urothelial carcinoma (UC): JAVELIN Bladder 100 phase III interim analysis. *J. Clin. Oncol.* **2020**, *38*, LBA1. [CrossRef]
33. Patel, M.R.; Ellerton, J.; Infante, J.R.; Agrawal, M.; Gordon, M.; Aljumaily, R.; Britten, C.D.; Dirix, L.; Lee, K.-W.; Taylor, M.; et al. Avelumab in metastatic urothelial carcinoma after platinum failure (JAVELIN Solid Tumor): Pooled results from two expansion cohorts of an open-label, phase 1 trial. *Lancet Oncol.* **2018**, *19*, 51–64. [CrossRef]
34. Rosenberg, J.E.; O'Donnell, P.H.; Balar, A.V.; McGregor, B.A.; Heath, E.I.; Yu, E.Y.; Galsky, M.D.; Hahn, N.M.; Gartner, E.M.; Pinelli, J.M.; et al. Pivotal Trial of Enfortumab Vedotin in Urothelial Carcinoma After Platinum and Anti-Programmed Death 1/Programmed Death Ligand 1 Therapy. *J. Clin. Oncol.* **2019**, *37*, 2592–2600. [CrossRef] [PubMed]
35. Tagawa, S.T.; Faltas, B.M.; Lam, E.T.; Saylor, P.J.; Bardia, A.; Hajdenberg, J.; Morgans, A.K.; Lim, E.A.; Kalinsky, K.; Simpson, P.S.; et al. Sacituzumab govitecan (IMMU-132) in patients with previously treated metastatic urothelial cancer (mUC): Results from a phase I/II study. *J. Clin. Oncol.* **2019**, *37*, 354. [CrossRef]
36. Loriot, Y.; Necchi, A.; Park, S.H.; Garcia-Donas, J.; Huddart, R.; Burgess, E.; Fleming, M.; Rezazadeh, A.; Mellado, B.; Varlamov, S.; et al. Erdafitinib in Locally Advanced or Metastatic Urothelial Carcinoma. *N. Engl. J. Med.* **2019**, *381*, 338–348. [CrossRef] [PubMed]
37. EMA Press Release. EMA Restricts Use of Keytruda and Tecentriq in Bladder Cancer. Available online: https://www.ema.europa.eu/en/news/ema-restricts-use-keytruda-tecentriq-bladder-cancer (accessed on 17 July 2020).

38. FDA Press Release. FDA Limits the Use of Tecentriq and Keytruda for Some Urothelial Cancer Patients. Available online: https://www.fda.gov/drugs/resources-information-approved-drugs/fda-limits-use-tecentriq-and-keytruda-some-urothelial-cancer-patients-:~{):text=FDA%20has%20limited%20the%20use,eligible%20for%20cisplatin%2Dcontaining%20therapy.&text=approved%20test%2C%20or-,Are%20not%20eligible%20for%20any%20platinum%2Dcontaining,regardless%20of%20PD%2DL1%20status (accessed on 30 July 2020).
39. FDA Press Release. Pembrolizumab (Keytruda): Advanced or Metastatic Urothelial Carcinoma. Available online: https://www.fda.gov/drugs/resources-information-approved-drugs/pembrolizumab-keytruda-advanced-or-metastatic-urothelial-carcinoma (accessed on 27 July 2020).
40. Bellmunt, J.; De Wit, R.; Vaughn, D.J.; Fradet, Y.; Lee, J.-L.; Fong, L.; Vogelzang, N.J.; Climent, M.A.; Petrylak, D.P.; Choueiri, T.K.; et al. Pembrolizumab as Second-Line Therapy for Advanced Urothelial Carcinoma. *N. Engl. J. Med.* **2017**, *376*, 1015–1026. [CrossRef]
41. PD-L1 IHC 22C3 pharmDx Interpretation Manual—NSCLC. Available online: file:///Users/leyj2601/Google%20Drive/Publishing/Reviews/Molecular%20ther.%20MIBC/ICIs/PD-L1%20biomarker/ihc-22C3-pharmdx-interpretation-manual.pdf. (accessed on 10 August 2020).
42. Balar, A.V.; Castellano, D.; O'Donnell, P.H.; Grivas, P.; Vuky, J.; Powles, T.; Plimack, E.R.; Hahn, N.M.; De Wit, R.; Pang, L.; et al. First-line pembrolizumab in cisplatin-ineligible patients with locally advanced and unresectable or metastatic urothelial cancer (KEYNOTE-052): A multicentre, single-arm, phase 2 study. *Lancet Oncol.* **2017**, *18*, 1483–1492. [CrossRef]
43. Merck Press Release. Merck Provides Update on Phase 3 KEYNOTE-361 Trial Evaluating Keytruda (pembrolizumab) as Montherapy and in Combination with Chemotherapy in Patients with Advanced or Metastatic Urothelial Carcinoma. 9 June 2020. Available online: https://investors.merck.com/news/press-release-details/2020/Merck-Provides-Update-on-Phase-3-KEYNOTE-361-Trial-Evaluating-KEYTRUDA-pembrolizumab-as-Monotherapy-and-in-Combination-with-Chemotherapy-in-Patients-with-Advanced-or-Metastatic-Urothelial-Carcinoma/default.aspx (accessed on 12 July 2020).
44. FDA Press Release. FDA Alerts Health Care Professionals and Oncology Clinical Investigators about an Efficacy Issue Identified in Clinical Trials for Some Patients Taking Keytruda (pembrolizumab) or Tecentriq (atezolizumab) as Monotherapy to Treat Urothelial Cancer with Low Expression of PD-L1. Available online: https://www.fda.gov/drugs/drug-safety-and-availability/fda-alerts-health-care-professionals-and-oncology-clinical-investigators-about-efficacy-issue. (accessed on 4 August 2020).
45. FDA Press Release. Nivolumab for Treatment of Urothelial Carcinoma. Available online: https://www.fda.gov/drugs/resources-information-approved-drugs/nivolumab-treatment-urothelial-carcinoma-:~{):text=On%20February%202%2C%202017%2C%20the,containing%20chemotherapy%20or%20have%20disease. (accessed on 27 July 2020).
46. Sharma, P.; Retz, M.; Siefker-Radtke, A.; Baron, A.; Necchi, A.; Bedke, J.; Plimack, E.R.; Vaena, D.; Grimm, M.O.; Bracarda, S.; et al. Nivolumab in metastatic urothelial carcinoma after platinum therapy (CheckMate 275): A multicentre, single-arm, phase 2 trial. *Lancet Oncol.* **2017**, *18*, 312–322. [CrossRef]
47. PD-L1 IHC 28-8 pharmDx. Available online: https://www.agilent.com/cs/library/packageinsert/public/P04672EFG_04.pdf. (accessed on 7 August 2020).
48. Massard, C.; Gordon, M.S.; Sharma, S.; Rafii, S.; Wainberg, Z.A.; Luke, J.; Curiel, T.J.; Colon-Otero, G.; Hamid, O.; Sanborn, R.E.; et al. Safety and Efficacy of Durvalumab (MEDI4736), an Anti–Programmed Cell Death Ligand-1 Immune Checkpoint Inhibitor, in Patients With Advanced Urothelial Bladder Cancer. *J. Clin. Oncol.* **2016**, *34*, 3119–3125. [CrossRef]
49. Williams, G.H.; Nicholson, A.G.; Snead, D.R.; Thunnissen, E.; Lantuejoul, S.; Cane, P.; Kerr, K.M.; Loddo, M.; Scott, M.L.; Scorer, P.W.; et al. Interobserver Reliability of Programmed Cell Death Ligand-1 Scoring Using the VENTANA PD-L1 (SP263) Assay in NSCLC. *J. Thorac. Oncol.* **2020**, *15*, 550–555. [CrossRef]
50. FDA Press Release. Durvalumab (Imfinzi). Available online: https://www.fda.gov/drugs/resources-information-approved-drugs/durvalumab-imfinzi (accessed on 27 July 2020).
51. Baldini, C.; Champiat, S.; Vuagnat, P.; Massard, C. Durvalumab for the management of urothelial carcinoma: A short review on the emerging data and therapeutic potential. *OncoTargets Ther.* **2019**, *12*, 2505–2512. [CrossRef]

52. AstraZeneca Press Release. Update on Phase III DANUBE Trial for Imfinzi and Tremelimumab in Unresectable, Stage IV Bladder Cancer. Available online: https://www.astrazeneca.com/media-centre/press-releases/2020/update-on-phase-iii-danube-trial-for-imfinzi-and-tremelimumab-in-unresectable-stage-iv-bladder-cancer-06032020.html (accessed on 22 July 2020).
53. FDA Press Release. FDA Approves Avelumab for Urothelial Carcinoma Maintenance Treatment. Available online: https://www.fda.gov/drugs/drug-approvals-and-databases/fda-approves-avelumab-urothelial-carcinoma-maintenance-treatment. (accessed on 27 July 2020).
54. Leyton, J.V. Improving Receptor-Mediated Intracellular Access and Accumulation of Antibody Therapeutics—The Tale of HER2. *Antibodies* **2020**, *9*, 32. [CrossRef] [PubMed]
55. Challita-Eid, P.M.; Satpayev, D.; Yang, P.; An, Z.; Morrison, K.; Shostak, Y.; Raitano, A.; Nadell, R.; Liu, W.; Lortie, D.R.; et al. Enfortumab Vedotin Antibody-Drug Conjugate Targeting Nectin-4 Is a Highly Potent Therapeutic Agent in Multiple Preclinical Cancer Models. *Cancer Res.* **2016**, *76*, 3003–3013. [CrossRef] [PubMed]
56. Takai, Y.; Irie, K.; Shimizu, K.; Sakisaka, T.; Ikeda, W. Nectins and nectin-like molecules: Roles in cell adhesion, migration, and polarization. *Cancer Sci.* **2003**, *94*, 655–667. [CrossRef] [PubMed]
57. Hanna, K. Clinical Overview of Enfortumab Vedotin in the Management of Locally Advanced or Metastatic Urothelial Carcinoma. *Drugs* **2019**, *80*, 1–7. [CrossRef] [PubMed]
58. FDA Press Release. FDA Grants Accelerated Approval to Enfortumab vedotin-ejfv for Metastatic Urothelial Cancer. Available online: https://www.fda.gov/drugs/resources-information-approved-drugs/fda-grants-accelerated-approval-enfortumab-vedotin-ejfv-metastatic-urothelial-cancer (accessed on 27 July 2020).
59. Rosenberg, J.; Sridhar, S.S.; Zhang, J.; Smith, D.; Ruether, D.; Flaig, T.W.; Baranda, J.; Lang, J.; Plimack, E.R.; Sangha, R.; et al. EV-101: A Phase I Study of Single-Agent Enfortumab Vedotin in Patients with Nectin-4–Positive Solid Tumors, Including Metastatic Urothelial Carcinoma. *J. Clin. Oncol.* **2020**, *38*, 1041–1049. [CrossRef]
60. Petrylak, D.P.; Rosenberg, J.E.; Duran, I.; Loriot, Y.; Sonpavde, G.; Wu, C.; Gartner, E.M.; Melhem-Bertrandt, A.; Powles, T. EV-301: Phase III study to evaluate enfortumab vedotin (EV) versus chemotherapy in patients with previously treated locally advanced or metastatic urothelial cancer (la/mUC). *J. Clin. Oncol.* **2019**, *37* (Suppl. S7), TPS497. [CrossRef]
61. Hoimes, C.J.; Rosenberg, J.E.; Petrylak, D.P.; Carret, A.-S.; Sasse, C.; Chaney, M.F.; Flaig, T.W. Study EV-103: New cohorts testing enfortumab vedotin alone or in combination with pembrolizumab in muscle invasive urothelial cancer. *J. Clin. Oncol.* **2020**, *38* (Suppl. S6), TPS595. [CrossRef]
62. Rosenberg, J.E.; Flaig, T.W.; Friedlander, T.W.; Milowsky, M.I.; Srinivas, S.; Petrylak, D.P.; Merchan, J.R.; Bilen, M.A.; Carret, A.-S.; Yuan, N.; et al. Study EV-103: Preliminary durability results of enfortumab vedotin plus pembrolizumab for locally advanced or metastatic urothelial carcinoma. *J. Clin. Oncol.* **2020**, *38* (Suppl. S6), 441. [CrossRef]
63. Moon, S.-J.; Govindan, S.V.; Cardillo, T.M.; D'Souza, C.A.; Hansen, H.J.; Goldenberg, D.M. Antibody Conjugates of 7-Ethyl-10-hydroxycamptothecin (SN-38) for Targeted Cancer Chemotherapy. *J. Med. Chem.* **2008**, *51*, 6916–6926. [CrossRef]
64. Shvartsur, A.; Bonavida, B. Trop2 and its overexpression in cancers: Regulation and clinical/ therapeutic implications. *Genes Cancer* **2014**, *6*, 84. [CrossRef]
65. Stepan, L.P.; Trueblood, E.S.; Hale, K.; Babcook, J.; Borges, L.; Sutherland, C.L. Expression of Trop2 Cell Surface Glycoprotein in Normal and Tumor Tissues. *J. Histochem. Cytochem.* **2011**, *59*, 701–710. [CrossRef] [PubMed]
66. Tagawa, S.T.; Petrylak, D.P.; Grivas, P.; Agarwal, N.; Sternberg, C.N.; Siemon-Hryczyk, P.; Goswam, T.; Loriot, Y. TROPHY-u-01: A phase II open-label study of sacituzumab govitecan (IMMU-132) in patients with advanced urothelial cancer after progression on platinum-based chemotherapy and/or anti-PD-1/PD-L1 checkpoint inhibitor therapy. *J. Clin. Oncol.* **2019**, *37* (Suppl. S7), TPS495. [CrossRef]
67. Cancer Genome Atlas Research Network. Comprehensive molecular characterization of urothelial bladder carcinoma. *Nature* **2014**, *507*, 315–322.
68. Turner, N.; Grose, R. Fibroblast growth factor signalling: From development to cancer. *Nat. Rev. Cancer* **2010**, *10*, 116–129. [CrossRef] [PubMed]

69. Hernandez, S.; Lopez-Knowles, E.; Lloreta, J.; Kogevinas, M.; Amorós, A.; Tardón, A.; Carrato, A.; Serra, C.; Malats, N.; Real, F.X. Prospective Study of FGFR3 Mutations as a Prognostic Factor in Nonmuscle Invasive Urothelial Bladder Carcinomas. *J. Clin. Oncol.* **2006**, *24*, 3664–3671. [CrossRef] [PubMed]
70. Roubal, K.; Myint, Z.W.; Kolesar, J.M. Erdafitinib: A novel therapy for FGFR-mutated urothelial cancer. *Am. J. Heal. Pharm.* **2020**, *77*, 346–351. [CrossRef] [PubMed]
71. FDA Press Release. FDA Grants Accelerated Approval to Erdafitinib for Metastatic Urothelial Carcinoma. Available online: https://www.fda.gov/drugs/resources-information-approved-drugs/fda-grants-accelerated-approval-erdafitinib-metastatic-urothelial-carcinoma (accessed on 6 August 2020).
72. Bardia, A.; Mayer, I.A.; Diamond, J.R.; Moroose, R.L.; Isakoff, S.J.; Starodub, A.N.; Shah, N.C.; O'Shaughnessy, J.; Kalinsky, K.; Guarino, M.; et al. Efficacy and Safety of Anti-Trop-2 Antibody Drug Conjugate Sacituzumab Govitecan (IMMU-132) in Heavily Pretreated Patients with Metastatic Triple-Negative Breast Cancer. *J. Clin. Oncol.* **2017**, *35*, 2141–2148. [CrossRef]
73. Bahleda, R.; Italiano, A.; Hierro, C.; Mita, A.C.; Cervantes, A.; Chan, N.; Awad, M.M.; Calvo, E.; Moreno, V.; Govindan, R.; et al. Multicenter Phase I Study of Erdafitinib (JNJ-42756493), Oral Pan-Fibroblast Growth Factor Receptor Inhibitor, in Patients with Advanced or Refractory Solid Tumors. *Clin. Cancer Res.* **2019**, *25*, 4888–4897. [CrossRef]
74. Andrews, A. Treating with Checkpoint Inhibitors—Figure $1 Million per Patient. *Am. Heal. Drug Benefits* **2015**, *8*, 9.
75. Pichler, R.; Loidl, W.; Pichler, M. High economic burden of immunotherapy underlines the need of predictive biomarkers for the individual therapy algorithm in metastatic bladder cancer. *Transl. Androl. Urol.* **2018**, *7* (Suppl. S6), S738–S740. [CrossRef]
76. Verma, V.; Sprave, T.; Haque, W.; Simone, C.B.; Chang, J.Y.; Welsh, J.W.; Thomas, C.R. A systematic review of the cost and cost-effectiveness studies of immune checkpoint inhibitors. *J. Immunother. Cancer* **2018**, *6*, 128. [CrossRef] [PubMed]
77. Renner, A.; Burotto, M.; Rojas, C. Immune Checkpoint Inhibitor Dosing: Can We Go Lower Without Compromising Clinical Efficacy? *J. Glob. Oncol.* **2019**, *5*, 1–5. [CrossRef] [PubMed]
78. Witjes, J.A.; Babjuk, M.; Bellmunt, J.; Bruins, H.M.; De Reijke, T.M.; De Santis, M.; Gillessen, S.; James, N.; Maclennan, S.; Palou, J.; et al. EAU-ESMO Consensus Statements on the Management of Advanced and Variant Bladder Cancer-An International Collaborative Multistakeholder Effort(dagger): Under the Auspices of the EAU-ESMO Guidelines Committees. *Eur. Urol.* **2020**, *77*, 223–250. [CrossRef] [PubMed]
79. Sarfaty, M.; Hall, P.; Chan, K.K.; Virik, K.; Leshno, M.; Gordon, N.; Moore, A.; Neiman, V.; Rosenbaum, E.; Goldstein, D.A. Cost-effectiveness of Pembrolizumab in Second-line Advanced Bladder Cancer. *Eur. Urol.* **2018**, *74*, 57–62. [CrossRef] [PubMed]
80. Slater, R.L.; Lai, Y.; Zhong, Y.; Li, H.; Meng, Y.; Moreno, B.H.; Godwin, J.L.; Frenkl, T.; Sonpavde, G.P.; Mamtani, R. The cost effectiveness of pembrolizumab versus chemotherapy or atezolizumab as second-line therapy for advanced urothelial carcinoma in the United States. *J. Med. Econ.* **2020**, *23*, 967–977. [CrossRef]
81. National Institute for Health and Care Excellence. Pembrolizumab for Treating Locally Advanced or Metastatic Urothelial Carcinoma after Platinum-Containing Chemotherapy [ID1536]. Available online: https://www.nice.org.uk/guidance/indevelopment/gid-ta10466. (accessed on 6 August 2020).
82. Gupta, S.; Kamat, A.M. NICE's rejection of pembrolizumab for platinum-refractory urothelial carcinoma: Is there a greater good? *Nat. Rev. Urol.* **2020**, *17*, 491–492. [CrossRef]
83. Ren, S.; Squires, H.; Everson-Hock, E.S.; Kaltenthaler, E.; Rawdin, A.; Alifrangis, C. Pembrolizumab for Locally Advanced or Metastatic Urothelial Cancer Where Cisplatin is Unsuitable: An Evidence Review Group Perspective of a NICE Single Technology Appraisal. *PharmacoEconomics* **2018**, *37*, 1073–1080. [CrossRef]
84. Lai, Y.; Zhong, Y.; Li, H.; Patterson, K.; Hale, O.; Meng, Y.; Frenkl, T.L.; Godwin, J.L.; Mamtani, R. Cost-effectiveness of pembrolizumab as first-line treatment of locally advanced or metastatic urothelial carcinoma ineligible for cisplatin-based therapy in the United States. *J. Clin. Oncol.* **2019**, *37* (Suppl. S27), 93. [CrossRef]
85. Scottish Medicines Consortium. Atezolizumab 1,200 mg Concentrate for Solution for Infusion (Tencentriq). 2018. Available online: https://www.scottishmedicines.org.uk/media/3850/atezolizumab-tecentriq-final-oct-2018.pdf (accessed on 11 August 2020).

86. NICE. Final Appraisal Determination Atezolizumab for Untreated Locally Advanced or Metastatic Urothelial Cancer where Cisplatin is Unsuitable. 2017. Available online: https://www.nice.org.uk/guidance/ta492/documents/final-appraisal-determination-document (accessed on 11 August 2020).
87. Kongnakorn, T.; Bharmal, M.; Kearney, M.; Phatak, H.; Benedict, A.; Bhanegaonkar, A.; Galsky, M. Budget Impact Of Including Avelumab As A Second-Line Treatment For Locally Advanced or Metastatic Urothelial Cancer In The United States: Commercial And Medicare Payer Perspectives. *Clin. Outcomes Res.* **2019**, *11*, 659–672. [CrossRef]
88. Grimm, S.E.; Armstrong, N.; Ramaekers, B.L.T.; Pouwels, X.; Lang, S.; Petersohn, S.; Riemsma, R.; Worthy, G.; Stirk, L.; Ross, J.; et al. Nivolumab for Treating Metastatic or Unresectable Urothelial Cancer: An Evidence Review Group Perspective of a NICE Single Technology Appraisal. *PharmacoEconomics* **2018**, *37*, 655–667. [CrossRef]
89. NICE Website. Durvalumab for Treating Metastatic Urothelial Bladder Cancer after Chemotherapy ID1172. Available online: https://www.nice.org.uk/guidance/indevelopment/gid-ta10394. (accessed on 29 July 2020).
90. NICE. Erdafitinib for Treating Metastatic or Unresectable FGFR-Positive Urothelial Cancer [ID1333]. Available online: https://www.nice.org.uk/guidance/indevelopment/gid-ta10252. (accessed on 7 August 2020).
91. Stuhler, V.; Maas, J.M.; Bochem, J.; da Costa, I.A.; Todenhoefer, T.; Stenzl, A.; Bedke, J. Molecular predictors of response to PD-1/PD-L1 inhibition in urothelial cancer. *World J. Urol.* **2019**, *37*, 1773–1784. [CrossRef] [PubMed]
92. Scheel, A.H.; Dietel, M.; Heukamp, L.C.; Jöhrens, K.; Kirchner, T.; Reu, S.; Rüschoff, J.; Schildhaus, H.-U.; Schirmacher, P.; Tiemann, M.; et al. Harmonized PD-L1 immunohistochemistry for pulmonary squamous-cell and adenocarcinomas. *Mod. Pathol.* **2016**, *29*, 1165–1172. [CrossRef] [PubMed]
93. Sapre, N.; Herle, P.; Anderson, P.; Corcoran, N.M.; Hovens, C.M. Molecular biomarkers for predicting outcomes in urothelial carcinoma of the bladder. *Pathology* **2014**, *46*, 274–282. [CrossRef]
94. Rosenberg, J.E.; Ballman, K.V.; Halabi, S.; Watt, C.; Hahn, O.M.; Steen, P.D.; Dreicer, R.; Flaig, T.W.; Stadler, W.M.; Sweeney, C.; et al. CALGB 90601 (Alliance): Randomized, double-blind, placebo-controlled phase III trial comparing gemcitabine and cisplatin with bevacizumab or placebo in patients with metastatic urothelial carcinoma. *J. Clin. Oncol.* **2019**, *37*, 4503. [CrossRef]
95. Petrylak, D.P.; De Wit, R.; Chi, K.N.; Drakaki, A.; Sternberg, C.N.; Nishiyama, H.; Castellano, D.; A Hussain, S.; Fléchon, A.; Bamias, A.; et al. Ramucirumab plus docetaxel versus placebo plus docetaxel in patients with locally advanced or metastatic urothelial carcinoma after platinum-based therapy (RANGE): Overall survival and updated results of a randomised, double-blind, phase 3 trial. *Lancet Oncol.* **2020**, *21*, 105–120. [CrossRef]
96. Hussain, M.H.; MacVicar, G.R.; Petrylak, D.P.; Dunn, R.L.; Vaishampayan, U.; Lara, P.N., Jr.; Chatta, G.S.; Nanus, D.M.; Glode, L.M.; Trump, D.L.; et al. Trastuzumab, paclitaxel, carboplatin, and gemcitabine in advanced human epidermal growth factor receptor-2/neu-positive urothelial carcinoma: Results of a multicenter phase II National Cancer Institute trial. *J. Clin. Oncol.* **2007**, *25*, 2218–2224. [CrossRef] [PubMed]
97. Oudard, S.; Culine, S.; Vano, Y.-A.; Goldwasser, F.; Theodore, C.; Nguyen, T.; Voog, E.; Banu, E.; Vieillefond, A.; Priou, F.; et al. Multicentre randomised phase II trial of gemcitabine+platinum, with or without trastuzumab, in advanced or metastatic urothelial carcinoma overexpressing Her2. *Eur. J. Cancer* **2015**, *51*, 45–54. [CrossRef]
98. Wu, A.M.; Senter, P.D. Arming antibodies: Prospects and challenges for immunoconjugates. *Nat. Biotechnol.* **2005**, *23*, 1137–1146. [CrossRef]
99. Paquette, M.; Vilera-Perez, L.G.; Beaudoin, S.; Ekindi-Ndongo, N.; Boudreaut, P.L.; Bonin, M.A.; Battista, M.C.; Bentourkia, M.H.; Lopez, A.F.; Lecomte, R.; et al. Targeting IL-5Ralpha with antibody-conjugates reveals a strategy for imaging and therapy for invasive bladder cancer. *Oncoimmunology* **2017**, *6*, e1331195. [CrossRef]
100. Vlachostergios, P.J.; Jakubowski, C.D.; Niaz, M.J.; Lee, A.; Thomas, C.; Hackett, A.L.; Patel, P.; Rashid, N.; Tagawa, S.T. Antibody-Drug Conjugates in Bladder Cancer. *Bladder Cancer* **2018**, *4*, 247–259. [CrossRef]

MDPI
St. Alban-Anlage 66
4052 Basel
Switzerland
Tel. +41 61 683 77 34
Fax +41 61 302 89 18
www.mdpi.com

International Journal of Molecular Sciences Editorial Office
E-mail: ijms@mdpi.com
www.mdpi.com/journal/ijms

www.ingramcontent.com/pod-product-compliance
Lightning Source LLC
LaVergne TN
LVHW070428100526
838202LV00014B/1549
* 9 7 8 3 0 3 6 5 4 3 5 3 6 *